Atlas of Common Subluxations of the Human Spine and Pelvis

Second Edition

William J. Ruch, D.C.

Life West Press
Life Chiropractic College West
25001 Industrial Blvd.
Hayward, CA 94545

LIFE CHIROPRACTIC
COLLEGE WEST

Atlas of Common Subluxations of the Human Spine and Pelvis

Second Edition

Second Printing

Library of Congress Control Number: 2014942383

ISBN 978-0-578-14382-8

DEDICATION

This book is dedicated to the memory of Norman N. Goldstein, Ph.D.

His gift was guidance, inspiration and encouragement, even in his final days.

FORWARD

The basis of everything chiropractors do involves anatomy. Chiropractors must learn and remember their anatomy.

Richard Stonebrink, D.C., D.A.B.C.O.
September 1975

What are we really doing? Why are we adjusting the patient and what is the adjustment doing?

During our education our teachers answer such questions. Often their answers are conflicting, anecdotal, prejudicial, misinformed, and even completely wrong.

In his search for answers, Dr. Ruch has engaged a unique approach: clinical anatomy. The results are this second edition of his pioneering book. Integrating clinical anatomy, advanced imaging, the pathophysiological response, and clinical observation, Dr. Ruch has amassed perhaps the most important reference text for chiropractic clinicians. His work also has great applications for other healthcare professionals, and for the medical legal arena.

The chiropractic profession owes Dr. Ruch a debt of gratitude for the immense amount of time and effort he expended in order to help our entire profession better understand the truth of spinal clinical anatomy and how it may be impacted by clinical practice.

Dan Murphy, D.C.

PREFACE

The purpose of this book is to help the chiropractic/medical/legal communities better understand the nature of the subluxation of the spine. The subluxation of vertebrae can have dramatic health consequences and can permanently alter an individual's quality of life. The goal of this book is to positively influence anatomically based rational intervention for spinal subluxations.

This book is the result of my work in the Life-West Chiropractic College Anatomy Laboratory. There I was able to dissect all or part of the spines of 240 individuals. The pictures herein are the result of the photographic record I made of 130 of those individuals.

As a chiropractic student, I received less instruction in the human spine and spinal cord in contrast to many classes on the heart and kidney. When I lecture to practicing chiropractors, I find they know more about the internal workings of the kidney than about the motion of the spinal cord in the canal with normal postural changes. Care of the spine should be based on the most comprehensive understanding possible. Knowledge of the anatomical and dynamic facets of the human spine and pelvis is limited in the teaching institutions of this country, both chiropractic and medical. One world renowned medical school has the cadavers remain supine for the entire human dissection course. When asked about instruction of the anatomy of the back and spine, the instructor said "they can look in a book if they are interested." He went on to add that, "we are so pressed for time that the students are given the choice between dissecting and being tested on either the arm or the leg, not both, because the anatomy is similar." Most medical personnel throw pills at almost all musculoskeletal problems, because the teachers can't teach what they don't know. In chiropractic college I was told we couldn't look at the intervertebral discs because "we don't have time."

I went into the lab on my own time to learn what I needed to know. In one of the first specimens I sectioned, I found the spinal cord tethered against the whole anterior canal wall, obliterating the anterior spinal artery. Only months from graduating, I realized I was seriously undereducated for my profession. I was saddened and, to say the least, frightened.

My laboratory studies illustrated that vertebral column deformities can alter the shape of spinal cord tissue and its vascular structures. My work as a chiropractor has shown me that these conditions impair circulation and generate neurological loss of function. I have been fortunate to be able to combine the two experiences.

The need for this knowledge to be distributed to practicing doctors is essential. I see primitive treatment being done by chiropractors, physicians, and surgeons alike because of lack of understanding of the anatomy and dynamics of the human spine. My hope is that this book will help to remedy this deficiency.

PREFACE TO THE SECOND EDITION.

When the 1st edition of this book went out of print, I knew it was time to do a 2nd edition. There were a number of reasons for this. One reason was that I felt the chiropractic community, chiropractors and chiropractic students, needed it to see the adverse health affects of spinal subluxation. This book needs to be available to them for the benefit of their patients.

An additional reason the 2nd edition is necessary is to include new material. The role of the spinal joints of the rib cage in neck and shoulder pain and dysfunction are underappreciated. As a clinician I find most patients with shoulder and neck pain complaints have subluxated ribs that are causing the muscles of the neck and shoulder to be rigid from neuromuscular guarding reflexes.

I am also including a small study I've done on the effects of vertebral subluxation and the autonomic nervous system. In the first edition I tried to show how serious the effects of vertebral subluxation can be on the central nervous system. These effects continue into adversely affecting the autonomic structures as well.

And finally I wanted to show the difficulty in imaging the pelvic girdle so that a true diagnostic picture is developed of someone's injuries. The focus by medicine and chiropractic on the discs of the lumbar spine producing low back pain and leg pain is for the most part misdirected. On a regular basis I have patients presenting to my office with persistent leg pain following all different types of interventions, mostly to the spine and including surgeries, which have neglected the pelvis and the injured leg. The experimentation that I've done on pubic symphysis imaging* shows how difficult it is, if not impossible, to determine the subluxation pattern of the pelvic bones from X-ray imaging. Physical examination of the position of the three bones, and the three joints in all three planes of space is needed to assess the injuries of our patients.

This book documents the damage to our spines in modern times. The majority of the spines in this study, in the high 80 percentile, have significant degenerative changes due to trauma. The international research organization, Bone and Joint Decade, reports that more than 1.75 billion people suffer from debilitating arthritis world wide. The National Council of Highway Safety is reporting that there were 16 1/2 million motor vehicle accidents in 2009. If we average four people per incident (my last accident included four vehicles and ten people) that's 66 million individuals exposed to spinal and other traumas per year in the USA. That's 100% exposure of the US population to spinal trauma just from motor vehicle accidents in 5 years. Nearly 100% of the students in the classes I teach at Life Chiropractic College West (LCCW) have reported having been in one or more accidents. Medicare is going broke because of arthritis. Eighty-five percent of Medicare claims are arthritis related. Social Security Disability (the agency you go to get Social Security before retirement age because of disability) is going broke because of arthritis claims, again it's 85%. This is a national and world wide problem.

I hope the second edition can help doctors understand how to better treat and prevent the damage depicted in these pages. The generous people that donated their bodies for science were almost invariably elderly and infirm. Only 15 to 20% of my patients are elderly. With most of my patients I am trying to prevent what I know are the expected outcomes without care. These pages show those expected outcomes. I am grateful for the support and publication of this second edition in color by LCCW. I hope this work will keep chiropractic focused on correcting the spine by adjusting subluxations.

---

* An Analysis of Pubis Symphysis Misalignment Using Plain Film Radiography
Journal of Manipulative & Physiological Therapeutics
Volume 28, Issue 5, Pages 330ñ335, June 2005
http://www.jmptonline.org/article/S0161-4754(05)00133-8/abstract

ACKNOWLEDGEMENTS

I would like to thank Life Chiropractic College-West for allowing this project to take place, without the laboratory and cadavers this study could not have occurred. The Life Chiropractic College-West Library has been very helpful with my never ending requests. I would also like to thank the many students, now doctors, who gave their valuable time in the anatomy laboratory to help this project. Especially helpful were Drs. Gordon Partridge, Jim Zallaha, Peter Fisk, Alvin Dolley, Steve Milligan, Danielle and Martien Crozier. There were many more than I can name now but I hope they all get valuable use of this book and know that their work and efforts bore fruit. I deeply appreciate the doctors who reviewed the text, wrote valuable comments and supportive letters. They are: Drs. Walter Freeman, Chuck Masarsky, Glen Harrison, Don Harrison, and Gerald Clum. I also want to thank attorneys John Starbuck, Paul Silver and Jack Silver for their review comments, which were extremely helpful in clarifying the text. I would also like to thank: Dr. Linda Fraley for taking me back to school, Gary Lewis of X-Ray Systems Inc. of San Jose, Ca. for donating the X-ray equipment to the anatomy laboratory, Dr. Jane Robinson for surveying and organizing all the material, Mitchell Boyce for getting my whole computer system up and running and making it "dummy proof", Jacqueline Ellis for teaching me how to "double click" and all the rest, Deirdre McCarthy for showing me through Photoshop, Donna Robbins for all the typing, editing and support, Brian Lewis for his help with the terminology, Susan Davis for her work on the illustrations and Olivia Destandau for help with the graphics. Without any one of you this book could not have been finished. Invaluable work on the final phases of this book were the typesetting, picture editing, and indexing by Paul Marcus and Shereen Harris of General Eclectics. There were many people, over the years, who were encouraging and supportive. I have been so fortunate they are too numerous to name. I thank you all.

William J. Ruch, D. C.
Oakland, 1996

I would like to acknowledge the people that helped with this 2nd edition. Dr. Brian Kelly's enthusiasm for the first edition is the main reason we're able to get this second edition done. Without his support and encouragement this second edition would still be being discussed instead of published. I would also like to thank Dr. Steve James for the dissections of the autonomic nervous system. Susan Davis, again, has provided us with her excellent illustrations. Paul Marcus has again lent his technical skills to getting this book published. I would also like to thank the reviewers, Drs. Malik Slosberg, Chris Kent, Roger Coleman, Loretta O'Brien, Bryan Gatterman and Dan Murphy for their reviews, comments and direction to help with clarity, and Dr. Ted Hunt for his extensive and meticulous editorial work. I thank you all.

William J. Ruch, D. C.
Oakland, 2014

INTRODUCTION

Subluxation of the vertebrae consists of injury to the ligaments, discs, cartilage, joint capsules, tendons, and other supporting tissues. Its occurrence initiates inflammation, muscle spasms, pain and immobility. Subluxation of the vertebrae is the etiology of spinal osteoarthritis and can influence the shape of the spinal cord and brainstem and alter nervous system blood supply. This book illustrates the future degenerative consequences of subluxation. Deterioration of the vertebral column following loss of normal alignment can impair circulation of blood and cerebral spinal fluid in the spinal cord leading to pain and loss of neurological control. Today's trauma can be a serious health factor twenty years from now.

This book is organized into six chapters. The first two chapters detail the principles and anatomical and physiological facts used in the next four chapters. The atlases of chapters 3, 4 and 5 are primarily paired pictures of a specimen with the X-rays I took of that specimen. Most of the dissections of the spines involved sagittal sectioning of the cervical spine and the thoracic spine. The remaining lumbar-pelvic section was dissected to show the combined muscular and nervous tissues that cross the whole region. The sections were cut in a mid-sagittal plane (as close as we could get) and X-rayed from the lateral view. A-P X-rays were also taken before sectioning but are not part of this presentation. There are characteristic patterns of subluxations and I have tried to classify these and document the more common types of changes that occur in all the structures of the spine. The pictures are arranged in the order of progressive severity of subluxation and degeneration. There are many ways in which the spine can subluxate (deviate) from normal. The normal spine has an architecture that can be described in the X-Y-Z planes (the Cartesian coordinate system). This book focuses on deviation in the Z plane (anterior to posterior direction) but there are some Y plane problems pointed out (inferior to superior direction). The sixth chapter, on the pelvis, deals with innominate rotation around the X axis (flexion/extension subluxations) and shearing dislocations in the Z and Y planes.

The book also contains advanced imaging (CT Scan and MRI) of sections of the spine and pelvis, some with their associated X-rays. These X-rays, CT Scans, and MRIs are of my patients, and I am grateful for their kind cooperation in allowing these images to be used for educational purposes.

I believe there are a number of professions that can benefit from this book besides chiropractic. Medical personnel need to know the biomechanics of the spine in emergency rooms, as well as orthopedic and neurosurgeons in operating rooms. Legal personnel evaluating injured claimants can have graphic material that shows the extent of soft tissue damage, as well as future degenerative conditions that can be expected post traumatically. Insurance personnel and nursing supervisors can get a more accurate picture of the future health care needs of their policy holders.

The chiropractic profession needs to have a better understanding of the dynamic principles and anatomic structures of the human spine and pelvis to better serve their patients. I hope this book can contribute to our abilities to understand the pathology of subluxations and to adjust them.

An Atlas Of Common Subluxations Of The Human Spine And Pelvis

IN THE ANTERIOR TO POSTERIOR VIEW
WITH MID-SAGITTAL SECTIONS OF SPECIMENS AND X-RAYS.

TABLE OF CONTENTS

FRONT MATTER

Dedication iii
Forward v
Preface vi
Preface to the Second Edition vii
Acknowledgements viii
Introduction ix
Table of Contents xi

CHAPTER ONE

Normal Spinal Anatomy: Structure and Dynamics

Discussion 1
The Three Spinal Systems 2
- The Vertebral Column 2
- The Thecal Sac 3
- The Spinal Cord 7

Normal Relationships of the Upper Cervical Anatomy 10
Motion of the Vertebral Column 11

CHAPTER TWO

The Pathophysiology of Subluxation

Discussion 13
- Spinal Subluxation and the Central Nervous System 13
- Spinal Cord Deformation 22
- Inflammation of the Meninges 24
- The Expected Outcomes 26

CHAPTER THREE
An Atlas of Cervical Subluxations

Discussion 29
Expanded Table of Contents of the atlas of cervical subluxations 35
Section I: Subluxations with lordotic cervical curve 38
Section II: Subluxations with loss of lordotic curve (straight or military neck) 54
Section III: Subluxations with reversed or kyphotic curve 60
Upper cervical subluxations 60
Mid-Cervical subluxations 66
Lower cervical subluxations 70

CHAPTER FOUR
An Atlas of Thoracic Subluxations

Discussion 85
Expanded Table of Contents of the atlas of thoracic subluxations 96
Section I: Subluxations with a normal thoracic curve 98
Section II: Subluxations with a reversed upper curve 100
Section III: Subluxations with a reversedlower curve 106
Section IV: Subluxations with anterolisthesis of the upper and lower thoracic vertebrae . . . 112
Section V: Hyperkyphosis of the thoracic curve 118
Additional MRIs and X-rays 124

CHAPTER FIVE
An Atlas of Lumbar Subluxations

Discussion 129
Expanded Table of Contents of the atlas of lumbar subluxations 139
Section I: Subluxations of the lumbar spine with a normal lordotic curve 142
Section II: Subluxations of the lumbar spine with a loss of lordotic curve 170
Section III: Subluxations of the lumbar spine with a reversed lordotic curve 182
Additional X-ray/MRI comparison 190

CHAPTER SIX
An Atlas of Subluxations of the Pelvic Girdle

Discussion 193
Section I: Physiological or rotational subluxations of the Innominate 205
Section II: Non-physiological subluxations of the Innominate 206
Section III: Intra-sacral subluxations 216

BACK MATTER

Endnotes/References 219
Glossary 225
Index 239
Biographical Information 244

CHAPTER ONE

Normal Human Spine

This chapter will discuss the normal spinal column as a complex and dynamic structure. The normal physiology and anatomy must be studied before one can understand the pathological effects of subluxation complexes. Emphasis will be placed on the physiology of the motion of the central nervous system and its supporting tissues within the normal spinal column.

The shape of the spinal column and canal, posture, and the pressures on the spinal cord are intimately related. Poor posture is not merely a reflection of personality or character. It can be a reflection of altered spinal curves and misplaced body masses. Examples are displacement of the head in relation to the rib cage, and displacement of the rib cage in relation to the pelvis. The displacements deform the spinal column and result in joint dysfunction. What is not commonly understood is the resulting disruption of the spinal cord, which brings with it impaired motor, sensory and autonomic function.

The spinal column has three integrated systems. Under normal conditions, each system moves differently and has distinct dynamic qualities from the others (**see Figure 1-1**). When healthy and normal, the three systems move synchronously and in harmony. Several of the causes which change the spinal column from the normal state are car accidents, compulsory education, and deforming our bodies to modern life.

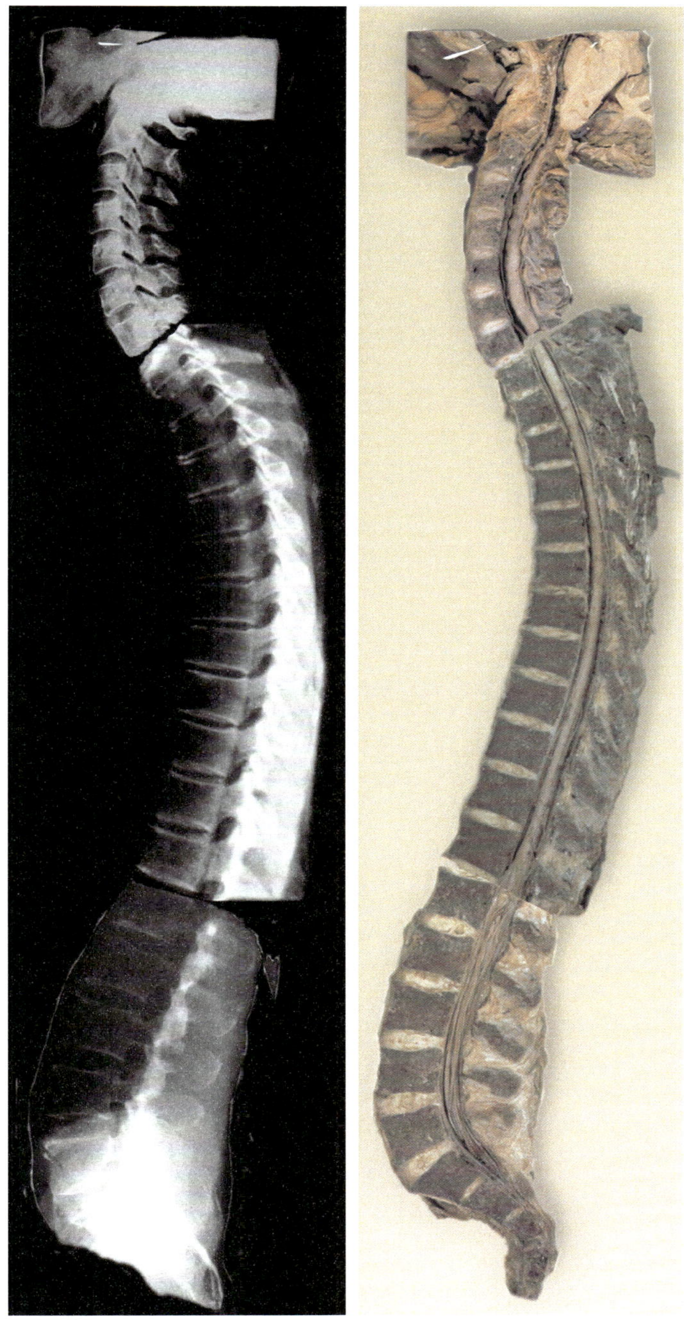

Figure 1-1
NEAR NORMAL SPINE
The normal spinal column has lordotic curves in the cervical and lumbar regions and kyphotic curves in the thoracic and sacral regions; these are essential architectural features. The pons, brainstem and spinal cord are all a continuous structure. There is space in the spinal canal between the spinal cord and the front of the canal in the neutral postion. There is slight disc degeneration in the anterior of every disc. Disc height is normal with some very slight anterior disc bulging. Note the presence of hydrated, healthy discs in an elderly individual.

THE THREE SPINAL SYSTEMS

The three spinal systems are:

- the vertebral column itself with the vertebrae, discs, ligaments, facets, capsules, cartilage and muscles.
- the thecal sac—the dura mater-arachnoid mater tube or envelope of the central nervous system.
- the brain stem, spinal cord and nerve roots ("pons-cord tissue tract"as Dr. Alf Breig calls the lower central nervous tissue). This is from the clivus of the occiput to the spinal canal and to the sacrum and coccyx. It is continuous tissue from the pons to the conus medularis and caudae equinae.[1]

Each system (**see Figure 1-2**) has a different way of moving based on its structure. Structure and function go together, and each has completely different tissues and handles motion in a unique way. We will discuss the structure and motion of each system in conjunction with the absolute or global motion of the normal spinal column.

The Vertebral Column

The first system is the vertebral column. One aspect of the vertebral column not well appreciated is the "3 point weight bearing" system of most of the vertebrae (**see Figure 1-3**). The occipital-atlas is a 2-point-joint system, as is essentially the atlanto-axial joint. The C2-C3 joints become a 3-point weight bearing system and thus it remains down to the L5-sacral joints. Studies indicate that the normal vertebral body/disc unit bears about 36% of the body weight and each of the two facets bear about 32%.[2] Altered weight bearing changes this relationship and causes altered bone remodeling. We know that gravitational force is involved with normal physiology (space travel causes osteoporosis).[3,4] Therefore, altered gravitational forces (altered weight bearing) create altered bone. Subluxations change the weight bearing of the involved joints. Altered posture and reduced viability are reflections of the subluxations.

The vertebral column is a much investigated system. Studies attempt to describe vertebral column motion with various terms, but all will agree that the motion between each vertebrae accumulates to give overall or absolute motion. This motion involves compression of the cartilaginous interfaces between the vertebrae at all the joint structures. Normal motion acts as a pump to promote the physiological forcing of fluid exchange, nutrient supply and waste elimination. When motion is prevented, pathology results.[5,6,7]

Segmental motion combines to give global or "absolute motion," like bending forward. The motion of the vertebra varies with the section of

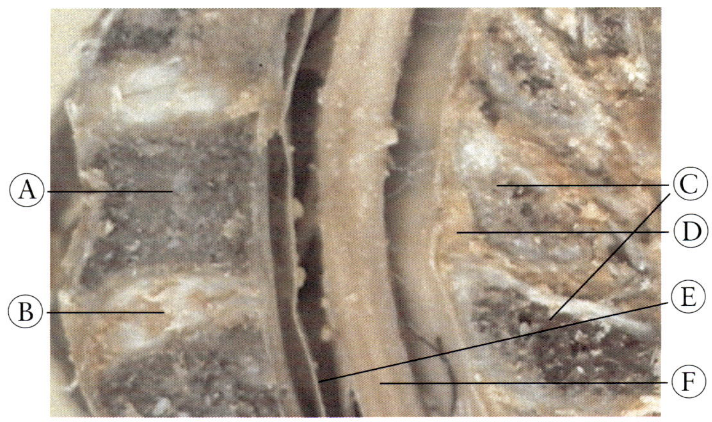

Figure 1-2
THE THREE SYSTEMS OF THE HUMAN SPINE:

1 -THE VERTEBRAL COLUMN
(A) Vertebral body
(B) Disc
(C) Spinous process
(D) Ligamentum flavum

2-THE MENINGES OR THECAL SAC
(E) Thecal wall

3-PONS-CORD TISSUE TRACT
(F) Spinal cord

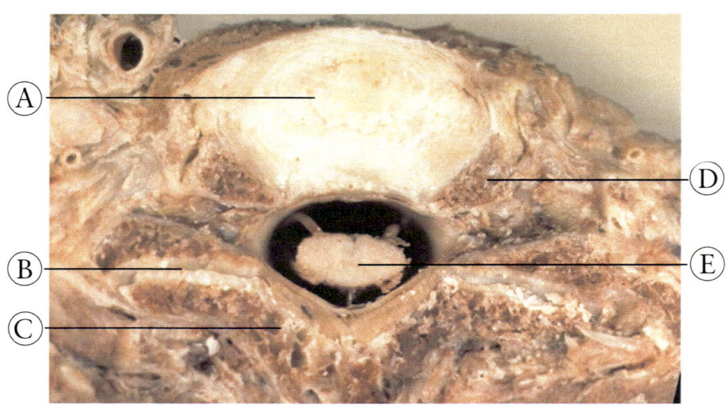

Figure 1-3
THREE POINT WEIGHT BEARING
Three point weight bearing in the cervical spine. The posterior articulations or facets provide weight bearing support as well as the body and disc.
(A) Disc
(B) Posterior articulation or facets
(C) Lamina
(D) Uncinate process
(E) Spinal cord

the vertebral column. Because the cartilaginous facets are in different planes of orientation, and the discs are of different sizes and shapes, the cervical vertebrae move differently than the thoracic vertebrae, which in turn move differently than the lumbar vertebrae. The motion between each pair of vertebrae, (segmental motion) such as C4 and C5, T4 and T5 or L4 and L5, is unique, each contributing to flexion, extension and twisting of the whole spine (global or absolute motion).

The Thecal Sac

The second system, the thecal sac, is connected to the top, bottom, and right and left sides of the spinal canal, surrounding and changing shape during motion[8] (**see Figure 1-4**). The changes of the spinal canal in normal motion are transmitted to the thecal sac as deforming forces. A common example is when pulling on a balloon (motion) one expects it to change shape (deform).

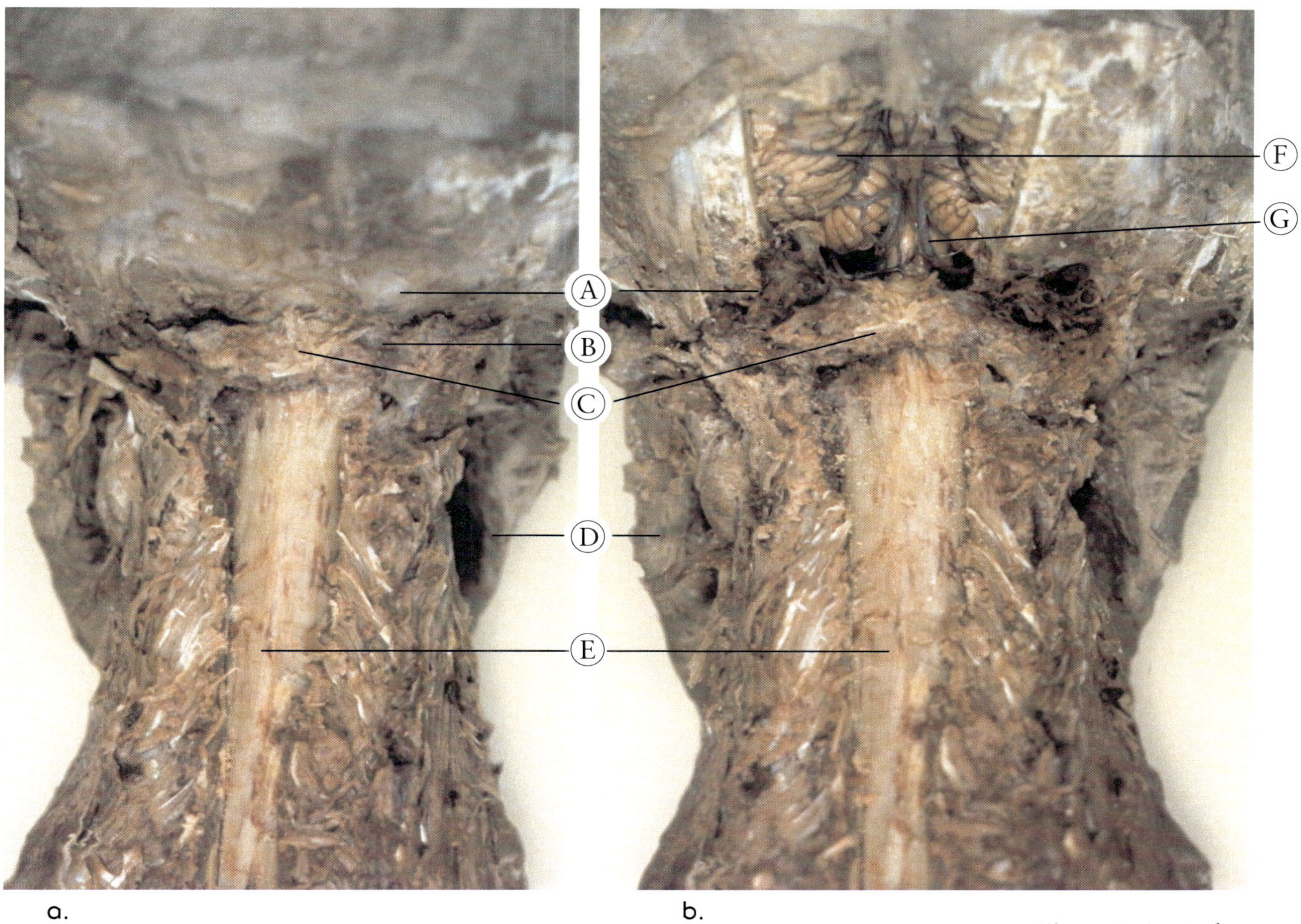

Figure 1-4 a & b

NORMAL ANATOMICAL RELATIONSHIPS OF THE SKULL AND VERTEBRAL COLUMN

Photo (a). Laminectomized specimen with skin removed from back of skull, to show relationships of structures. (Posterior view.)

(A) Base of Skull (Occiput)
(B) Vertebral artery
(C) Atlas
(D) Mandible
(E) Thecal Sac

Photo (b). Same specimen with occiput partially removed to show the cerebellum.

(F) Cerebellum
(G) Posterior Inferior Cerebellar Artery

The term "thecal" or "theca" is used to describe the combined dura/arachnoid mater and other supportive structures. The dura mater is the tough enclosing membrane of the sac. The arachnoid mater is the inner lining of the sac. The "subdural space," between the dura and arachnoid mater, is a potential space (**see Figure 1-5**). This space doesn't really exist in a normal spinal column. That is why the term "theca" is used to describe this seemingly single structure with the dura mater on one side and the arachnoid mater on the other. Pathological conditions can separate these structures, but normally they act or function as a single structure.

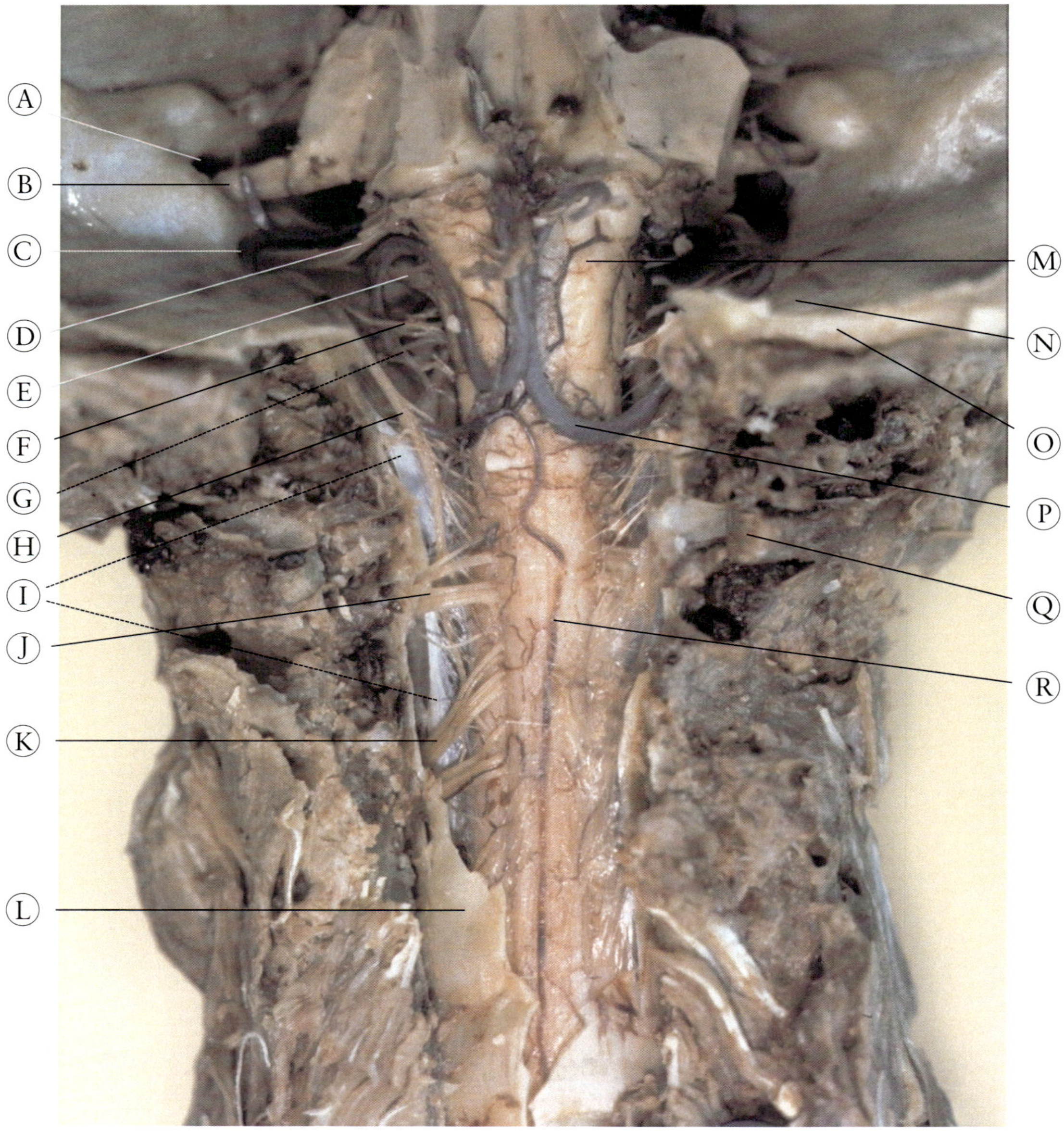

Figure 1-5
NORMAL ANATOMICAL RELATIONSHIPS, continued

Photo (c). Same specimen with occiput opened and cerebellum removed, with the skull in the neutral position relative to the neck.

(A) Internal Auditory Meatus
(B) Acoustic Nerve(VIII)
(C) Jugular Foramen
(D) Glossopharyngeal Nerve(IX)
(E) Vagus Nerve(X)
(F) Hypoglossal Nerve (XII)
(G) C1 nerve rootlets
(H) Spinal Accessory Nerve (XI)
(I) Dentate Ligament
(J) C2 Nerve rootlets
(K) C3 Nerve rootlets
(L) Thecal sac (dural side)
(M) Brainstem
(N) Cerebellar Fossa
(O) Occiput (cut edge)
(P) Posterior Inferior Cerebellar Artery
(Q) Arch of Atlas
(R) Dorsal Spinal Vein

"Meninges" is a collective term used to describe all the supporting tissue of the central nervous system. This includes; the thecal sac (theca), the pia mater, the dentate ligaments (AKA denticulate), arachnoid trabeculae, a web of fibers in the subarachnoid space attaching to the arachnoid mater, and pia mater that holds the cerebral spinal fluid (CSF) as a cushion for the spinal cord. The median septum is a single sheet of tissue in the posterior canal between the cord and the theca. The meninges provide support and confer shape to the cord tissue.

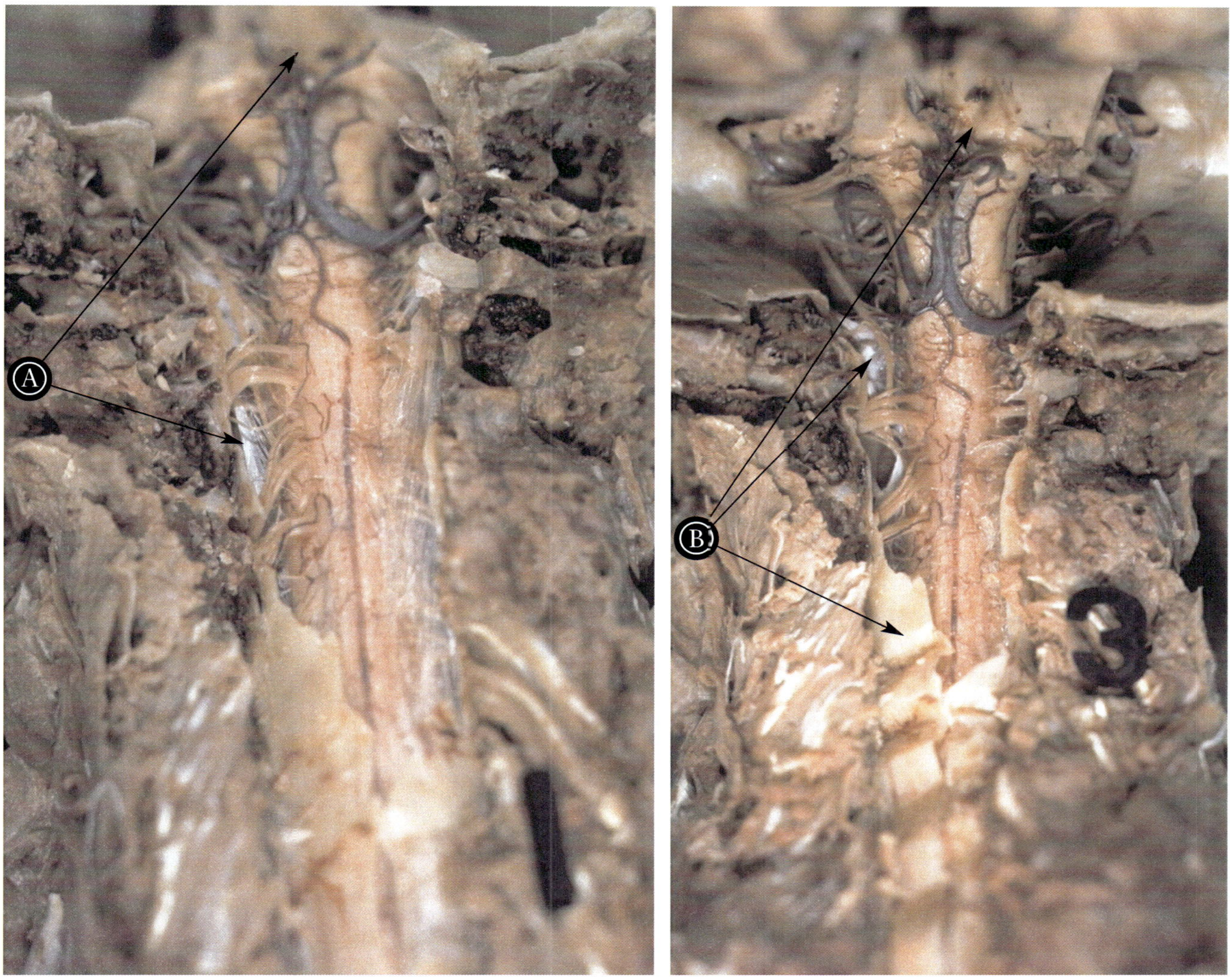

a. b.

Figure 1-6 a & b

EFFECTS OF HEAD FLEXION AND EXTENSION ON THE CENTRAL NERVOUS SYSTEM

(a). Flexion(head tipped forward) increases the distance between the occiput and the coccyx, therefore lengthening the neural canal and the stretching the cord and brainstem.

(A) Note stretching of the dentate ligament and the movement of the brainstem down toward the occiput. Note positions of Dentate Ligament, Brainstem, Base of Occiput, Arch of Atlas (refer to Fig. 1-5 for keys to anatomical structures)

(b). Extension (head tipped backward) decreases the distance between the occiput and the coccyx, shortening and relaxing the cord and brainstem.

(B) Note the relaxed left dentate ligament, the folded, relaxed dura mater (thecal sac), and the distance of the brainstem from the occiput. Note positions of Dentate Ligament, Brainstem, Base of Occiput, Arch of Atlas, Thecal sac.

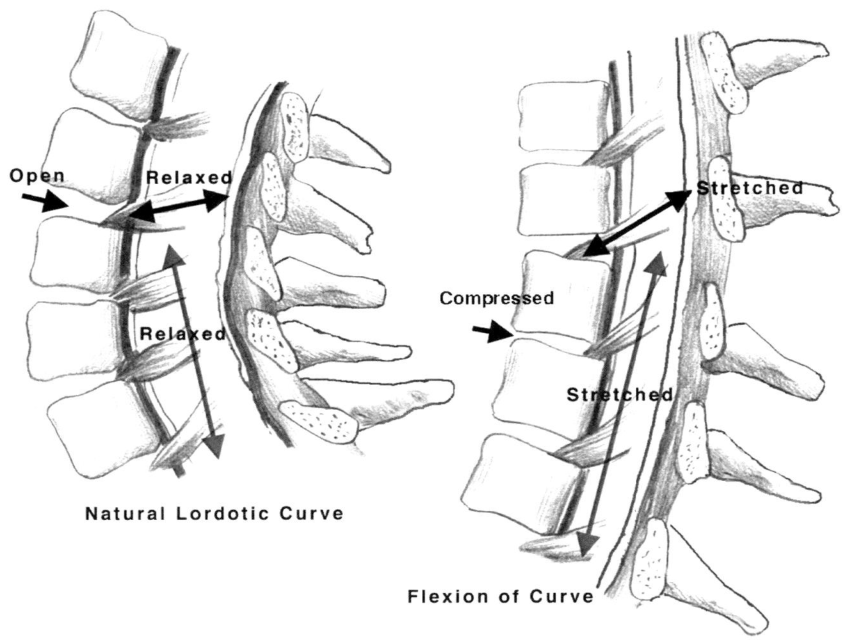

Figure 1-7
A normal ("natural") lordotic curve in comparison to flexion. The closeness of the lamina and spinous processes in extension shortens the posterior aspect of the canal. Compare the flexion position with the large space between each lamina and spinous process. The spinal cord and thecal sac go from being on the inside of a concavity to the outside of a convexity.

There are some significant effects of absolute motion on the spinal cord. Vertebral column flexion (bending forward) increases the length of the spinal canal and spinal cord.[9,10] The net increase in distance from the foramen magnum to the coccyx varies with each individual's spinal canal, but can be 2-3 inches (5-7cm) from extreme extension (shortened position) to extreme flexion (lengthened position).[11] (**See Figure 1-6.**) This is accomplished in the vertebral column by lamina and facet separation and posterior disc height increase (**see Figure 1-7**). Also, in lateral flexion, the concave side is shortened and the convex side is lengthened. For instance, in right lateral flexion, the right side of the spinal canal is shorter in length than the left side of the canal. Absolute motion changes the shape of the spinal canal.

The thecal sac is made of the same tissue from top to bottom and has normal tube dynamics. It deforms as a tube in flexion and extension. Its net length will vary inversely with its diameter. The longer the tube gets, the narrower it becomes while the shorter the tube gets, the wider it becomes. The volume remains relatively the same throughout the various positions the vertebral column can assume. Loss of the normal spinal architecture can change this relationship with mechanical and hydrualic pressures that result in pathology.[12]

The thecal sac in the normal spinal column should be attached to the foramen magnum and upper cervical spine and coccyx. In between, it should be free of attachment to the vertebrae. This is not strictly true because the nerve root sheath of every nerve root is an extension of the thecal sac which attach to the intervertebral foramen (IVF) and distal tissue (**see Figure 1-8**). These other attachments create slightly different dynamics than independent tubular structures.

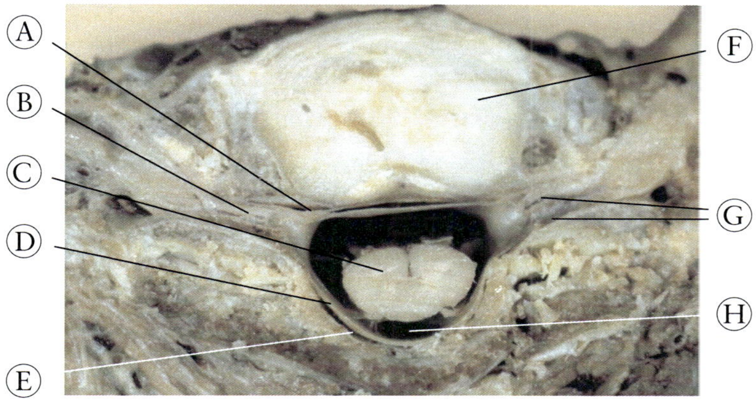

Figure 1-8
NORMAL ANATOMICAL RELATIONSHIPS-AXIAL VIEW
Axial section through the C7-T1 disc. See how the epineural sheath around the nerve root in the I.V.F. is an extension of the thecal sac. This shape and position of spinal cord is normal.
(A) Nerve root sheath
(B) Nerve root
(C) Spinal cord
(D) Thecal sac
(E) Epidural space
(F) Disc
(G) Intervertebral foramen (I.V.F.)
(H) Subarachnoid space

THE SPINAL CORD

The third system, the "pons-cord tissue tract," includes the entire spinal cord from the conus medularis to the brain stem and the pons.[13] It also includes the nerve rootlets that gather to form the nerve roots. This is all continuous tissue. The spinal cord is attached to the thecal sac via the pia mater, spinal nerve rootlets, dentate ligaments, arachnoid mater, and the filum terminale, collectively called the meninges. The spinal cord and much of the nervous tissue of the central nervous system is actually an amorphous, gelatin-like substance; its shape is controlled by the supporting (meningal) structures.

As the thecal sac changes in shape with normal position change of the individual, the pons-cord tissue tract also changes in shape and position. In forward flexion, the cord moves anteriorly in the canal and increases in overall length. This motion can change the relationship between the nerve roots and the foraminae. The anterior to posterior diameter of the cord decreases and the right-to-left diameter increases. This makes the spinal cord look oval on cross section, while it should be round, or nearly round.[14] The dentate ligaments, attaching to the pia mater on the right and left side of the cord, cause a different action in lateral flexion and rotation. As the person bends and/or rotates to one side, the dentate ligament on the concave or shortened side relaxes while the dentate ligament of the convex side is stretched. This pulls the cord to the convex or longer side of the canal away from the compressing side of the spine. This change in the shape of the cord changes the shape of the tiny arteries, arterioles and capillaries. The continual motion of the vertebral column acts as a pump. This normal pumping action pushes the blood cells and nutrients through the cord tissue, facilitating the blood flow that occurs in the lower central nervous system.[15]

As stated earlier, when the spinal column is healthy, the three systems move in harmony. Segmental vertebral column motion is unique, differing with the section under observation. Deforming forces of the vertebral column during normal motion are transmitted through the thecal sac as a uniform motion. Despite the uneven, unique inter-segmental motion of the vertebrae, the motion of the thecal sac, under normal conditions, transmits a uniform force to the spinal cord. This is a very important point. Standing with just cranial flexion will stretch the meninges and cord all the way to the caudae equinae.[16,17] The spinal cord needs and requires uniform distribution of this motion along its entire length for normal function. This leads to a distribution of forces to the whole pons-cord tissue tract, thus helping to reduce the occurrence of deforming forces severely affecting one part of the cord and causing nervous tissue injury. The nervous tissue also needs this motion and changing shape to deliver adequate nutrients, because the motion acts as a pump for the whole CNS.[18,19,20]

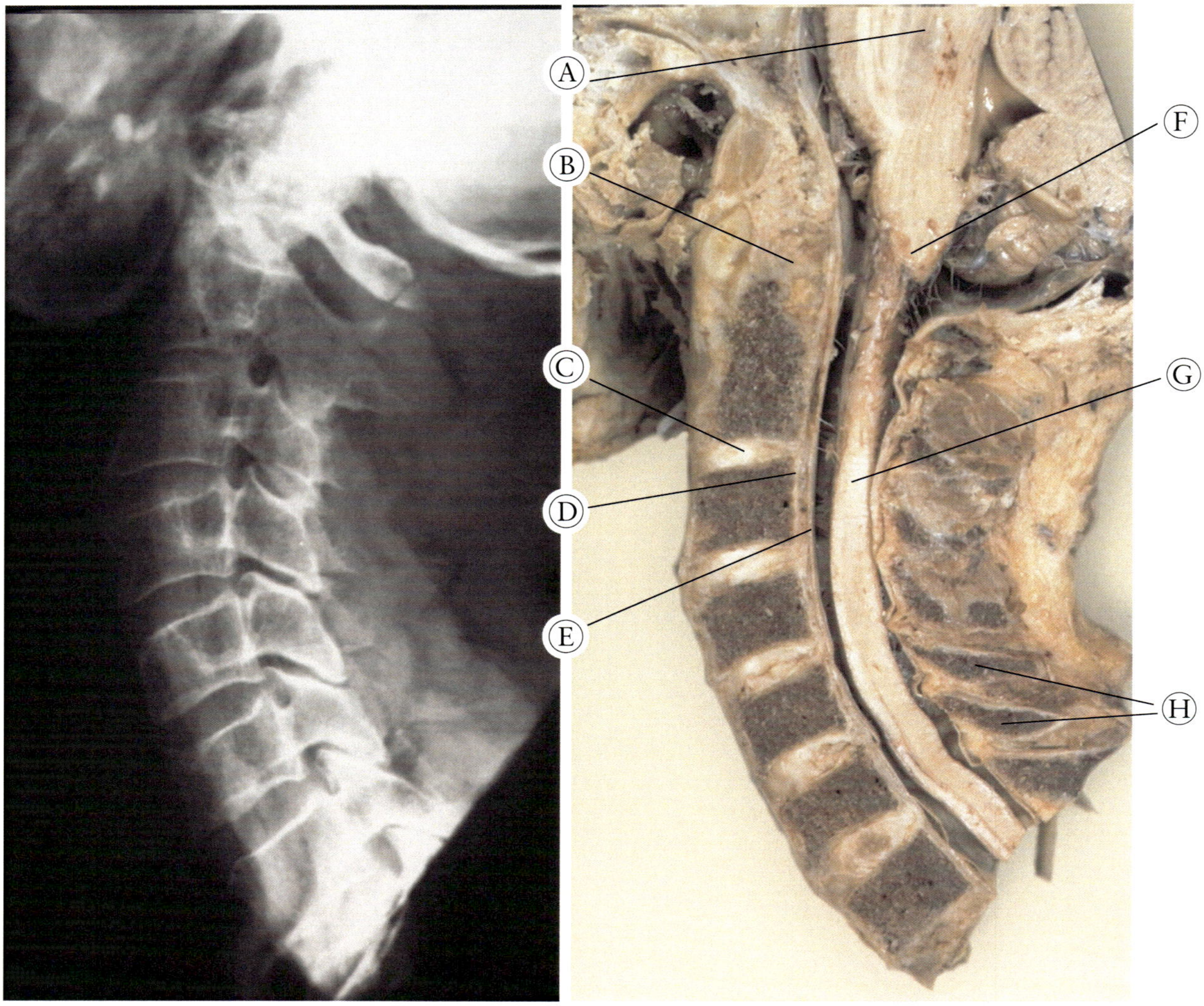

Figure 1-9

NORMAL SPINAL CORD - CANAL RELATIONSHIP

In this individual, the spinal cord does not completely fill the vertebral canal. Minor posterior disc bulging (as at C5-C6 and C6-C7) has occurred without directly impinging on the cord, so this individual may have experienced only minor symptoms or none at all. Note the healthy cervical curve.

(A) Pons
(B) Dens of C2
(C) Disc of C2-C3
(D) Posterior longitudinal ligament
(E) Thecal sac
(F) Brainstem
(G) Spinal cord
(H) Spinous processes

There are individual differences or variations in the diameter of the spinal cord and in the diameter of the vertebral canal (**see Figures 1-9 and 1-10**). A canal diameter of 10 mm or less is considered narrow and any canal larger than 13 mm is unlikely to have stenosis.[21] Being born with a narrow canal is called congenital canal stenosis. This anatomical variation can manifest itself as different symptoms with the same diagnosis or trauma.[22] Different individuals can have completely different responses to similar injuries. They can have different symptoms, complaints, and recovery times. This is the basis for using "syndromes" to describe the range of effects of types of injuries. Some of the symptoms will be present in certain people and not in others even in the same accident. To illustrate the differences in spinal canal diameter and its relationship to disc bulging please look at **Figure 3-3** and **Plate 3-3B**. In **Figure 3-3** we see a mild disc bulge in contact with the spinal cord because of the narrow canal. In **Plate 3-3B** we see a large canal with a more significant disc bulge without spinal cord contact.

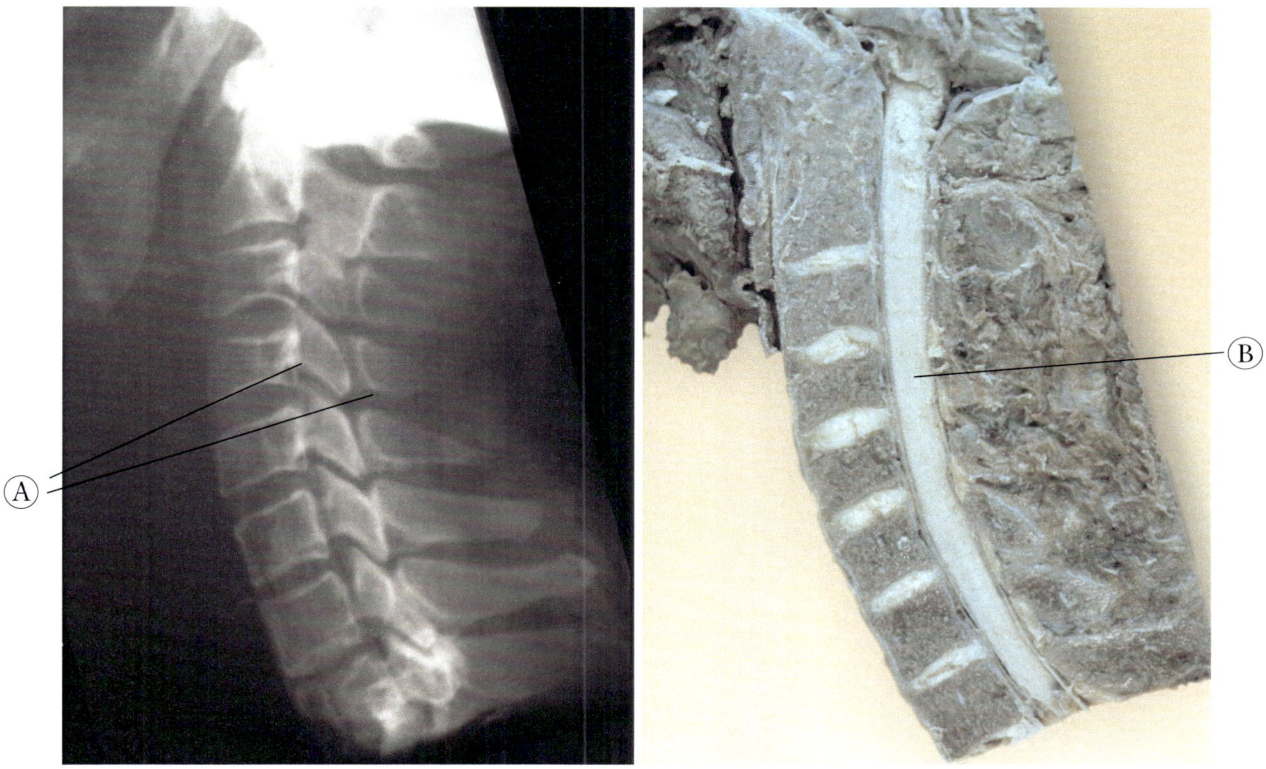

Figure 1-10
CERVICAL SPINAL CANAL NARROWING OR STENOSIS.
The relationship between the size of the canal and spinal cord can vary between individuals. In this specimen the spinal cord occupies the entire canal. Any changes in the shape in the wall of the canal can have significant neurological consequences. (A) narrow spinal canal, (B) spinal cord.

NORMAL RELATIONSHIPS OF THE UPPER CERVICAL ANATOMY

The upper cervical spine, with the occiput and the head and brain to support, has important structural significance. All the neurological and vascular components of the head go through this region. Distortion or rearrangement of any components will have adverse affects on other components as well as itself.[23] Local peripheral neurological structures include the superior sympathetic ganglion, and the main parasympathetic nerve, the vagus. **Figure 1-11** shows the close relationship of the occiput, vertebrae and the contents of the jugular foramen. Subluxation of the upper cervical vertebrae and or occiput subluxation will distress any or all of these neurological structures. Profound health problems could be initiated by interfering with and stressing these neurological structures.[24,25] Symptoms would be gradual and insidious. Duration of irritation is a critical factor in neurological problems.[26,27] In **Figure 1-11** note the connection of levator scapula to the C1 transverse process. A shoulder or rib cage injury can have an adverse affect on the alignment of the upper cervical spine. These types of relationships; structures going from one region to the next, make study by regions (this book) difficult. The muscle, levator scapula, attaches to the medial angle of the scapula and ascends medially to the upper cervical spine and attaches to the transverse processes of C1 to C3 or more, (I have found, in one individual, the levator scapula attached to every cervical vertebrae down to C7). A rib cage injury will cause serratus anterior muscle guarding (serratus anterior attaches to the anterior surface of the scapula and goes forward and laterally to the side of the rib cage). This would move the scapula away from the midline and the levator scapula would then pull laterally and posteriorly on the upper cervical spine. This action would provoke a persistent pulling and tension to the upper cervical spine and base of the occiput. Motor vehicle accidents are a typical source of this common type of tension headache.

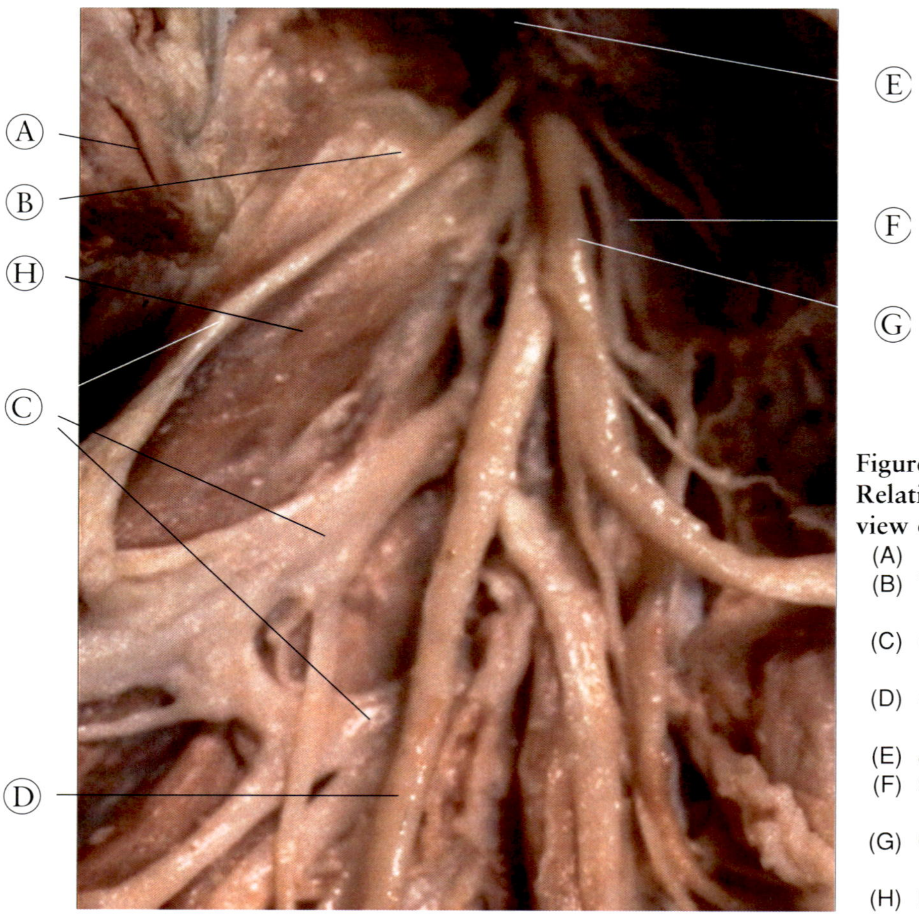

Figure 1-11
Relationships in the lateral view of the upper cervical area.
(A) Mastoid process
(B) Tip of transverse process of C1
(C) Cervical nerve roots 1, 2 and 3
(D) Cranial nerve X, the vagus nerve
(E) Jugular foramen
(F) Superior sympathetic ganglion
(G) Cranial nerve IX, the glossopharyngeal nerve
(H) Levator scapulae

Motion of the Vertebral Column

The discs of the vertebral column are for allowing flexibility of the spinal column so the head and eyes can interact with the environment[28,29]. This flexibility is essential to vascular flow in the capillaries of the spinal cord. The bending, twisting and turning an individual does is important for the nutrient and oxygen delivery to the axons and neurons of the central nervous system[30,31]. Muscles need motion for proper circulation. When at rest the muscles have "tone," a state of mild sequential contraction to aid capillary blood flow. When tone is lost in stroke or spinal cord injury, circulation to the muscles is impaired. This motion is also essential to the health of the discs and ligaments of the vertebral column[32]. Neither the discs or spinal cord have tone in their tissues. They also require motion for nutrient and oxygen exchange.[33] Studies show forced immobility initiates degenerative changes of the joint tissues.[34,35] So the discs allow motion in the spinal column. Their primary function is not a shock absorbing function.[36] The flexibility they exhibit is necessary for their health as well as that of the nervous tissue.

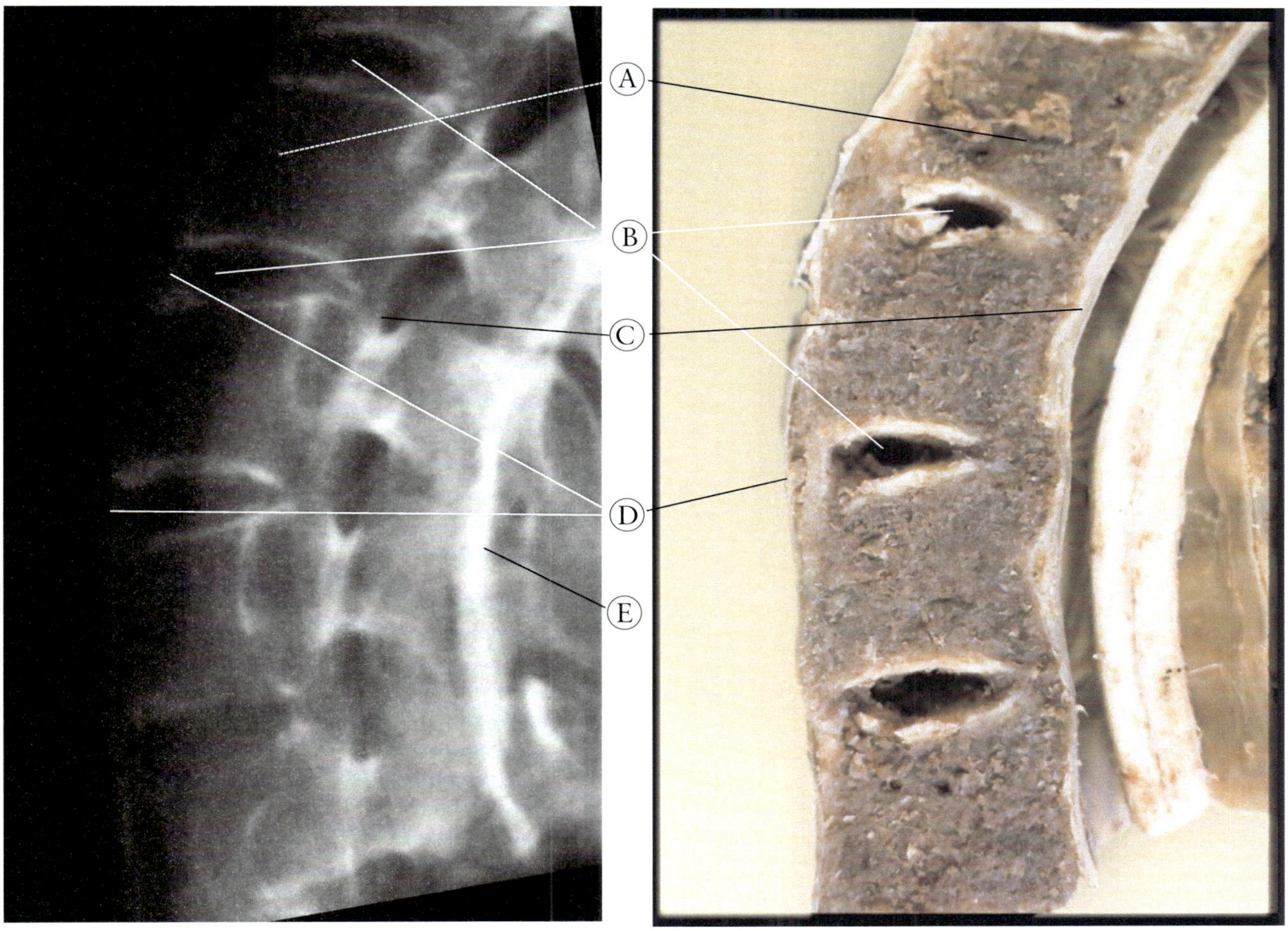

a. b.

Figure 1-12 a & b

LOSS OF MOTION RESULTS IN LOSS OF JOINT TISSUE

An X-ray and specimen of a cervical spine with fusion of all the ligaments and resulting loss of the discs and other joint tissues

(A) Vertebral bodies
(B) Disc spaces
(C) Calcified posterior longitudinal ligament
(D) Calcified anterior longitudinal ligament
(E) Facets or zygopophyseal joints are fused.

CHAPTER TWO

Pathophysiology Of The Human Spine

Spinal Subluxation and the Central Nervous System

Subluxation is a term used to describe the loss of normal joint integrity. A luxation is a complete loss of integrity or dislocation. A displacement that is less than a dissociation of two adjacent bones joined by an articulation is a subluxation. In the case of the human spine a subluxation involves two adjoining vertebrae, the disc and two pairs of facets or zygopophyseal joints. This loss of normal integrity results in stress of the connecting soft tissues, spasmodic contractions consisting of "guarding responses" to joint distress by the surrounding musculature.[1,2,3,4] Joint spaces often become reduced, and range of motion becomes limited, often accompanied by pain and inflammation.[5,6]

In the mid-sagittal plane of the human spine, the most common patterns of subluxation are a

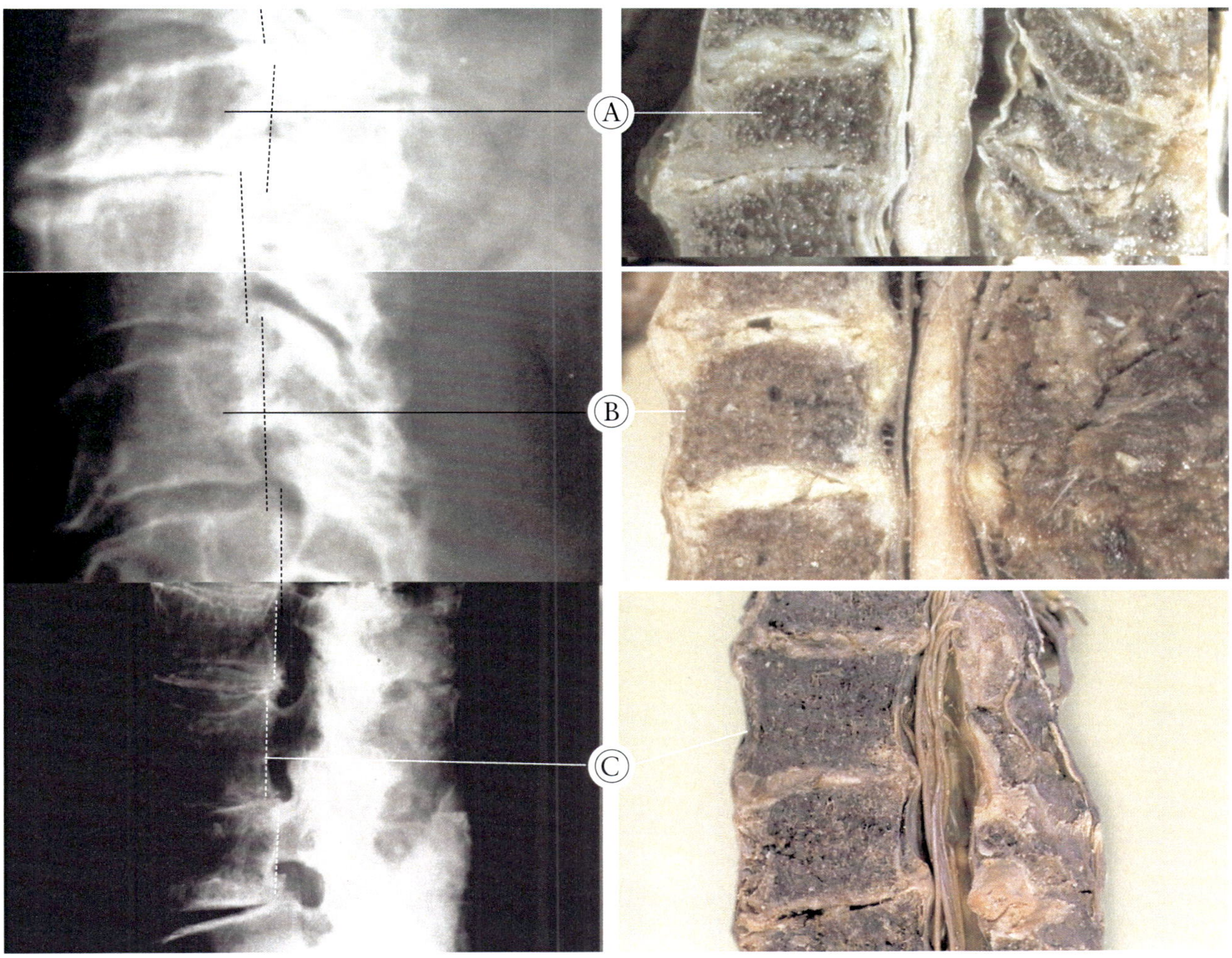

Figure 2-1
TYPES OF COMMON SUBLUXATIONS
Subluxation of vertebrae involve the three joints of two adjacent vertebrae: a disc and two zygopophyseal joints. Note the pathological changes of the zygopophyseal joints as well as the discs.

(A) A retrolisthesis: the body of this vertebra is posterior to both the superior and inferior segments.
(B) Stair stepped anterolisthesis: this vertebra is posterior to the superior vertebra but anterior to the inferior.
(C) An anterolisthesis: this vertebra is anterior to both the superior and inferior segments.

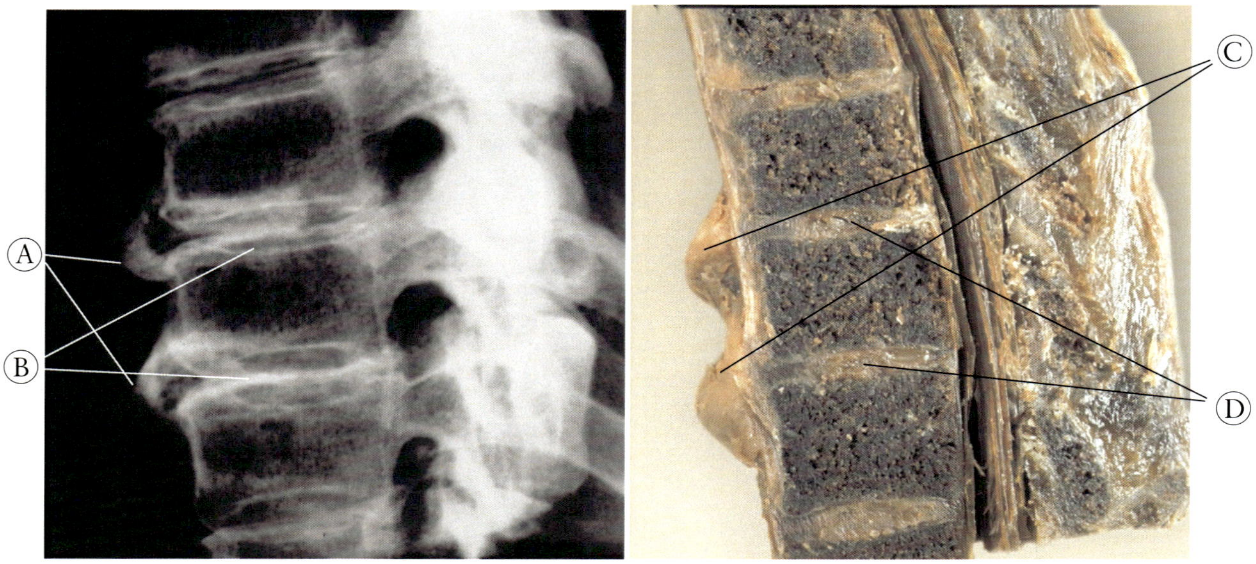

Figure 2-2
This illustrates disc bulging and endplate changes.
The endplate damage indicates trauma that has healed but has left injured soft tissues. The instability and altered mechanics of the injured joints results in chronically degenerative changes. Pictured here is a pair of bulging discs with their X-rays indicating calcification of the anterior longitudinal ligament (A.L.L.) and discs.

(A) Osteophytes
(B) Damaged endplates
(C) Bulging discs
(D) Dessicated discs.

complete retrolisthesis (**see Figure 2-1**), a retrolisthesis, stairstepped anterolisthesis and a anterolisthesis.[7] These occur in all combinations to form subluxation complexes when more than two vertebrae are involved. This is a major cause of osteoarthritis of the spine, degenerative joint disease and spondylosis.[8] Loss of normal joint integrity alters weight bearing of the joints, puts abnormal stress on soft tissues and bones and initiates degenerative processes.[9,10,11,12] In time the vertebral body develops "spurs" or "osteophytes" of various types.[13,14,15,16]

We are used to looking at vertebral bodies from two dimensions, the A-P and lateral X-ray. The endplate changes are three dimensional and are the responses to the loss of normal weight bearing (**see Chapter 1**). The subluxation of a vertebra can do one of two things to a joint: hyperload the joint or unload the joint. Both conditions will cause the bone and joint tissue to change. Normal motion is interrupted causing abberant mechanoreception, sympathetic reflexes which increases muscular tone that leads to decreased blood and nutrient flow causing deterioration of all avascular structures, ligaments, cartilage, and other connective tissue.[17] This is also true for the facets or zygopophyseal joints. A retrolisthesis hyperloads at least one disc and puts shearing forces on the anterior longitudinal ligament (A.L.L.), the posterior longitudinal ligament (P.L.L.), the annular rings, nucleus pulposus, cartilage plates and capsular ligaments.[18,19,20] The bulging, twisting, and straining tissue attached to the end plates pull, push, and stretch it. It worsens with time, becoming irreversible (**see Figure 2-2**). Pictured are two bulging discs in the anterior-lateral direction with calcification of part of the A.L.L. and end plate.

The retrolisthesis usually causes more disc degeneration, end plate changes, facet sclerosis, and spinal canal changes.[21] The stairstepped anterolisthesis is more common and associated with disc bulging, spinal curve and spinal canal changes.[22] The anterolisthesis is not as common and can be associated with either or both of the other types.

The change from normal alignment in the cervical spine can also have vascular consequences. The shape of the vertebral artery can become longer and more narrow than normal from kyphotic deformity of the cervical spine.[23,24] Mechanical distress can generate a sympathetic "storm," and a regional vasoconstriction causing irritation of the arterial wall of the vertebral artery and its tributaries, the sinu-vertebral nerves.[25] In **Figure 2-4** an axial cut was made at the middle of the body of C2 below the superior articulating facets but above the transverse processes. Viewed from below, it is apparent that C1 is rotated relative to C2 and the inferior articulating facet of C1 on the left is contacting and compromising the vertebral artery. The vertebral arteries are the blood supply to the cervical spinal cord, brainstem, and cerebellum, and any impairment can have adverse results.[26] Poor vascular circulation from pressure and increases in reflex sympathetic tone on the arteries that supply the spinal cord and pressure on the spinal tissue itself, is a natural consequence of subluxation of the spine.[27] Pain can be only one of the many results of hypoxia of the spinal cord tissue.

Multiple subluxations of the vertebral column can have a profound effect on the quality of movement, nutrition, and general health of the central nervous system. This effect occurs due to the basic anatomical fact that the shape of the vertebral column affects the shape of the spinal canal (the basic size is congenital) which in turn affects the shape of the lower central nervous system (spinal cord, brainstem and nerve roots). Subluxation of the vertebrae changes the shape of the vertebral canal. Usually this change is an increase in length of the canal. The more change, the greater the effect on the central nervous system and the spinal cord.[28]

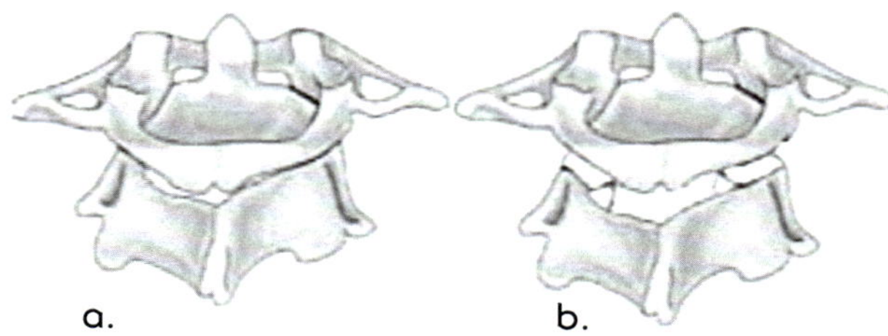

Figure 2-3 a & b

(a). Posterior view of C1 and C2.
(b). Plane of cut Fig. 2-4 has through C1 and C2. Fig. 2-4 is top section looking from underneath.

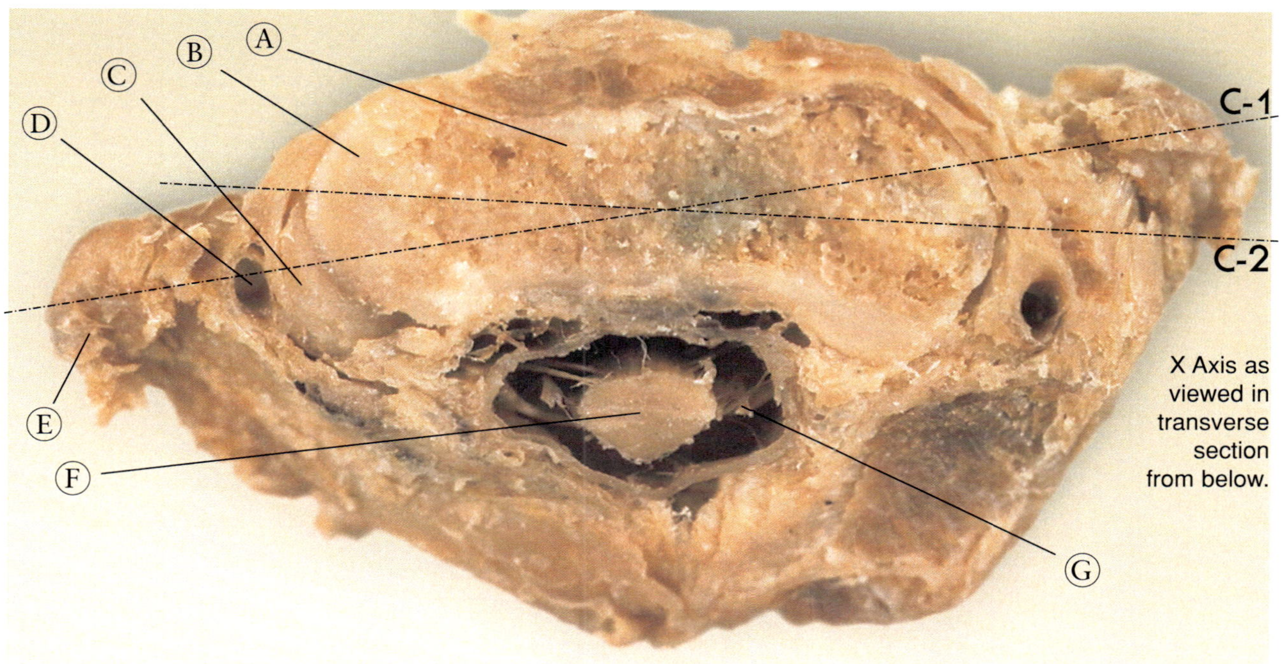

Figure 2-4
SUBLUXATION OF C1-2

Rotation of C1 to C2 with occlusion of the vertebral artery by C1 inferior facet.

(A) Body of C2
(B) Superior articulating facet of C2
(C) Inferior articulating facet of C1
(D) Vertebral artery/ foramen transversari
(E) Transverse process of C1
(F) Spinal cord
(G) Dentate Ligament

The amount of change due to subluxation can vary with the individual, the number of vertebrae involved, and how the curves are altered. There seems to be substantial natural variation between the diameter of the canal and diameter of the spinal cord. The space between the bony canal and the spinal cord can also vary with individuals (**see Chapter 1**). The degenerative changes observed with vertebral subluxation are commonly considered age related. The degree or amount of degeneration is definitely time related. As time elapses from the date of injury the joint(s) are subject to more altered weight bearing and aberrant motion from the subluxation. So time and age are related, but if an individual has a trauma at age three, then at 28 they can have 25 years of degeneration. It is difficult to tell a young patient with advanced arthritis that their problem is they are old.

This explains how some people can tolerate more change due to subluxation than others. In some cases this space, or forgiveness of the system, can explain why relatively minor subluxations can cause distress on one person's nervous system, while a second person can tolerate radical changes in the vertebral column with little or no distress. In the case of this second person one might be able to elicit some symptoms on exam but generally in the second case the person seems to enjoy good health.

The normal architectural features of lordotic and kyphotic curves are an essential component of the human spine (**see Figures 2-5 and 2-6**). In **Figure 2-5** there are near normal curves so that the multiple misalignments and bulging discs are not seriously impinging the cord. The increased thoracic curvature and reduced cervical and lumbar curves have tractioned the thoracic section of the spinal

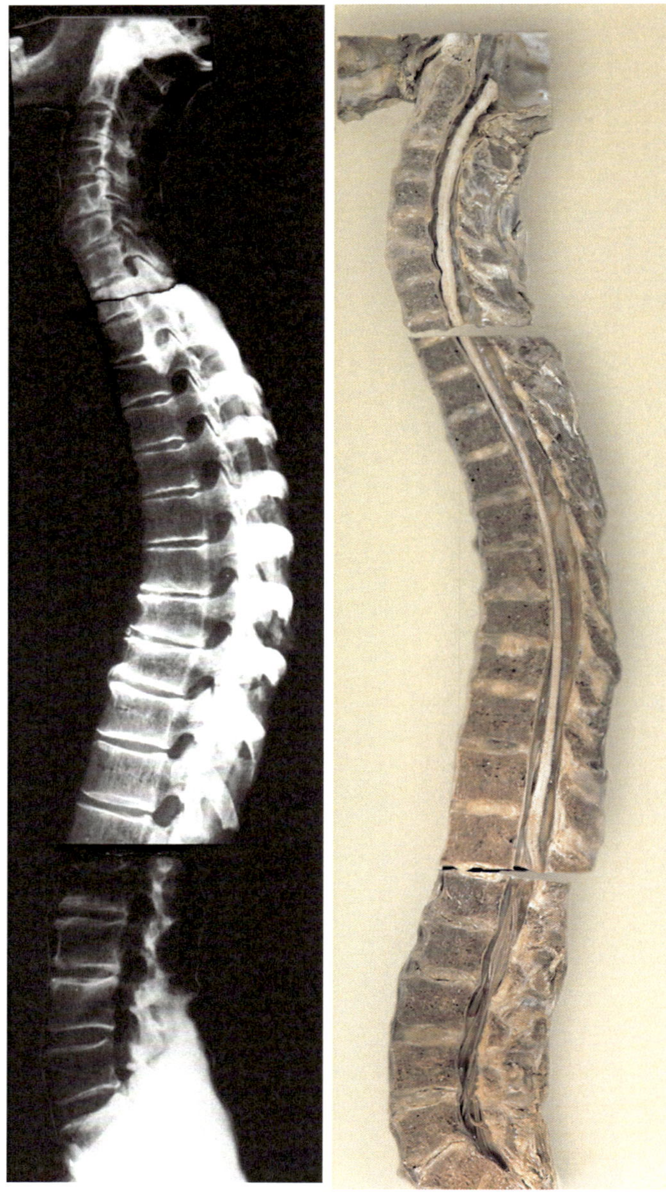

Figure 2-5
VERTEBRAL COLUMN WITH MULTIPLE SUBLUXATIONS WITH CURVES MAINTAINED

NOTE: This study shows discs don't have degeneration unless there are subluxations or they have suffered some architectural disturbance. Healthy discs occur next to pathological ones, so age can't be a factor. There is a reduced cervical curve with posterior and anterior disc bulging and loss of disc height.

1. Note: cord impressions without significant stenosis.
2. Tractioned cord in upper thoracic despite almost "normal" curve; all discs with various levels of degeneration.
3. Reduced lumbar curve and loss of disc height and hydration.

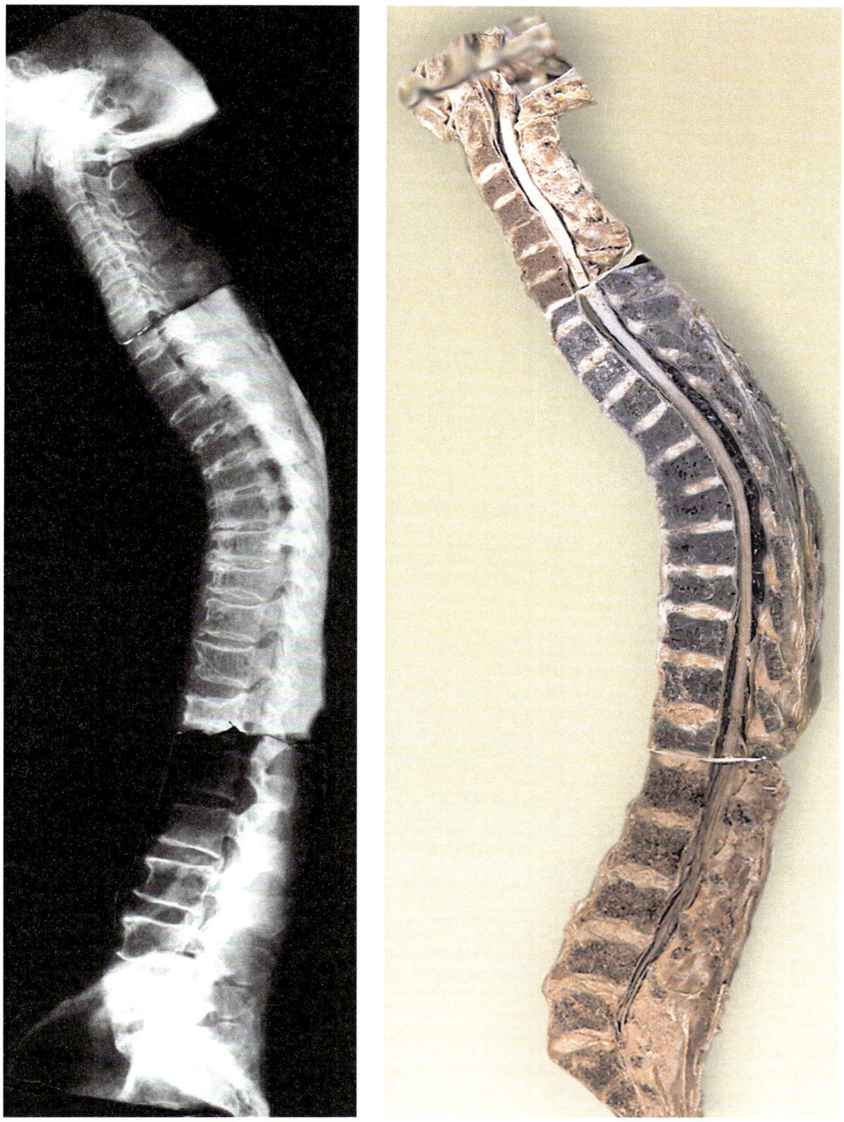

Figure 2-6
VERTEBRAL COLUMN WITH MULTIPLE SUBLUXATIONS AND LOSS OF CURVES

Here we see a reversal of cervical curve with canal stenosis and cord contact at C5-C6. The thoracic spine has progressive anterior spurring with hyperkyphosis from altered weight bearing and osteoporosis. Increased thoracic curve changes due to compression fractures T6-T12.

Note cord/canal contact T5-T9. Discs have dark brown areas that correspond to calcified appearance on X-ray. Loss of lumbar curve adds to flexion deformity of entire vertebral column and resulting poor posture.

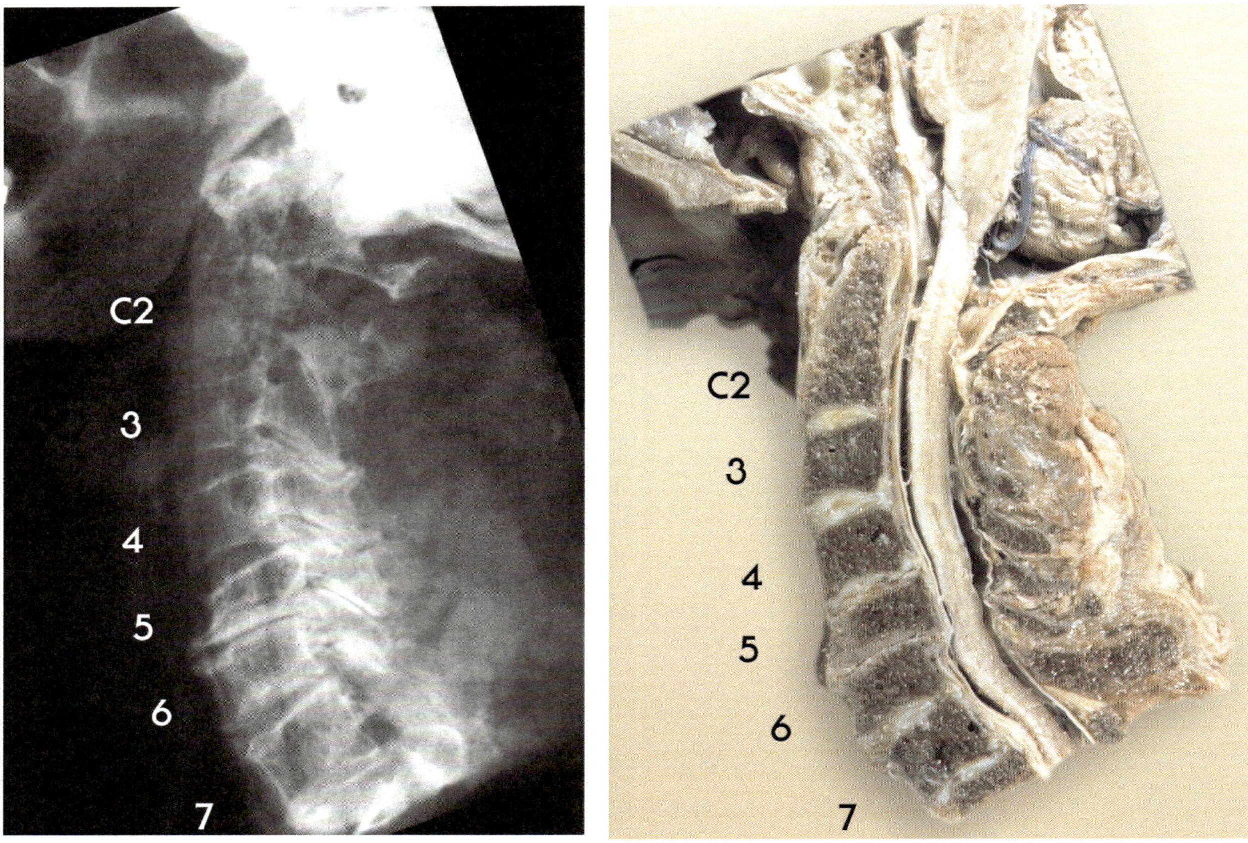

Figure 2-7
MULTIPLE SUBLUXATIONS WITH CURVE REDUCTION AND CORD CONTACT
The lower cervical spine has by far the most injuries and degenerative changes of any section of the spine. Both in the cadavers and in our patients in clinical practice, the C4-C5 and C5-C6 segments show the greatest relative anteroposterior displacement in the entire cervical spine (Hadley, 1964). They are also remote from the head, and therefore are more vulnerable to whiplash than the upper segments.

cord into the anterior wall of the canal. One can observe the normal posture of this individual. In **Figure 2-6** there is altered curvatures of all sections and a resulting "poor posture," and a bent forward or flexion deformity of the spinal column. Note the canal stenosis of the cervical region as a result of the reversal of the lordotic curve and osteophytic changes. This change in the shape of the canal is an increase in its length. The anterior portion of the cervical spinal cord is in contact with the anterior wall of the canal as is the mid thoracic cord from T5 to T9. This condition is viewed in the neutral position. Any postural change into more flexion, such as sitting in a chair, increases the traction and vascular compromise of the cord and nerve roots.

Looking at **Figure 2-7**, we see a lateral cervical X-ray and specimen (a type called a mid-sagittal section). These figures have the discs, ligaments, and a central nervous system still intact. What we see is a change in the normal relationship of the vertebrae C3-C4, mostly C4-C5, C5-C6, and C6-C7. These are very common subluxation patterns. Notice the amount of change in only the subluxated segments. This cannot be completely explained due to age because C1, C2, C3 joint complexes are the same age as C4, C5, C6.

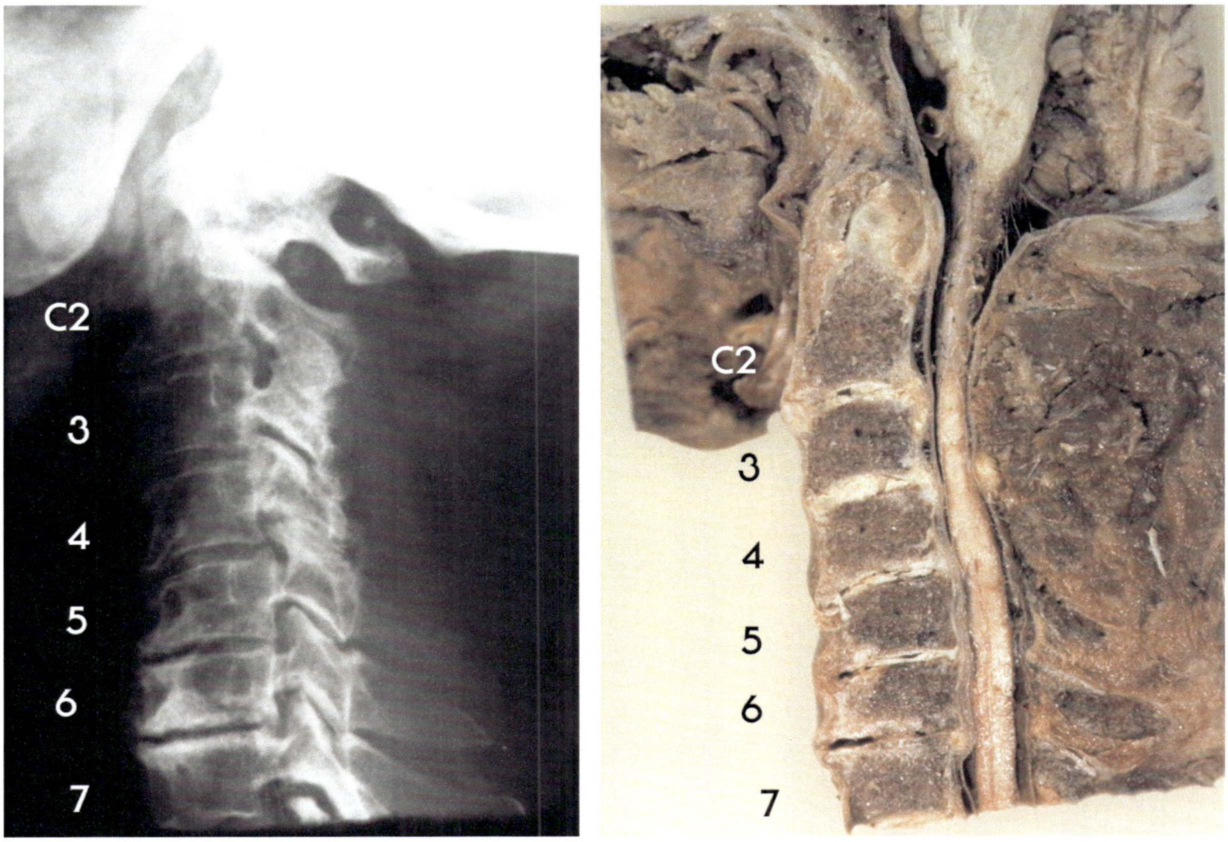

Figure 2-8
MULTIPLE SUBLUXATIONS WITH REVERSED CERVICAL CURVE
Loss of curve starts with C2-C3 and a complete retrolisthesis of C5 to C4 and C6, with cord compromise C4-C7. Vertebral body enlargement forms stenosis of the canal and significant anterior spurring of C4-C7. C6 retro to C7 with cavitation and near fusion of vertebrae.

The change in the position of the vertebrae C4, C5, C6 causes an alteration in the shape of the canal. The cervical cord has a normal enlargement, making it more susceptible to compression. The cervical spine cord is compressed in this region because the canal narrows due to the displacement of the vertebrae posterior to each other, coupled with the fact that the A to P diameter of C5's body has increased by almost 20%, due to the altered weight bearing. This example shows the C5 posterior inferior body being closer to the superior spinal laminar junction of C6. Many studies show that bone remodels to stress. When weight bearing or stress is altered, the bone changes its shape to accommodate the weight bearing.[29,30,31,32] The result will be disc degeneration and eventual fusion. This condition can lead to cervical myelopathy with various symptoms of the upper extremities, and may also have a serious effect on the rest of the spinal cord function.

Figure 2-8 is another specimen with its associated X-ray showing more advanced degeneration. Multiple subluxations of a long standing nature have a profound effect on the central nervous system and in the shape of the vertebral canal. We see in both specimens a radical change, especially in **Figure 2-8**'s X-ray. This is a result of the subluxations that have altered the curvature. These subluxations have created a flexion deformity of the cervical spine.

Figure 2-9 shows a cervical MRI and X-ray of a patient with multiple complaints. There are some similarities between **Figure 2-8** and **Figure 2-9**. The history of the patient is when working at a desk, with his cervical spine in persistant flexion. After sitting looking down for more than 2 hours he had parasthesia bilaterally from his shoulders to the fingers, weakness, diminished reflexes, shoulder and neck pain, and some pain in his arms. The MRI of this patient was taken in the recumbent position, not in the position that created the symptoms. He got relief by lying down on his back.

The patient in **Figure 2-10** has a similar problem, getting relief by laying down on her back. Here we have a mid-sagittal view of the entire spine seen in the position in which it was taken. The spinal cord is in the anterior portion of the canal from C3 to T10. The patient gets relief (head, neck, stomach and back pain) in this position. Her problem is aggravated while seated at her desk with her neck flexed forward. In both cases signs of spinal cord distress are seen while in a position that relieves symptoms. In both these cases, cervical flexion increased symptoms. The loss of the normal curve results in a longer than normal canal, flexion stretches the spinal cord and presses it into the bulging

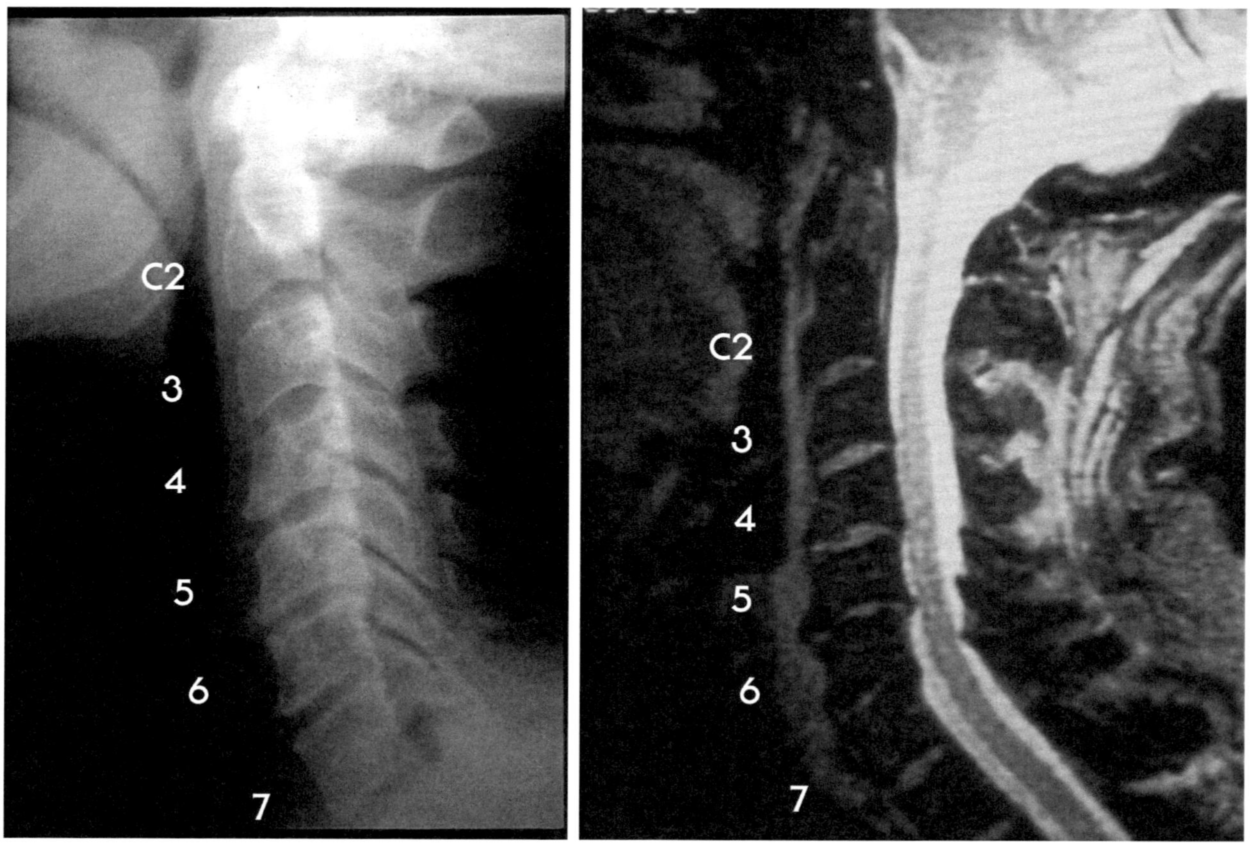

Figure 2-9

CERVICAL X-RAY AND MRI STUDY WITH LOSS OF LORDOSIS

The lateral X-ray of this patient clearly shows the loss of curvature, multiple subluxations, loss of disc height, and posterior osteophytes. This MRI shows loss of curvature ("military neck") resulting from posterior subluxations at C3 retro to C2; C4 retro to C3 and C5 retro to C6.

Note the loss of disc height and posterior spurring. The spinal cord is much smaller in diameter than the vertebral canal, but it is the tethering or stretching of the cord against C3-C5 that makes these significant problems. The posterior disc bulging and osteophytes of C3-C5 are actually in contact with the spinal cord in the neutral supine position, a position of relief for this patient of bilateral parasthesia in the upper extremities. His symptoms were brought on by sitting at his desk doing paper work. We have to extrapolate his changing positions to the changing length of the vertebral canal.

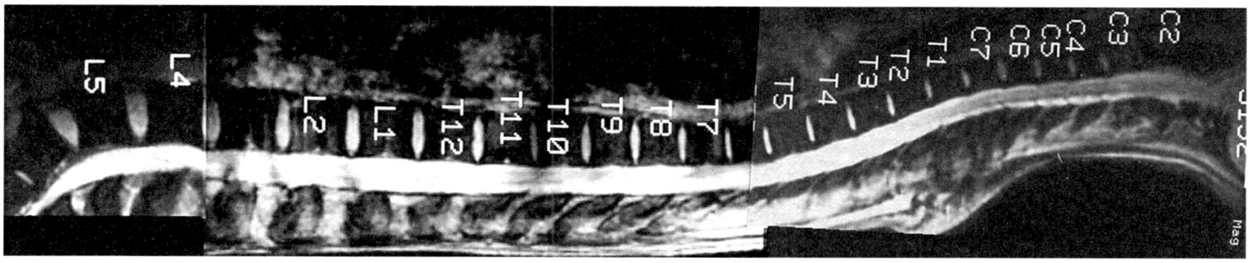

Figure 2-10
MIDSAGITTAL MRI STUDY OF THE ENTIRE VERTEBRAL COLUMN SEEN IN THE POSITION THE STUDY WAS TAKEN

The anteriority of the cord in the canal from C4 to T9 (tethering) shows the overall effect of the reverse curve is tethering of cord and the hypokyphotic curve of the thoracic spine in standing or supine views. Aligned segments with reduced curve. Anterior location of the spinal cord in the canal in the supine view through most of the thoracic spine.
Loss of lordotic curve in the lumbar spine is a flexion deformity or a lengthening of the canal.
Note sacral disc. Central nervous system tension is transferred to caudae equinae all the way to the IVF's. We need to extrapolate postural change from supine to flexed (seated or other) positions.
Note: Anterior cord displacement in the 'neutral position'. Patient actually gets relief in this position, all flexion irritates her condition.

discs and osteophytes. The cord is elevated to the anterior portion of the canal even in the recumbent position. This is not normal.[33] The anterior spinal artery can be compressed by the posterior osteophytes and bulging discs. This contact can be reduced when the patient is lying on his or her back and the cervical spine or lumbar spine is in extension (**see Figure2-11**). The reversal of the cervical curve (or kyphosis) can lengthen the canal in the cervical area and the entire spinal cord. Note the straight appearance of the spinal cord and brain stem, the increased distance between the spinous processes of C3-C7, the subluxation complex involving C3-C7, bulging discs of the involved segments, and the beginning of osteoarthritic changes of C5 and C6. The components of the cervical subluxation complexes alter lordotic curves. The resulting effects on the central nervous system cause profound health changes.[34]

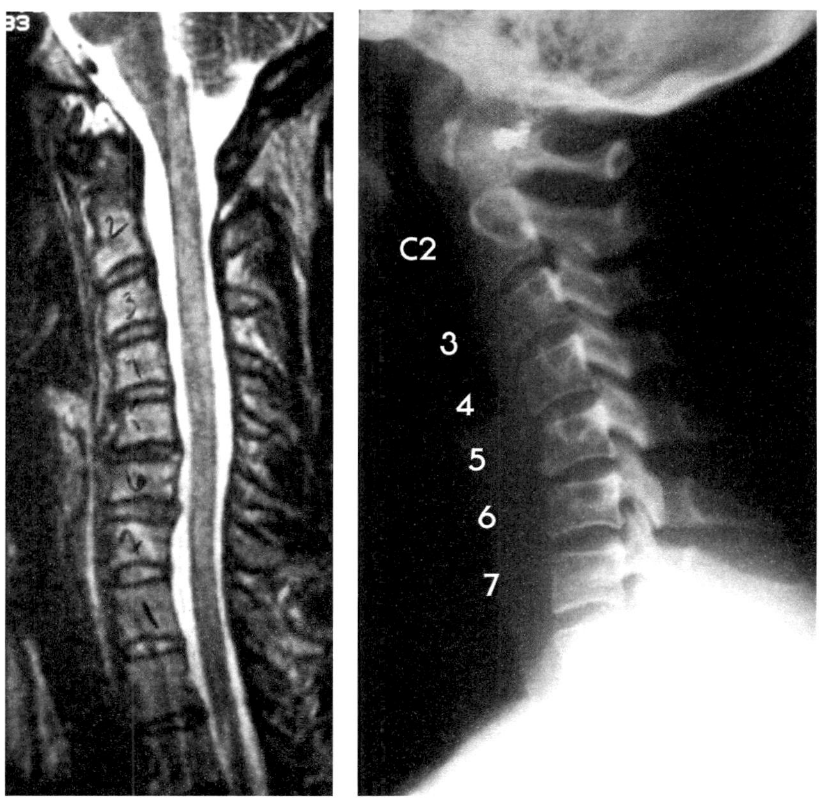

Figure 2-11
CERVICAL X-RAY AND MRI STUDY SHOWING REVERSAL OF CURVE

Cervical MRI and X-ray of same individual showing reversal of lordotic curve or a cervical kyphosis. Note the straightening of the brainstem to thoracic cord, a complete retrolisthesis of C5, large interspinous distance from C3-C7, enlargement of C5 body due to hyper loading and bulging discs. Consider the anatomic and physiologic changes with active, persistent cervical flexion as required by many jobs.

Spinal Cord Deformation

Alteration of the curves and shape of the vertebral column will deform the spinal cord. The changes in shape of the spinal cord are due to the affects of the dentate ligaments. The increase in left to right distance and the narrowing of the anterior to posterior distance of the spinal cord is due to dentate ligament tension. Dentate ligament tension is created by increasing the length of the spinal canal. Note in **Figure 2-12a** the normal position and shape of the spinal cord in this picture.

Figure 2-12b, which consists of a combination of cadaver studies and MRI studies, shows that significant deformation of the spinal cord can occur.

The animal studies are clear. When the cord is deformed, altered conductivity results.[35] When this happens, there are two main components; duration and intensity. How long a period the condition persists is important because the studies show decreased conductivity with increase in time of deforming force. The intensity is obviously a factor. When an increase in tethering or compression occurs, the conductivity decreases. There was a 70% incidence of all degrees and forms of cord deformation in the random population of 116 cadavers in this study. Another complication of the deforming effects of subluxation complexes of the vertebral column is inflammation and resulting adhesions.[36,37] In **Figure 2-13** you see epidural adhesions that have developed because of chronic inflammation. There are obvious subluxations with end stage disc degeneration. In

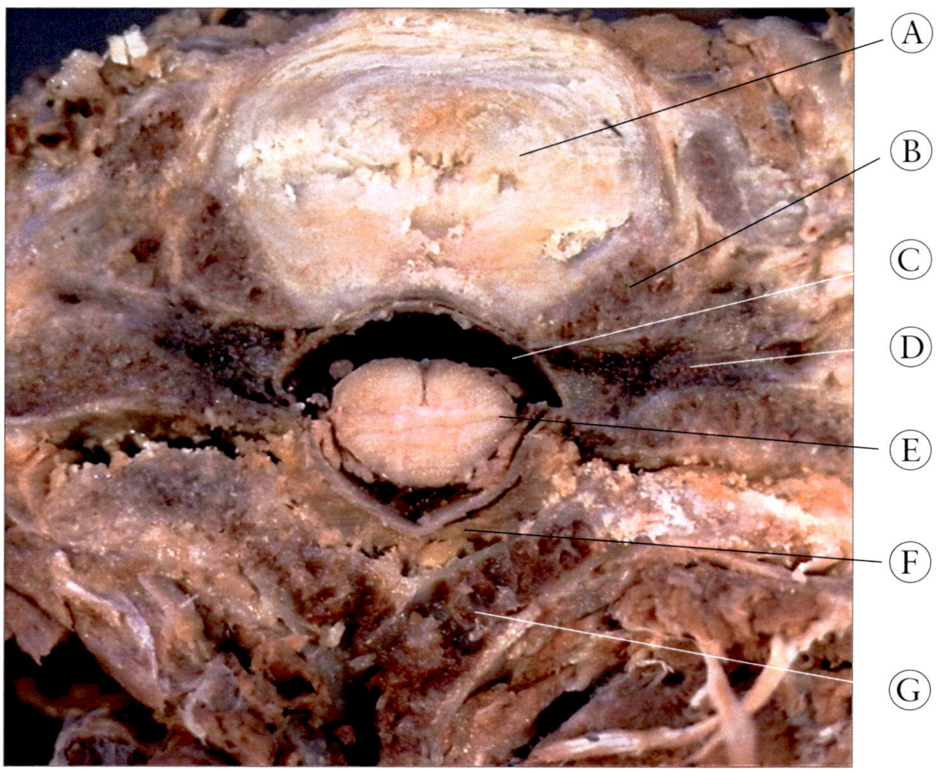

Figure 2-12a
CROSS SECTION OF NORMAL VERTEBRAL COLUMN

Note the spinal cord has a nearly round appearance or 1:1 ratio between the sagittal and coronal diameters. Also it is in the posterior aspect of the spinal canal indicating a relaxed lower central nervous system in the supine position, which is normal.

(A) Disc
(B) Uncinate process
(C) Spinal canal
(D) Dorsal root ganglion
(E) Lateral columns of spinal cord
(F) Ligamentum flavum
(G) Lamina

Figure 2-13a the dura mater (the outside of the thecal sac) is adhered to the P.L.L. This condition severely impairs the normal independent motions of the thecal sac and the vertebral column. (**see Chapter 1**). The adhesions can be extensive in the spinal canal. **Figure 2-13b** shows adhesions of the dura mater to the lamina and ligamentum flavum in the posterior wall of the canal. This has to be a further restrictive condition to normal motion and physiology. There are two main factors at work here; the degeneration of the disc and ligament tissue as essentially an inflammatory condition, and the abnormal mechanics of vertebral motion putting unusual stress on the thecal sac and other meningeal structures. This causes an inflammation of the meninges inside the subarachnoid space (**see Figures 2-14** and **2-15**). Here are two specimens with subarachnoid adhesions. In both cases the thoracic cord is tethered against the anterior wall of the canal. This condition, more than any other, chronically pulls or stretches the posterior elements of the thecal sac. The persistent irritation causes inflammation and adhesions of the pia mater, arachnoid mater, median septum, and the arachnoid trabeculae. In both cases the cervical curve is altered by subluxation complexes. The tractioning and irritation of the thoracic cord and meningeal tissues is one major result. Also there must be impaired CSF flow in this area along with the altered biomechanics of CNS.[38] See **Figure 2-16** for the MRI appearance in the thoracic spine. Note the imaging density of the adhesions is similar to that of the spinal cord. In situ the adhesions are dense and entrap arterioles and nerve rootlets.

As demonstrated, subluxation of the vertebral column has many aspects that interfere with normal health. The vertebral column is a complex structure with many types of tissues, that when healthy, work in harmony. Alteration of the normal architectural features of the vertebral column can have severe health consequences that can advance with increasing duration and intensity.

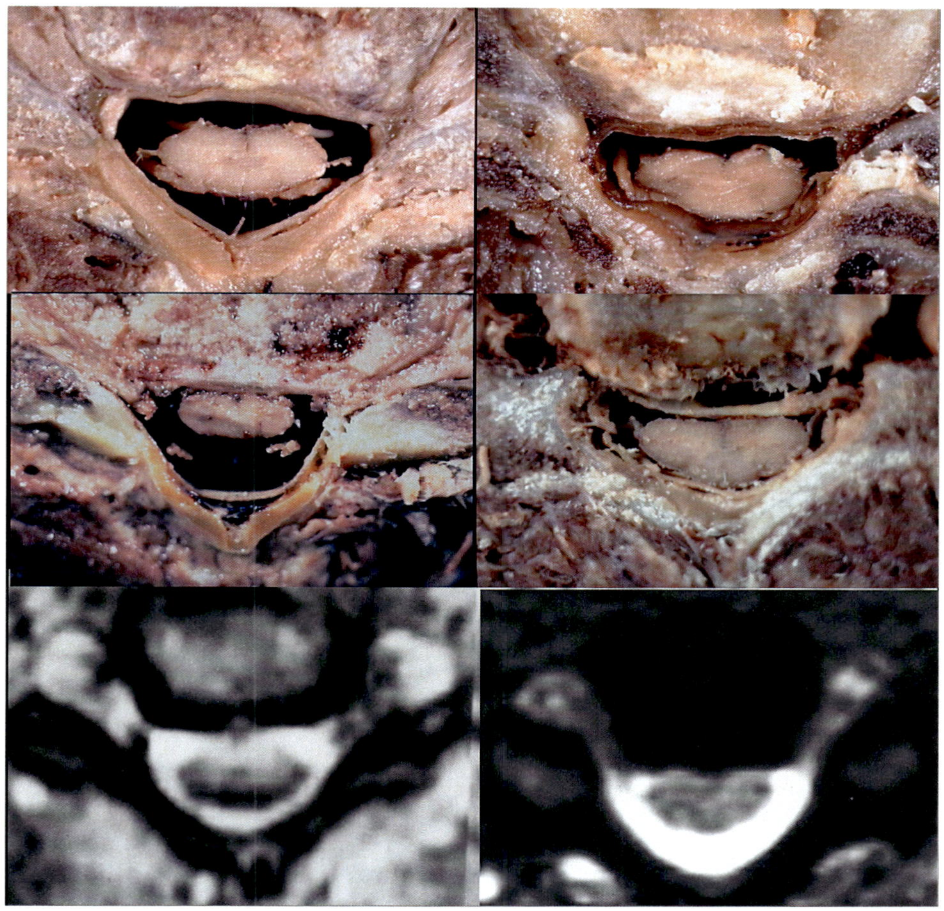

Figure 2-12b A SERIES OF VERTEBRAL COLUMN CROSS SECTIONS OF 6 INDIVIDUALS.

The top 4 are cadavers and the bottom 2 are patients' MRIs. All are in the supine position. Note the lack of 1:1 ratio of the saggital and coronal diameters of the spinal cords; the oval appearance is due to an increase in length of the spinal canal and therefore the spinal cord.

Both of the patients would lie down to get relief, which is the position the MRI was taken.

Inflammation of the Meninges

Little has been written about inflammation and adhesions of the meninges in the spinal canal. Inflammation and adhesions can occur inside and outside the thecal sac. **See Figures 2-13a, 2-13b, 2-14 and 2-15.** I only found intrathecal adhesions in the thoracic spine when the spinal cord was tractioned against the front of the canal. This would stretch the pia mater and the thecal sac. I think this is the cause of the adhesions; persistent stretching of the meninges as well as the spinal tissue. The appearance of intrathecal adhesions on MRI can be seen in **Figure 2-16.** Note the anteriorly displaced spinal cord, which can only be caused by tethering or stretching of the spinal cord.

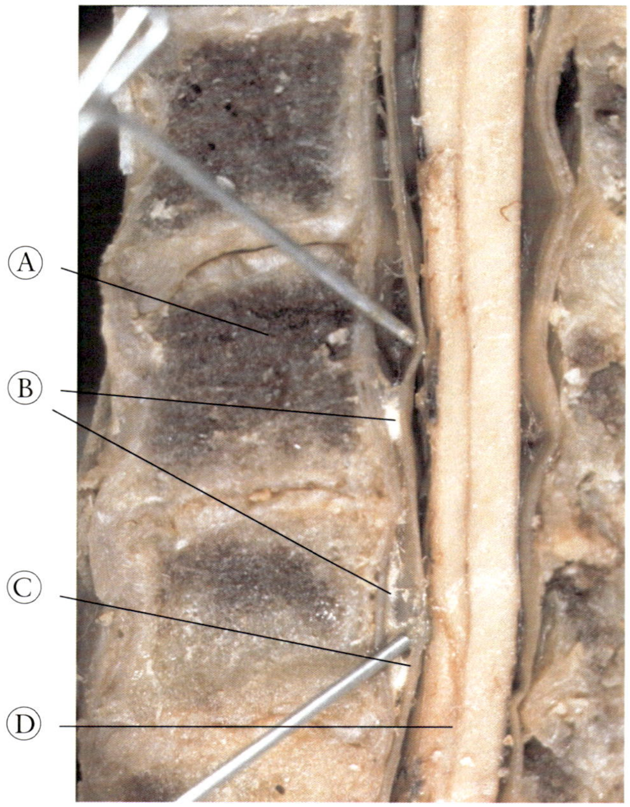

Figure 2-13a

EPIDURAL ADHESIONS/ANTERIOR WALL

Epidural adhesions between the anterior vertebral canal wall and the thecal sac (Dura Mater). These tissues are supposed to be freely moveable relative to each other. The adhesions are the result of chronic inflammation due the subluxations of the vertebra and end stage DJD.

(A) Body of vertebra
(B) Epidural adhesions
(C) Thecal wall
(D) Spinal cord

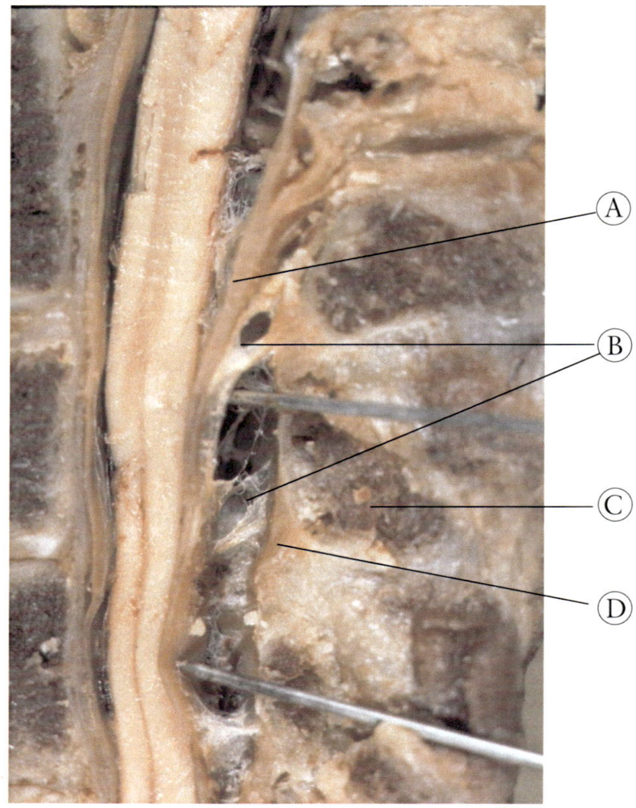

Figure 2-13b

EPIDURAL ADHESIONS/POSTERIOR WALL

Epidural adhesions in the posterior portion of the vertebral canal. These adhesions are the result of chronic inflammatory states in the posterior joints and soft tissues of the vertebral column in the thoracic region and even the thecal sac, pia mater, nerve rootlets and arteries.

(A) Thecal wall
(B) Epidural adhesions
(C) Spinous process
(D) Ligamentum flavum

Figure 2-14 Figure 2-15

INTRATHECAL OR SUBARACHNOID ADHESIONS *(on following page)*

Both of these specimens show posterior subarachnoid adhesions in the thoracic region of the vertebral column. They each have tethered the spinal cord with large contact areas against the canal wall. Since the posterior canal wall lengthens more, the stretch or irritation is greater in the posterior hemisphere of the thecal sac.

(A) Spinal cord
(B) Vertebral bodies
(C) Thecal wall
(D) Subarachnoid adhesions
(E) Ligamentum flavum,
(F) Spinous processes.

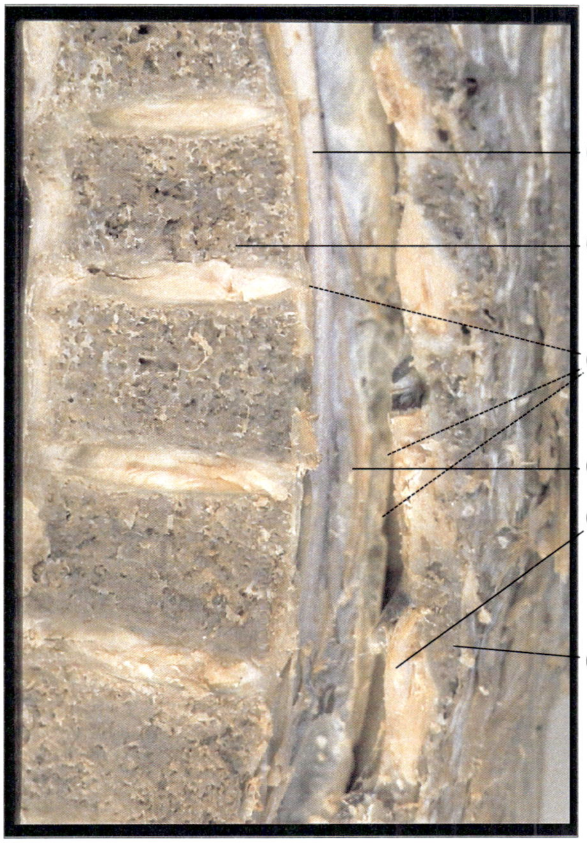

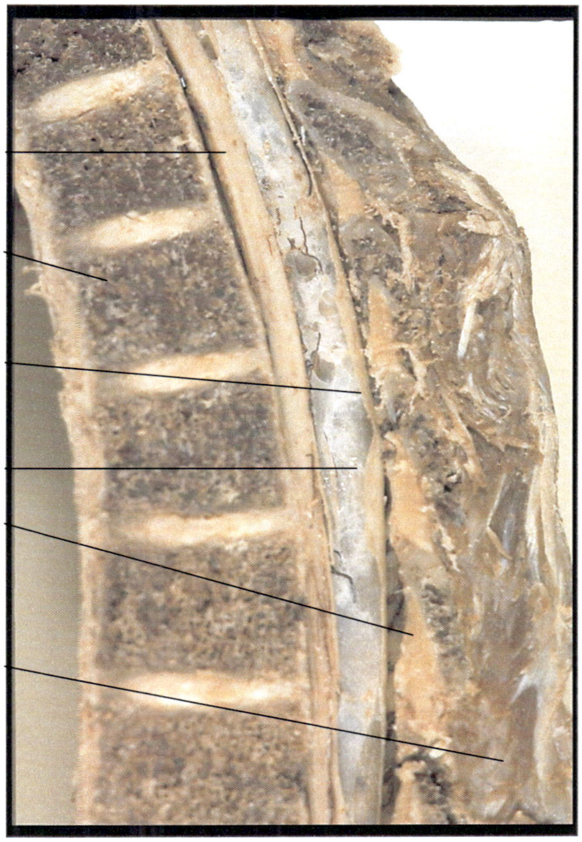

(see caption previous page) Figure 2-14

(see caption previous page) Figure 2-15

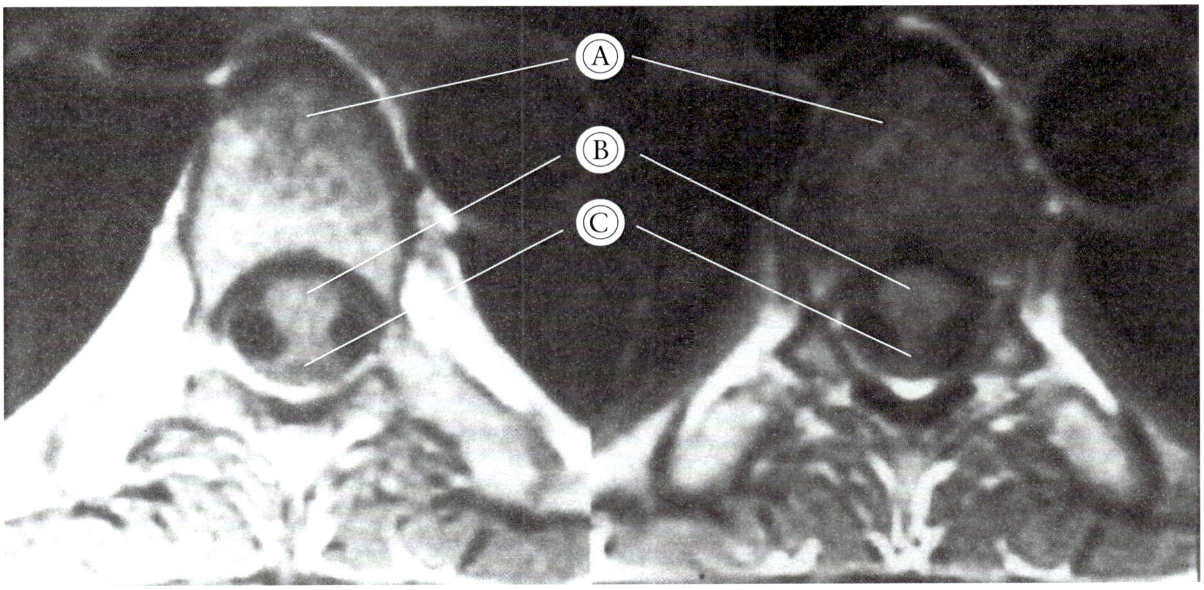

Figure 2-16

THORACIC SPINE: MRI AXIAL VIEWS OF TETHERED SPINAL CORDS

Note subarachnoid adhesions and cord-canal contact in the recumbent position, the spinal cord is in the wrong part of the canal for this position.

(A) Vertebral body (B) Spinal cord (C) Subarachnoid or intrathecal adhesions

Expected Outcomes

Joint injury causes inflammatory responses. Persistent joint dysfunction causes inflammation to continue. Tissue repair cannot occur with persistent inflammation. This condition is the basis for degenerative change that is called Degenerative Joint Disease (DJD) and Osteoarthritis. When trauma occurs to the spine (or any other joint complex), persistent subluxation and the passage of time the expected outcome is degenerative changes. The trauma creates unstable joint motion, the spinal cord reflexes induce the involved musculature to guard, or tighten.

The body's defensive mechanisms are the driving forces in the patient's symptoms of pain and stiffness, loss of motion, loss of disc height or bulging, bone spurs and entrapment syndromes. Deformation of the spinal canal causes deformation of the spinal cord.[39,40] In the series of **Figures 2-17** and **18** presented here are of a patient's MRI studies of his cervical spine shortly after his trauma and another study 16 years later. At age 28 he had a "modern injury," as I term it, being hit by a garbage truck weighing 24 tons.

In **Figure 2-17a** the initial post injury lateral cervical MRI with altered lordosis is shown. Notice the normal hydration and disc height indicating a recent injury. He suspended chiropractic care shortly after he was relieved of pain. In **Figure 2-17b** the patient's cervical MRI, now 44 years old, shows he has advanced

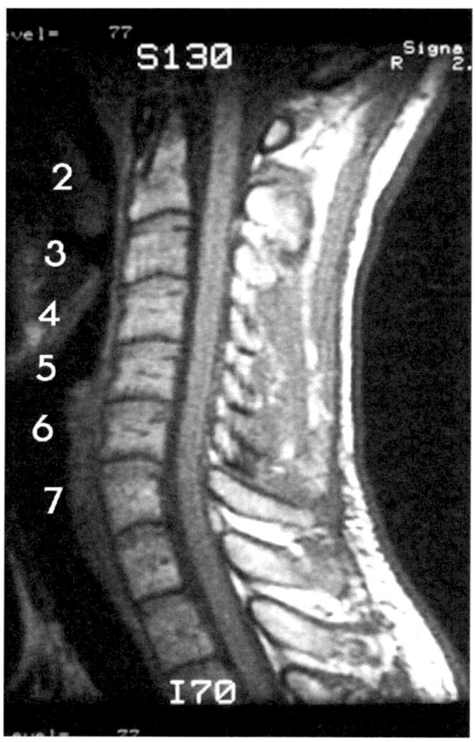

Figure 2-17a
MRI mid-sagittal study of the cervical spine of a person one week post injury.

He was struck as a pedestrian by a garbage truck. The radiographic report said it was a normal study. Note the subluxations of C4, C5 and C6. The appearance of hydration and normal disc height is an indication of a recent injury.

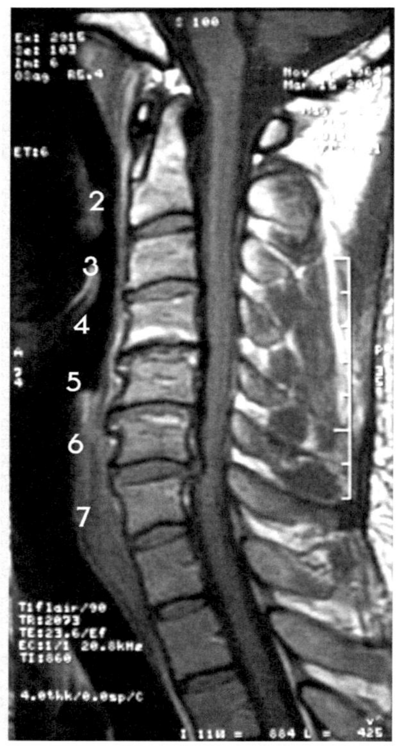

Figure 2-17b
The same individual 16 years later.

Note the degenerative changes where the subluxations which were noted in the previous study. Also note how the misalignment looks worse. Seen is the expected degeneration with bulging discs and loss of disc height, both indicating a passage of time. He has neurological and muscular changes in the left upper extremity.

degeneration of the mid-cervical spine. This is the expected outcome with the passage of 16 years and continued inflammation from the persistent subluxations. This condition was silent until he started weight lifting. During a particularly heavy lift he felt a "pop" in his neck with subsequent loss of strength and muscle mass of the left arm. In **Figure 2-18a** the spinal cord is oval and elevated off the back of the canal, indicating dentate ligament tension.

In **Figure 2-18b** the spinal cord deformation has increased and flattened it to the anterior wall of the spinal canal. There has to be compromise to the anterior spinal artery that supplies the anterior tracks of the spinal cord. The eccentric position of the cord to the left would correspond to the unilateral nature of his complaints.

Fortunately for him a "non-traditional" outcome has occurred. During cervical extension tractioning his grip strength increased by 15 pounds. While this was an indication he could respond to conservative care, the neurosurgeon that ordered the second MRI study recommended immediate surgery. However, with a short course of chiropractic care the negative neurological and muscle changes were reversed. Please notice in **Figures 2-17a** and **2-17b** the relatively good health of the IVD joints above and below the subluxations. These discs are all the same age and the only discs that are degenerating are the subluxated ones. This is more proof, for me, that the subluxation is the critical factor in joint health, not age.

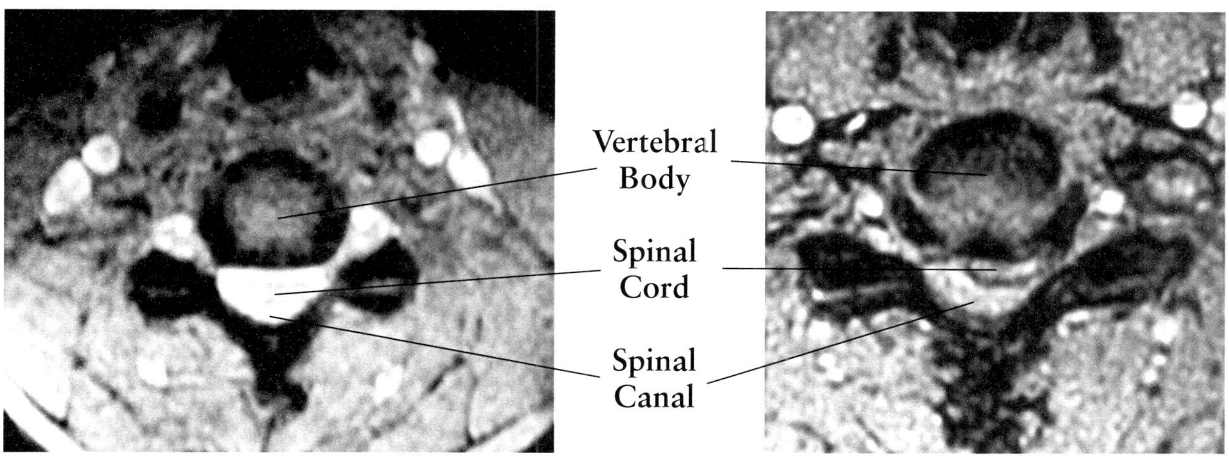

Figure 2-18
The same individual at the initial evaluation.

This is an axial view at the C5 level. Note the elevation of the spinal cord off the posterior aspect of the spinal canal. Also note the elliptical shape of the spinal cord indicating spinal cord tension. And dentate ligament stretching.

Figure 2-18b
The same individual 16 years post injury.

Note the spinal cord deformation and the displacement of the spinal cord to the left side of the canal and up against the anterior part of the canal. This shows increased adverse mechanical tension via the dentate ligaments throughout the entire spinal cord.

CHAPTER THREE

Subluxations Of The Cervical Spine

Discussion

The motion and support of the head are main features of the unique joint complexes of the cervical spine. The alteration of the normal architecture aligning the head with the thoracic spine is the primary mechanical cause of degenerative change.[1,2,3,4,5] The blood supply of the cervical spine, face, and lower head are controlled by the integrity of the vertebral column, rib cage and neck (**see Figure 3-1**). The changes caused by subluxation of the upper cervical vertebrae and rib cage can result in headaches as a patient complaint.[6] The cervicogenic or thoracogenic origins of most headaches are only partially appreciated by the health care community. Muscle guarding patterns of the suboccipital muscles is a common finding with "tension headache" complaints. Blood flow to vital parts of the upper central nervous system can alter due to subluxations of the cervical spine.[7,8] Headaches can also be caused by head to thorax misalignment which can include SCM (sternocleidomastoid muscle)spasm that can develop and compress the external jugular vein.[9] This decreases or stops blood drainage from the face, nasal sinuses, orbit of the eye, TMJ region, inner ear and side of the head.[10,11] Some headaches are caused by inflammation of the tendinous attachments of the SCM into the mastoid process due to chronic spasm.[12]

When the head is accelerated in a different direction from the thorax, the cervical spine will deform. This is commonly referred to as whiplash, but I prefer the term "buckling." Buckling is an engineering term that conveys partial collapse of an architectural structure, an accurate description of the results of the head being suddenly accelerated 20 miles an hour faster and in a different direction than the thorax.

The result is anterior to posterior as well as rotational misalignments. With preservation of the normal lordotic curve, the cervical spine undergoes less of the changes of osteoarthritis, even in old age.[13,14] Most osteoarthritis of the spine is the result of uncorrected subluxations and remolded bones and joints due to the chronically altered weight bearing according to Wolf's Law.[15,16]

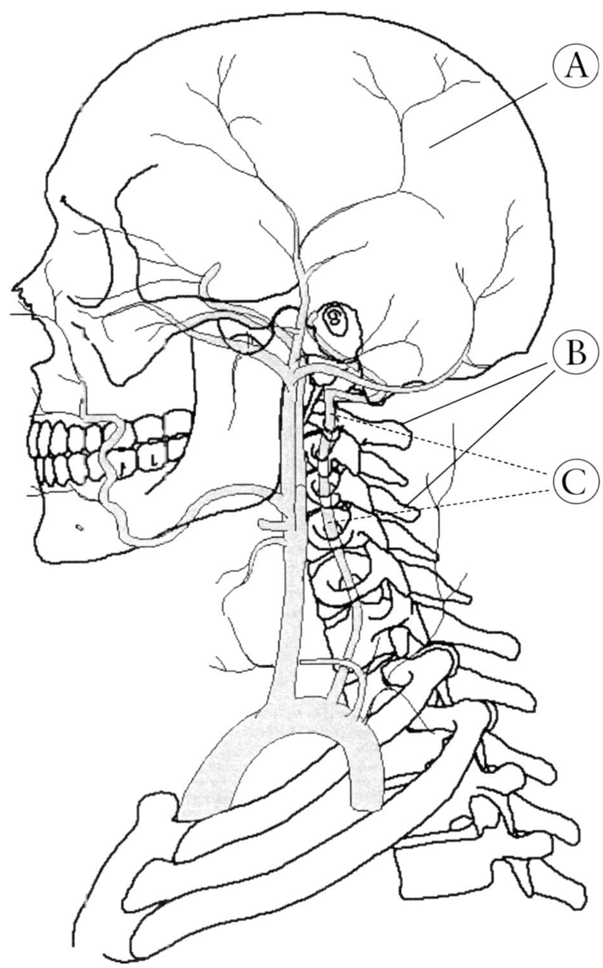

Figure 3-1
The head and cervical spine can misalign and have altered structure. The vertebral artery and other vascular and nervous system structures can suffer a change in function.
Note the position of the vertebral artery and its relationship to the cervical spine and the head. These arteries supply the spinal cord, vertebrae, ligaments and brainstem with blood.
(A) Head
(B) Cervical spine
(C) Vertebral artery.

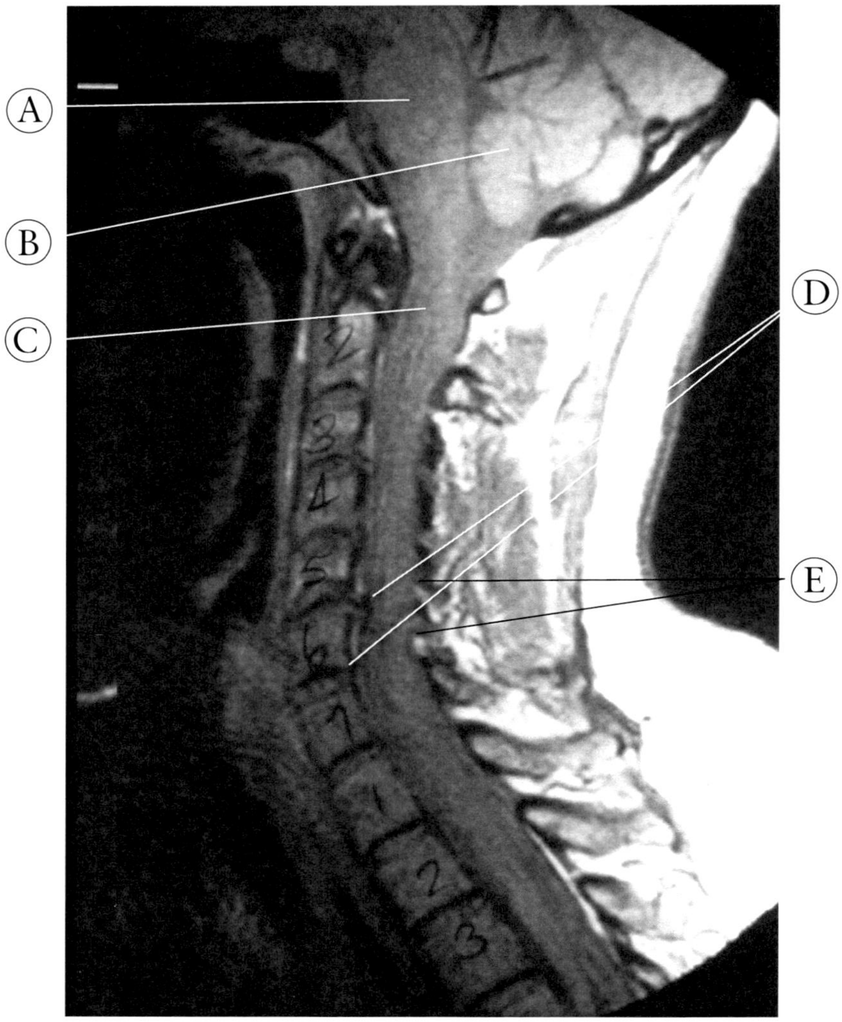

Figure 3-2
MRI study of cervical and upper thoracic spine.
The subluxated sixth vertebra has formed posterior osteophytes. The retrolisthesis of C6, the posterior osteophytes and the lamina of C7 have created a canal stenosis.
(A) Brainstem
(B) Cerebellum
(C) Spinal cord
(D) Posterior osteophytes
(E) Lamina

Osteoarthritic changes include: disc degeneration, spinal canal stenosis, intervertebral foramen narrowing, uncinate process hypertrophy and facetal sclerosis (**see Figure 3-2**). Loss of joint alignment or subluxation of the cervical vertebrae results in changes to all the tissues of the affected segments. This also has unfortunate consequences for areas of the central nervous system (**see Figure 3-3**). The subluxations alter the course of the vertebral arteries and tributaries and therefore alter the blood flow in those vascular structures[17,18,19,20] (**See Chapter 2**). The subluxations can change the shape of the spinal cord, brainstem and pons (**see Figure**

3-4). Altered shape and blood supply to the central nervous system changes its function. The factors that can lead to altered function include the type of anatomical relationships, the degree of change, and the time or duration of subluxation. Some patients have all factors working against them, while others are more fortunate.

The cervical spine has more capacity to change in length than the other portions of the spine.[21,22] The posterior cervical canal wall has more flexion-extension range of motion than any other part of the vertebral column. The center of the cervical canal can lengthen 3 cm. from full extension to full flexion. That is nearly half the total change possible for the whole spine.[23,24] The loss of the lordotic curve can add 1 to 2 cm. or more of length to the whole canal, permanently stretching the spinal cord, brainstem, pons, and nerve roots.[25,26] With certain flexed postures or positions, an overstretching of the lower CNS can take place.

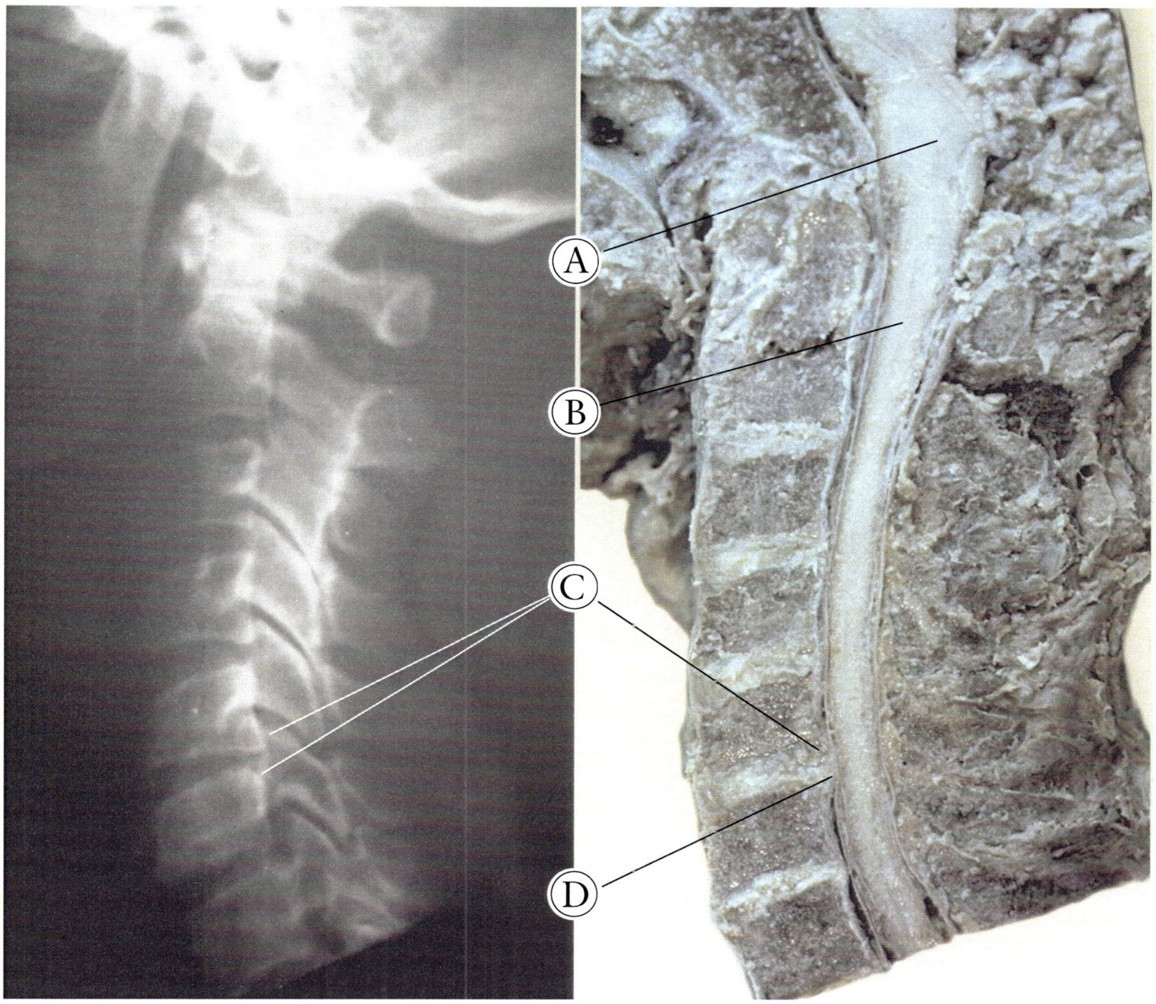

Figure 3-3
Cervical spine stenosis with disc bulge

This specimen has a reduced canal diameter and a large lower central nervous system. The combination has created a spinal canal stenosis. The brainstem is compressed and there is a hypolordotic or reduced cervical curve. The C5-6 disc bulge is a minor change in the anterior canal wall. C5 and C6 are subluxated and the disc and end plates have remolded and reduced the canal at that point. In this situation a small disc bulge can be clinically significant.

(A) Brainstem
(B) Spinal cord
(C) Endplate changes
(D) C5-C6 disc bulge.

Head to thorax misalignment can alter the shape of neurological and vascular structures of the neck and their function. This could also happen to the pharynx and larynx which are attached to the anterior longitudinal ligament at the back of the esophagus (see **Figure 3-5**).

The mandible is moved by the muscles of mastication. The inferior muscular groups hold the mandible in place by attachments to the hyoid bone and the sternum and clavicles. Subluxation of the cervical spine can alter that arrangement and normal mandibular motion will be impossible.[27,28,29]

The specimens presented are common patterns of subluxation, however, this is not a complete depiction of all types of subluxation.

In **Figure 3-6** we see the connection between the shoulder and thoracic spine and the cervical spine.

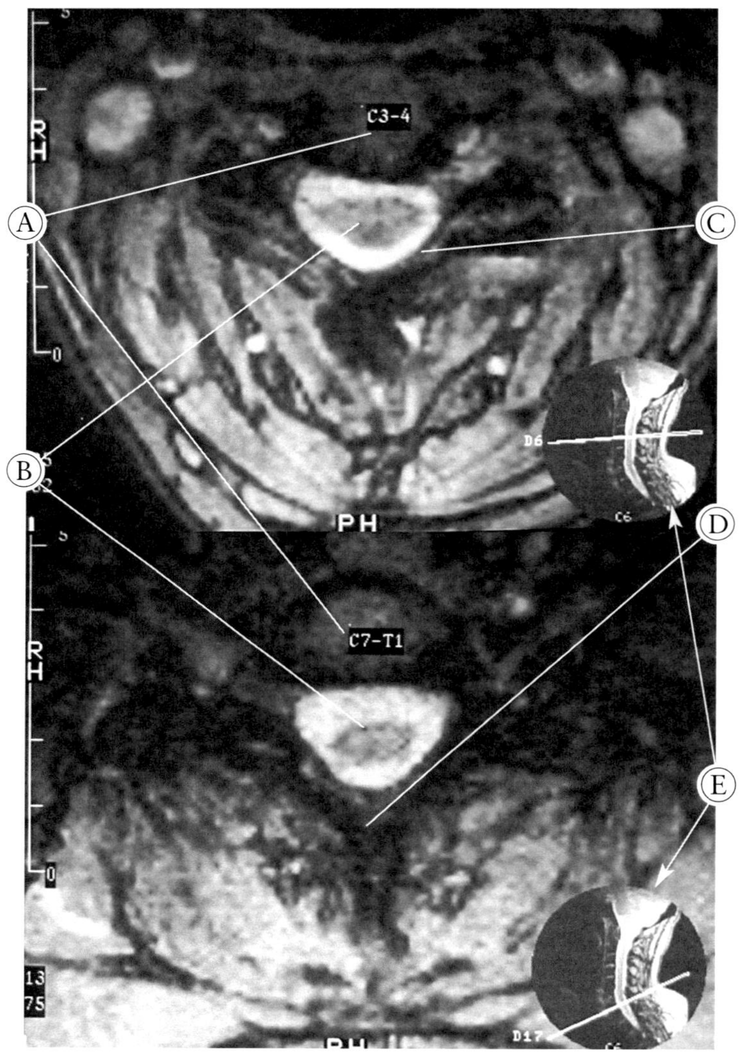

Figure 3-4
Two MRI axial views of the cervical spine. These views show a stretched spinal cord. The upper picture is a view at C3-C4. The left to right diameter of the spinal cord is elongated. The dentate ligaments have narrowed and pulled on each side of the spinal cord, making it wider. The lower picture is taken at the C7-T1 level and also shows a widened cord.
(A) Vertebral body
(B) Spinal cord
(C) Lamina
(D) Spinous process
(E) Picture key showing the level viewed and angle of scan

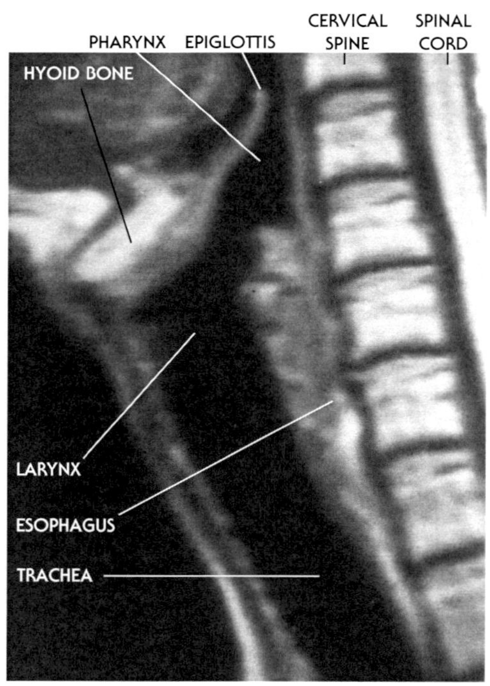

Figure 3-5
Cervical Spine/Soft-Tissue Attachments
The throat: esophagus, hyoid bone, larynx and other structures attach directly to the anterior of the cervical spine. These structures can be altered in shape and length with head-to-thorax misalignment.

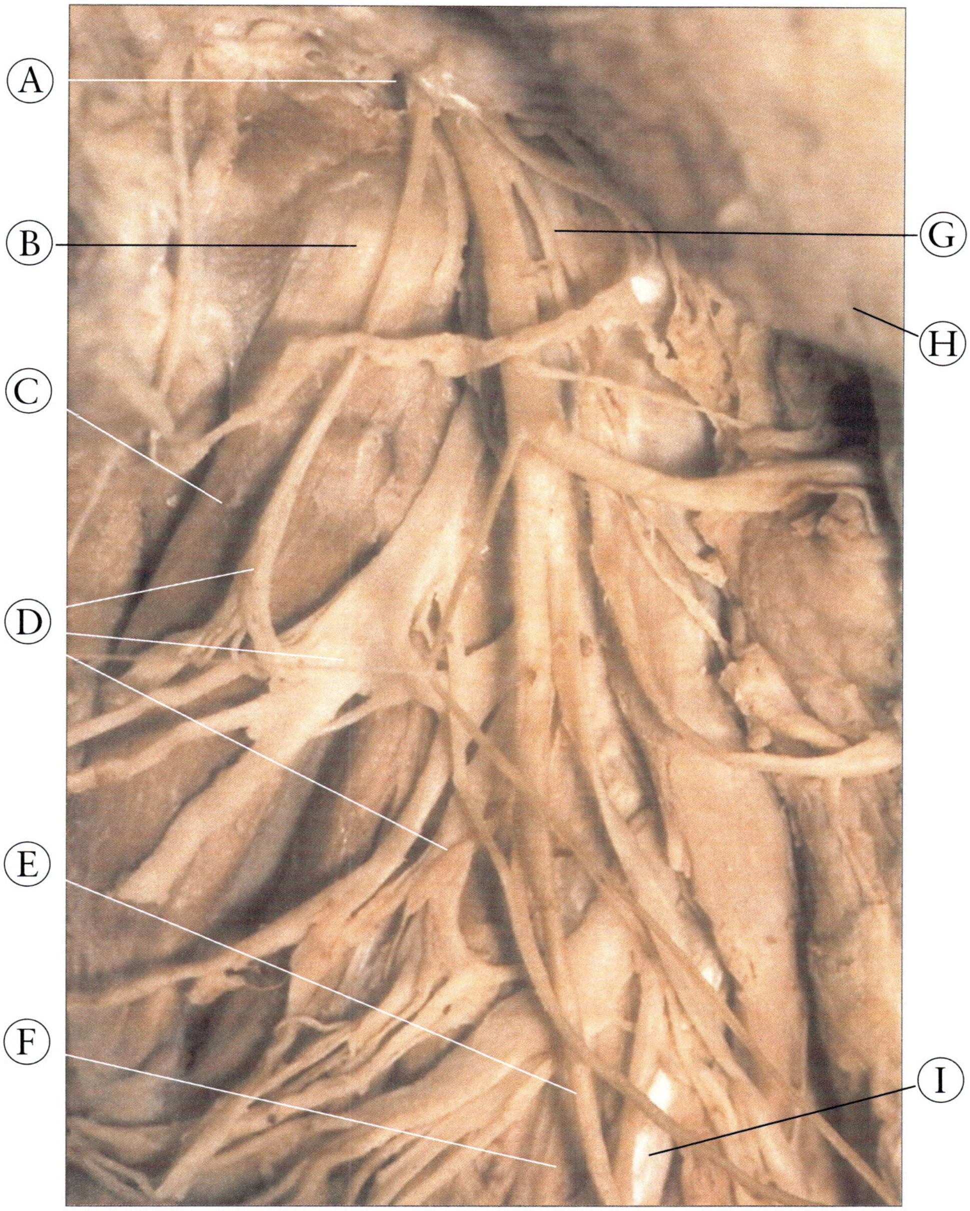

Figure 3-6
Lateral view of cervical spine.

Note the musculature that is shared with the thoracic region. Rib subluxation will make the scalene muscles tight and painful. The pain in the cervical region can be so severe as to give the mistaken impression that the entire problem is in the cervical spine. Note the number of neurological structures that can be entrapped with any rib cage subluxation pattern.

(A) Jugular foramen
(B) Tip of C1 transverse process
(C) Levator scapulae
(D) Cervical nerve roots 1, 2 and 3
(E) Vagus nerve
(F) Medial scalene
(G) Superior sympathetic ganglion
(H) Mandible
(I) Brachial plexus

CHAPTER THREE — EXPANDED TABLE OF CONTENTS

Atlas of Subluxations of the Cervical Spine

SECTION I:

Subluxations with lordotic cervical curve (8 pairs)

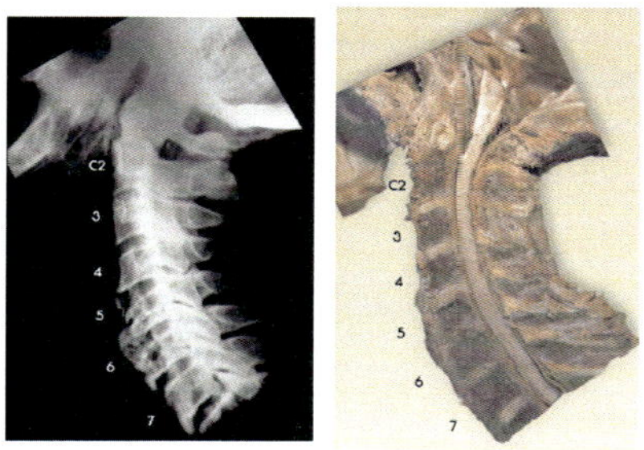

Plates 3-1 A & B
SUBLUXATIONS WITH LORDOTIC CERVICAL CURVE

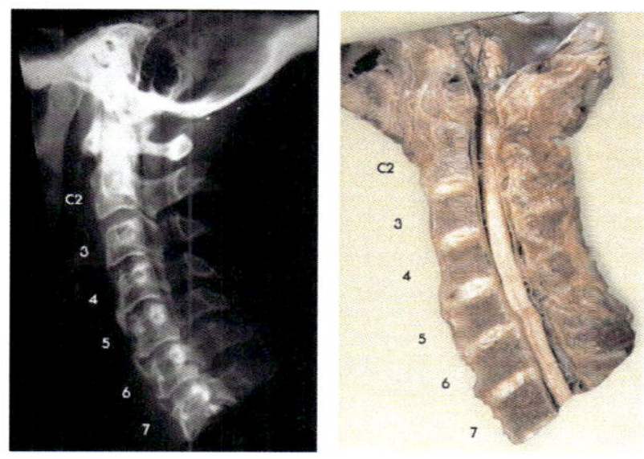

Plates 3-2 A & B
SUBLUXATIONS WITH LORDOTIC CERVICAL CURVE

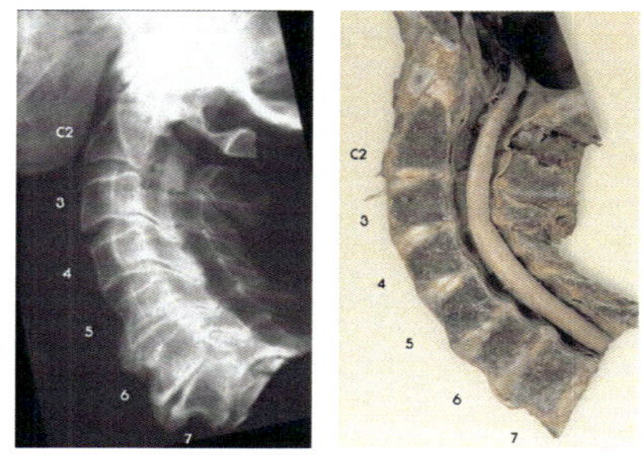

Plates 3-3 A & B
SUBLUXATIONS WITH LORDOTIC CERVICAL CURVE

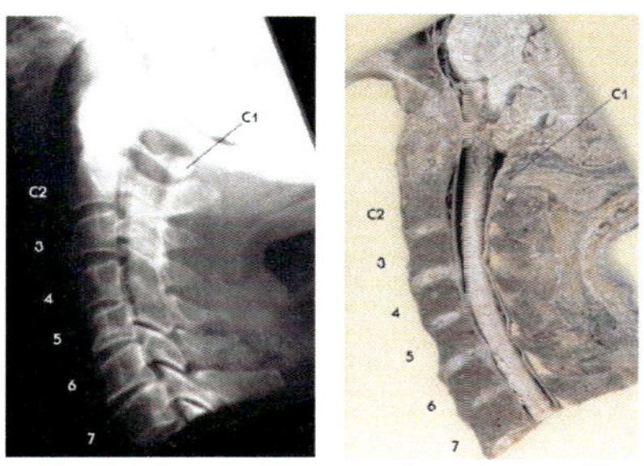

Plates 3-4 A & B
SUBLUXATIONS WITH LORDOTIC CERVICAL CURVE

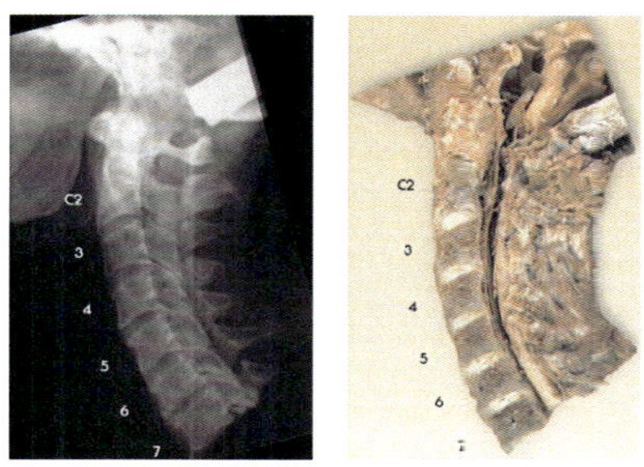

Plates 3-5 A & B
SUBLUXATIONS WITH LORDOTIC CERVICAL CURVE

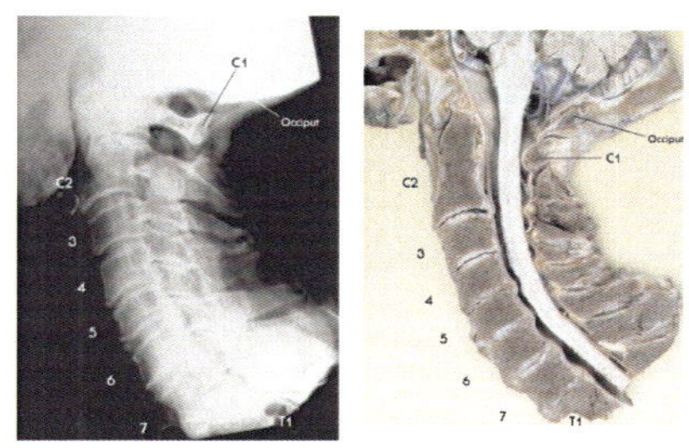

Plates 3-6 A & B
SUBLUXATIONS WITH LORDOTIC CERVICAL CURVE

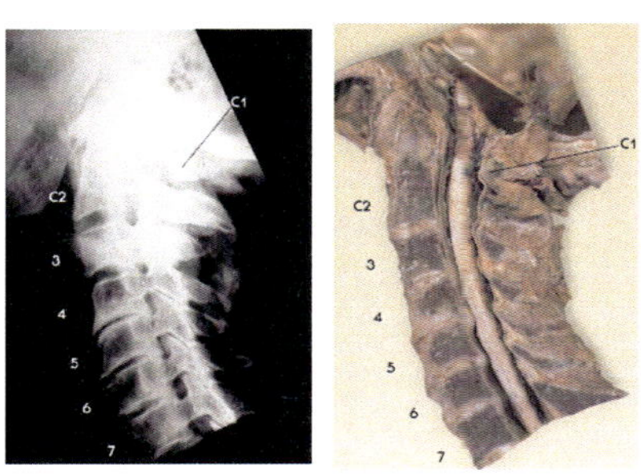

Plates 3-7 A & B
SUBLUXATIONS WITH LORDOTIC CERVICAL CURVE

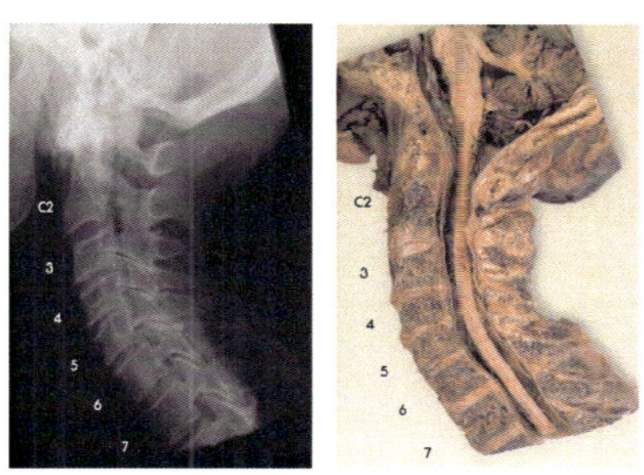

Plates 3-8 A & B
SUBLUXATIONS WITH LORDOTIC CERVICAL CURVE

CHAPTER THREE — EXPANDED TABLE OF CONTENTS

Atlas of Subluxations of the Cervical Spine

SECTION II:

Subluxations with loss of lordotic curve (straight or military neck) (3 **pairs**)

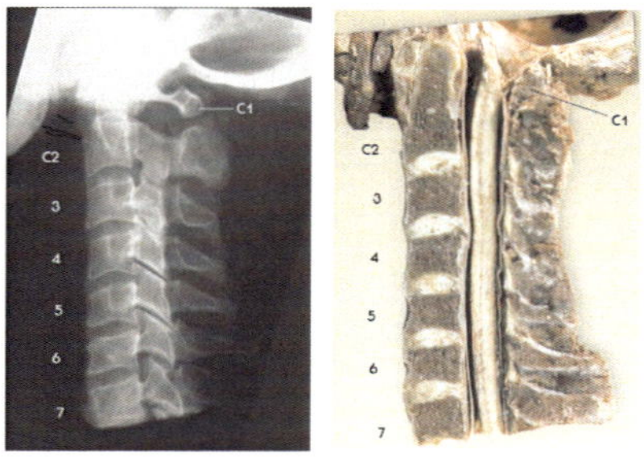

Plates 3-9 A & B
SUBLUXATIONS WITH LOSS OF LORDOTIC CURVE
(Straight or military neck)

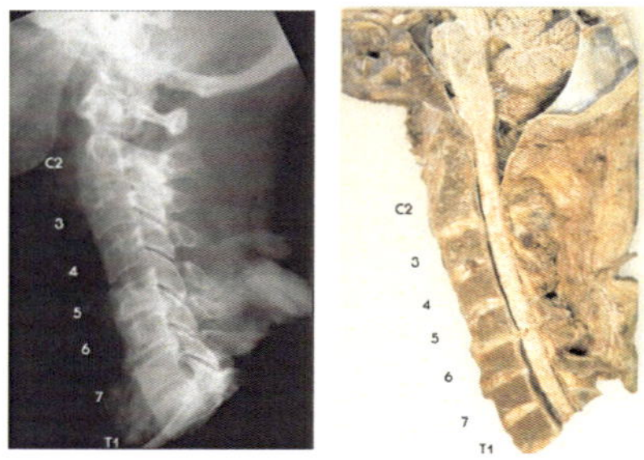

Plates 3-10 A & B
SUBLUXATIONS WITH LOSS OF LORDOTIC CURVE
(Straight or military neck)

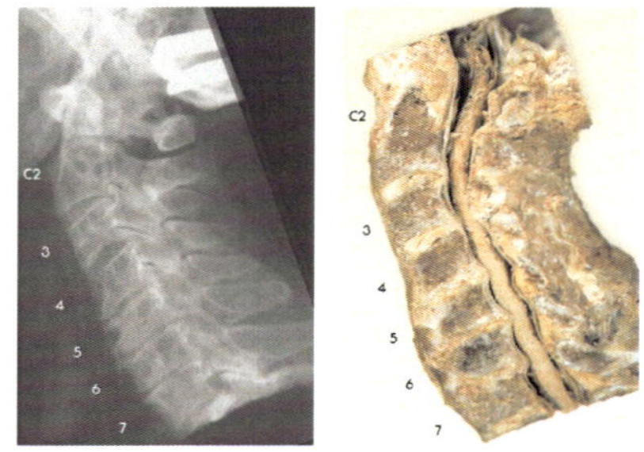

Plates 3-11 A & B
SUBLUXATIONS WITH LOSS OF LORDOTIC CURVE
(Straight or military neck)

SECTION III:

Subluxations with reversed or kyphotic curve (12 pairs)

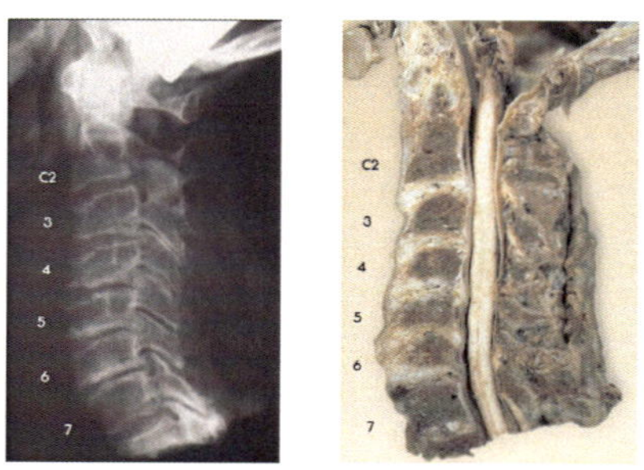

Plates 3-12 A & B
SUBLUXATIONS WITH REVERSED OR KYPHOTIC CURVE
Upper cervical subluxations

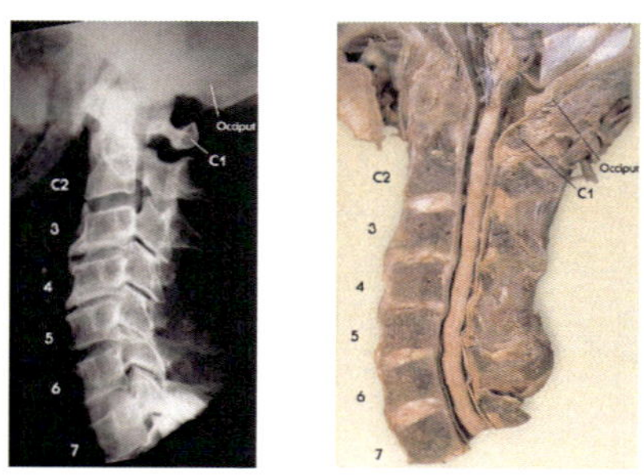

Plates 3-13 A & B
SUBLUXATIONS WITH REVERSED OR KYPHOTIC CURVE
Upper cervical subluxations

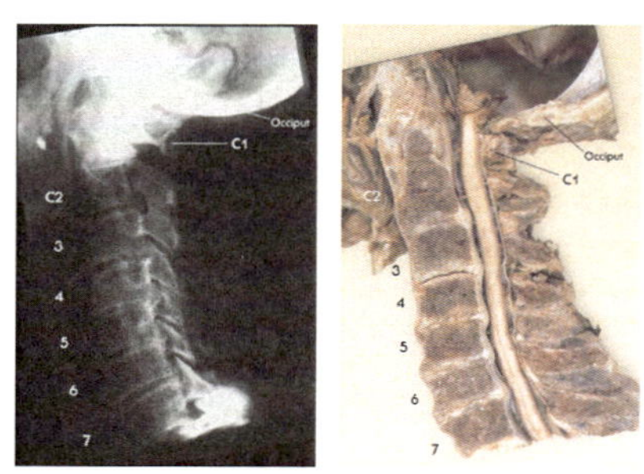

Plates 3-14 A & B
SUBLUXATIONS WITH REVERSED OR KYPHOTIC CURVE
Upper cervical subluxation

CHAPTER THREE — EXPANDED TABLE OF CONTENTS

Atlas of Subluxations of the Cervical Spine

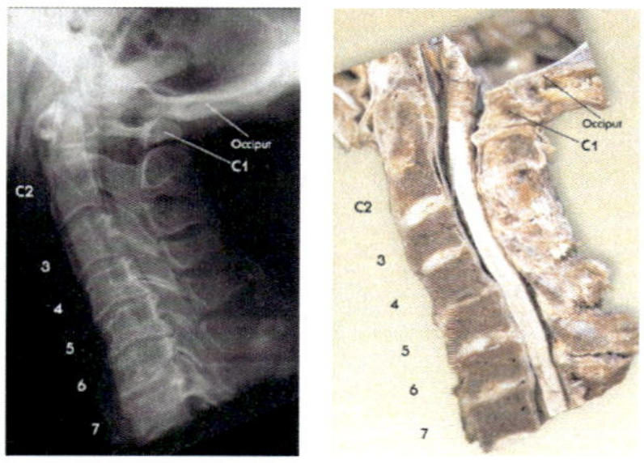

Plates 3-15 A & B
SUBLUXATIONS WITH REVERSED OR KYPHOTIC CURVE
Mid-cervical subluxations

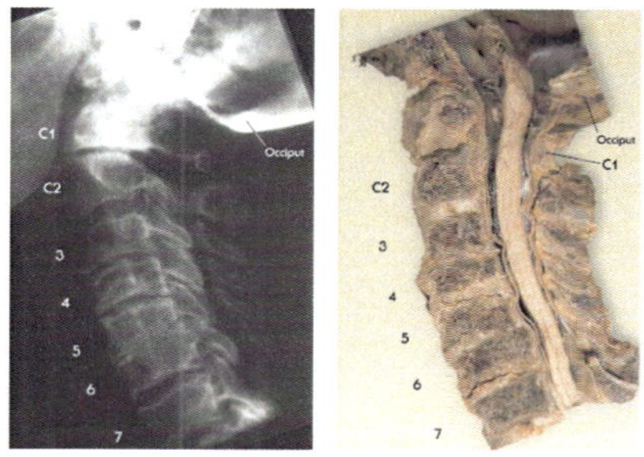

Plates 3-16 A & B
SUBLUXATIONS WITH REVERSED OR KYPHOTIC CURVE
Mid-cervical subluxations

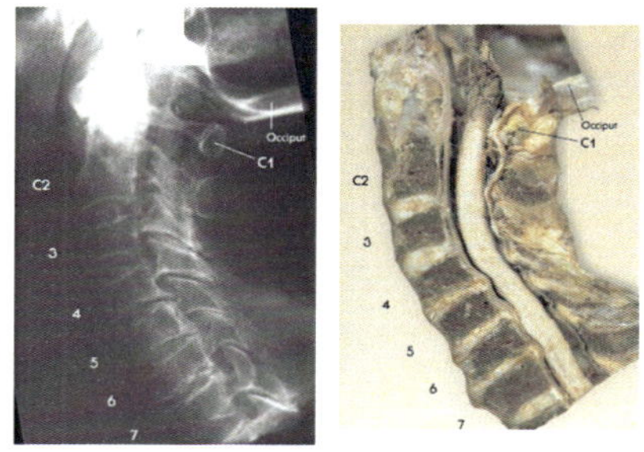

Plates 3-17 A & B
SUBLUXATIONS WITH REVERSED OR KYPHOTIC CURVE
Lower cervical subluxations

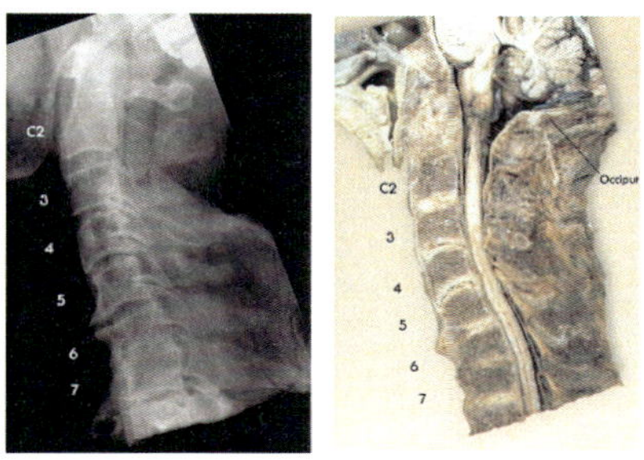

Plates 3-18 A & B
SUBLUXATION WITH REVERSED OR KYPHOTIC CURVE
Lower cervical subluxations

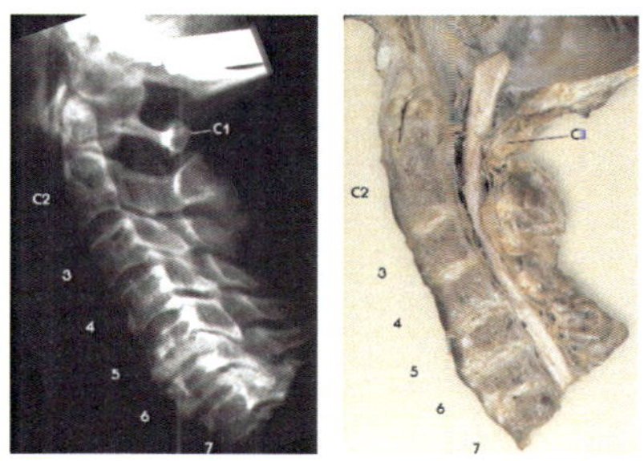

Plates 3-19 A & B
SUBLUXATIONS WITH REVERSED OR KYPHOTIC CURVE
Lower cervical subluxations

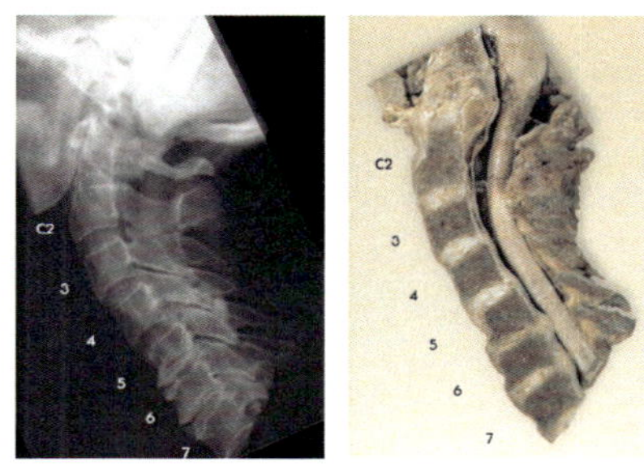

Plates 3-20 A & B
SUBLUXATIONS WITH REVERSED OR KYPHOTIC CURVE
Lower cervical subluxations

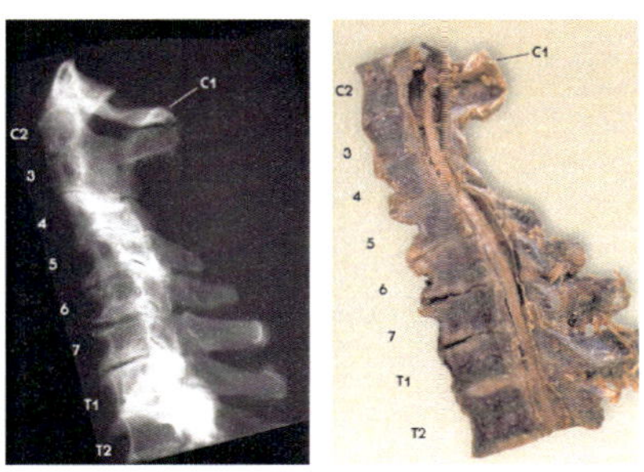

Plates 3-21 A & B
SUBLUXATIONS WITH REVERSED OR KYPHOTIC CURVE
Mid-cervical subluxations

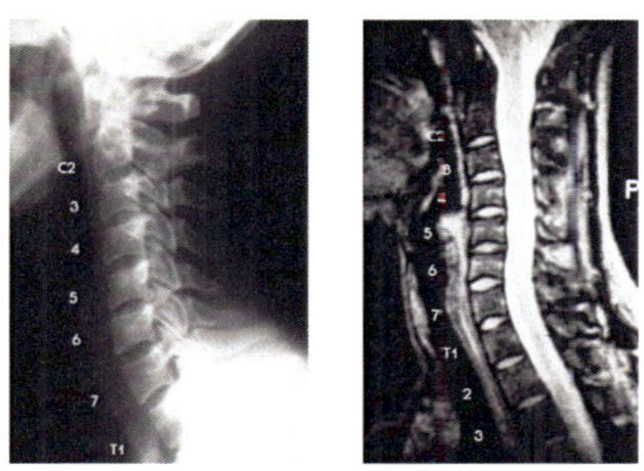

Plates 3-22 A & B
SUBLUXATION WITH REVERSED OR KYPHOTIC CURVE
An X-ray and MRI comparison

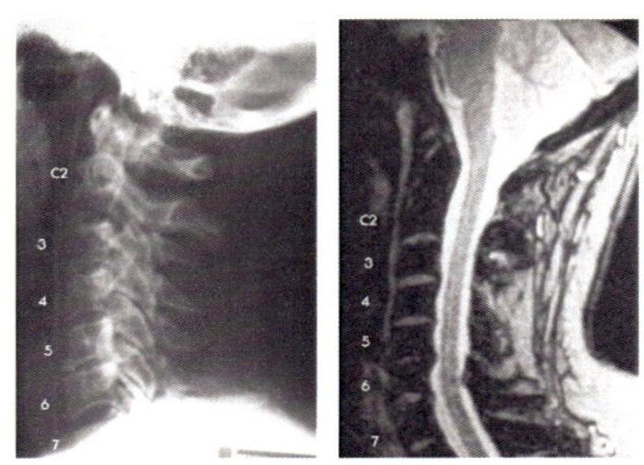

Plates 3-23 A & B
SUBLUXATION WITH REVERSED OR KYPHOTIC CURVE
An X-ray and MRI comparison

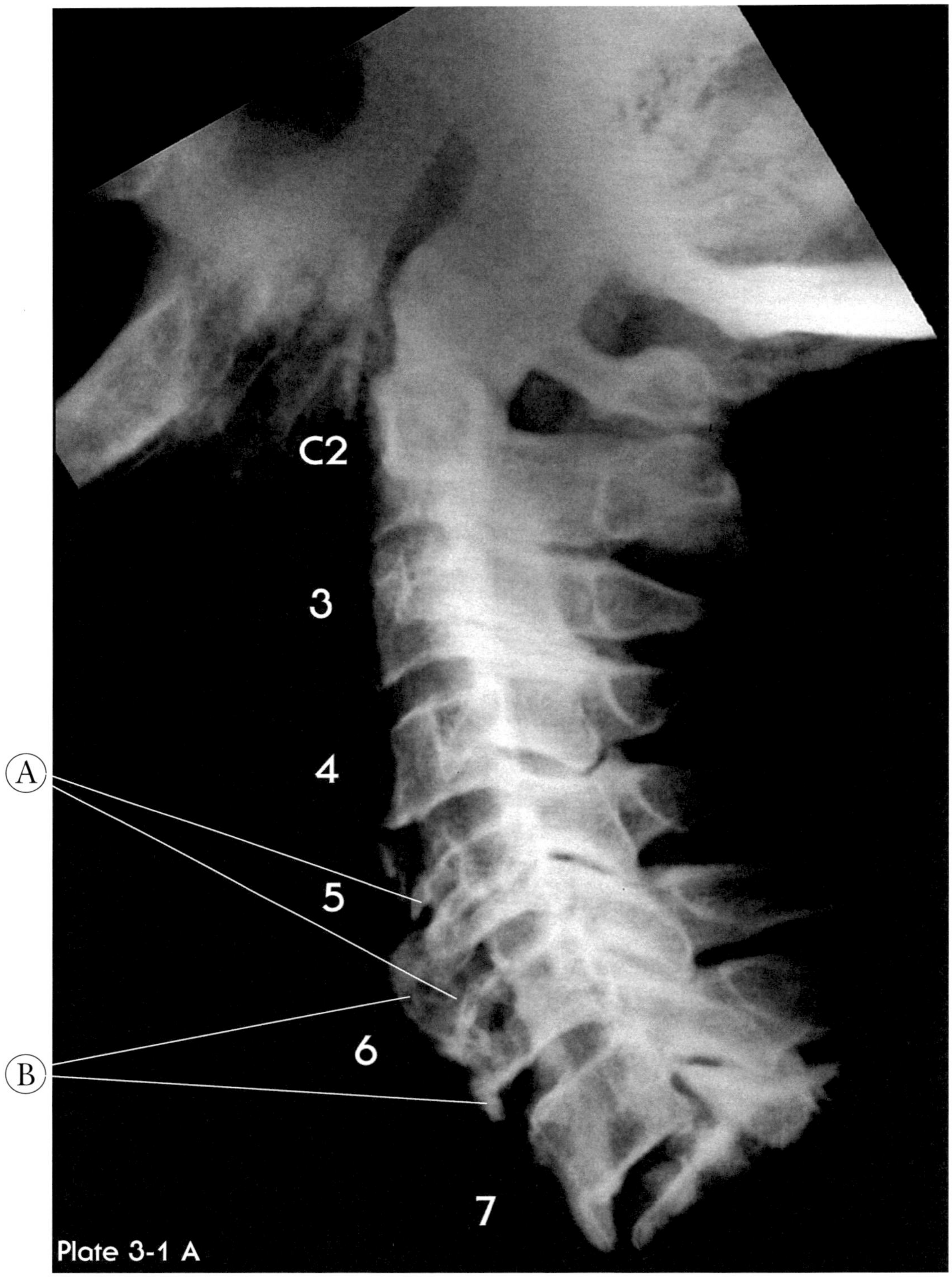

Plates 3-1 A & B

SUBLUXATIONS WITH LORDOTIC CERVICAL CURVE

This is an example of a modest lordotic cervical curve with signs of old trauma. Note the vertebral alignment, congenital stenosis, with virtually no posterior disc bulging. All of the cervical discs are substantial and hydrated despite the signs of old trauma. The discs had plenty of time to degenerate post accident but are healthy. Anterior bulging and spurring have occurred at C4-C5 and C5-C6, along with compression fractures of the C5 and C6 vertebral bodies.

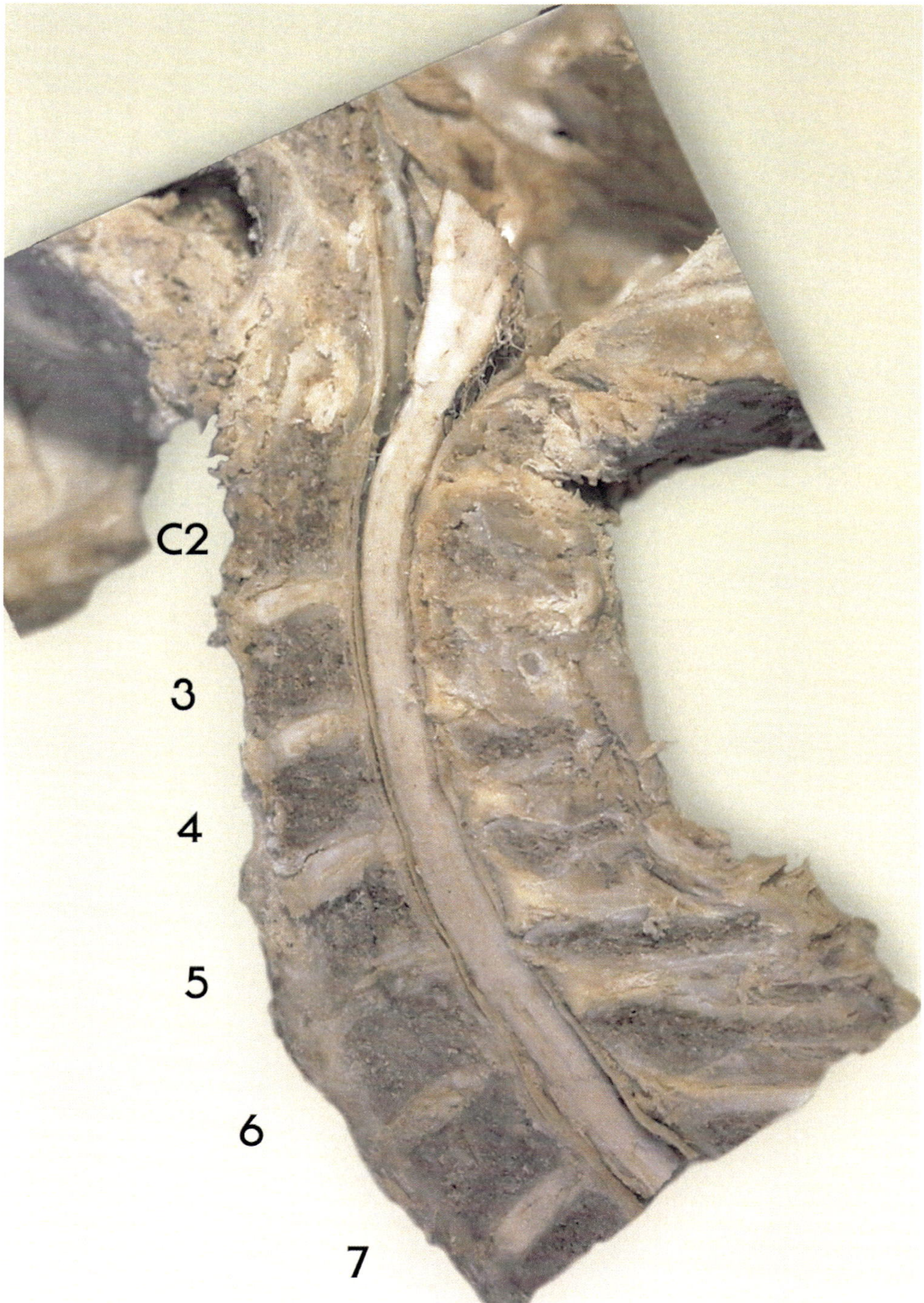

Plate 3-1 B

This type of injury is consistent with a fall where the individual lands on their buttocks with head flexing forward violently. (The lumbar damage in this specimen would support this). The main point is the lack of A-P misalignment. All segments except C1 and C2 show very slight stair stepped subluxation; C3 is retro to C4, C4 to C5 to C6 and C6 to C7. However, since the vertebral bodies still share weight-bearing with the facets, disc degeneration has not occurred to a pronounced degree in spite of the traumatic injury.

(A) Compression fractures of anterior vertebral bodies.

(B) Osseous repair and changes indicating old trauma

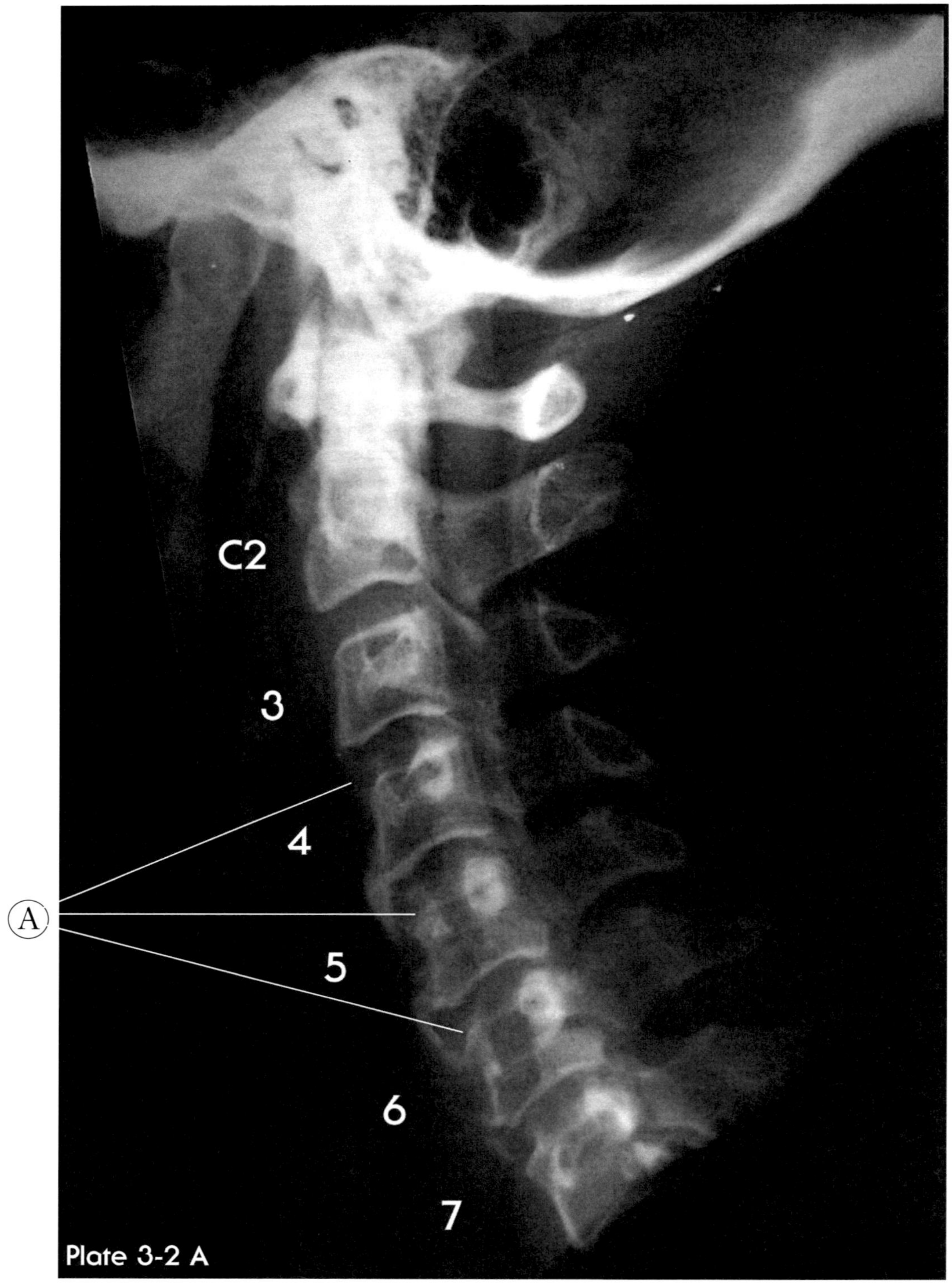

Plates 3-2 A & B
SUBLUXATIONS WITH LORDOTIC CERVICAL CURVE

The modest lordotic curve, despite the signs of trauma and subluxations, has allowed some normal weight bearing.

This specimen shows vertebral canal stenosis at the subluxated portion of the spine and stair stepped retrolisthesis from C3 through C5, with complete retrolisthesis of C6 (to C5 and C7).

(A) The vertebral bodies at C4, C5 and C6 appear to have been anteriorly crushed;

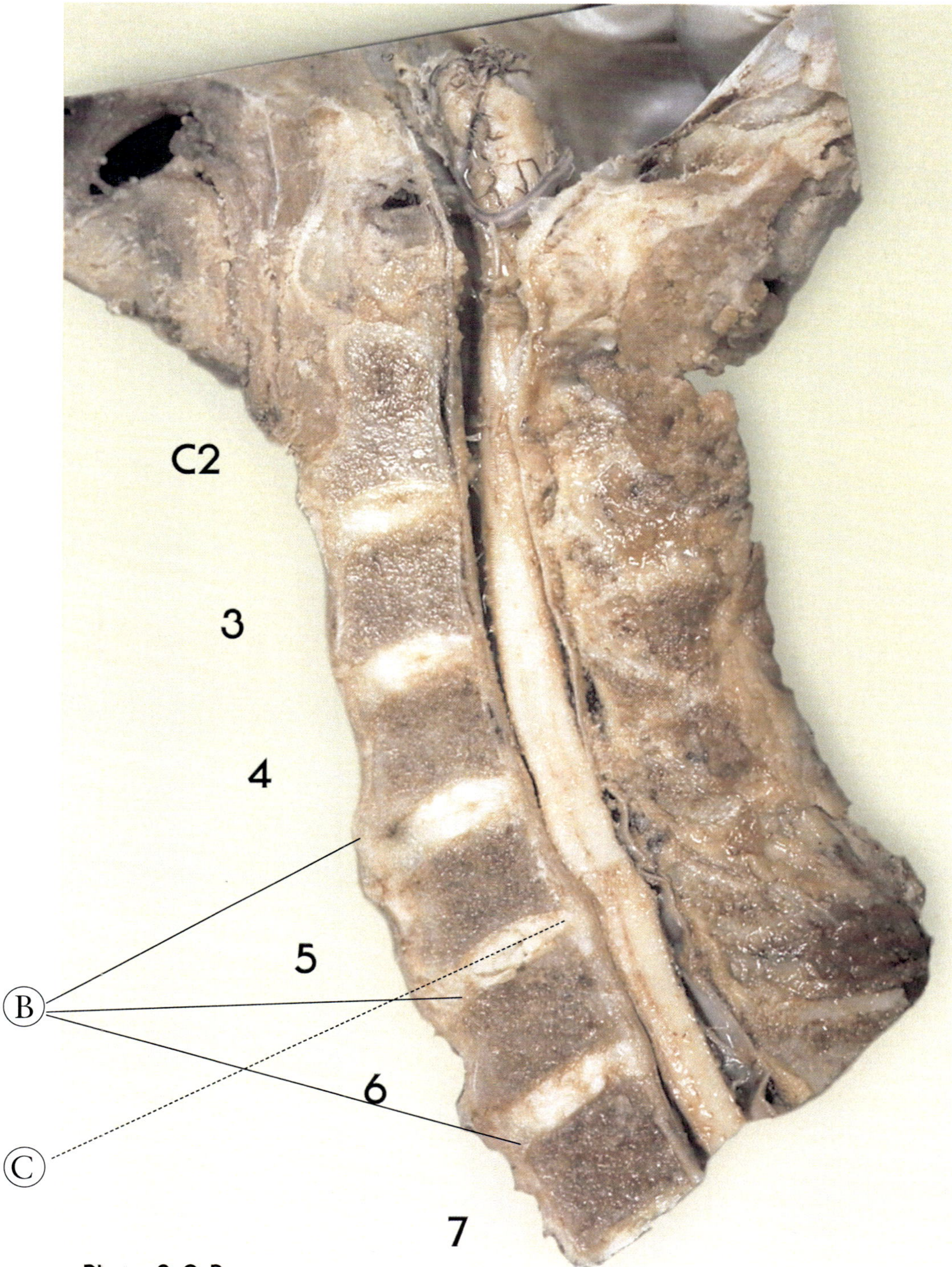

Plate 3-2 B

(B) The discs have bulged anteriorly and calcification of the anterior longitudinal ligament has occurred at C4-C5; C5-C6 and C6-C7. A traumatic event such as a collision may have caused these injuries.
In spite of the trauma, the discs are all present and hydrated.

(C) The only significant disc damage is at C5-C6, where tearing and posterior bulging have occurred. The bulge impinges dramatically on the spinal cord, so it was probably of clinical significance to the individual.

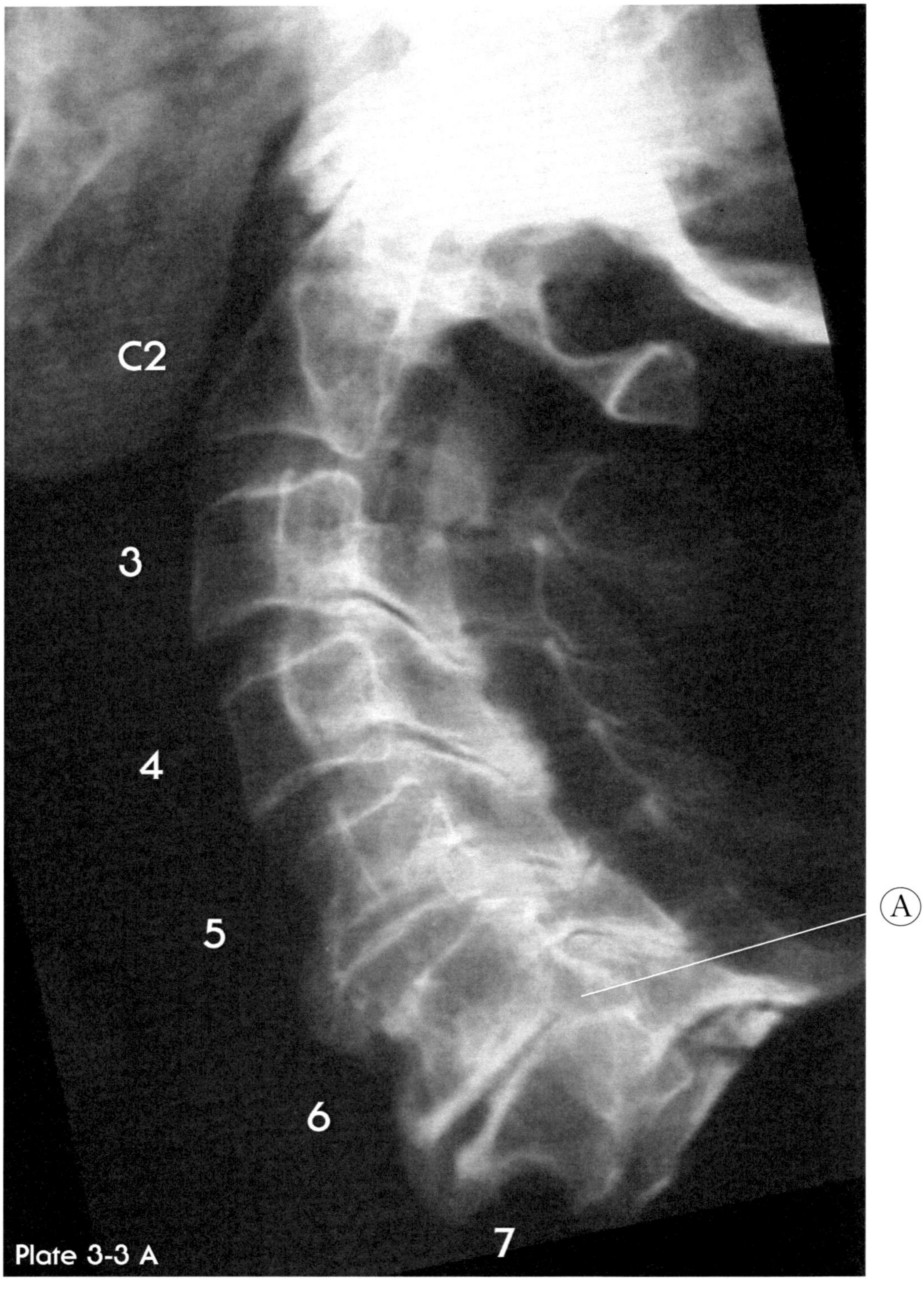

Plates 3-3 A & B

SUBLUXATIONS WITH LORDOTIC CERVICAL CURVE

In this view, the curve is maintained, with the subluxation and damage at each segment with disc bulging clinically insignificant because of the large central canal. There are slight subluxations at all levels with loss of posterior disc height at every segment and loss of facetal joint space with eburnation (hypertrophy) of facets. Note that the loss of

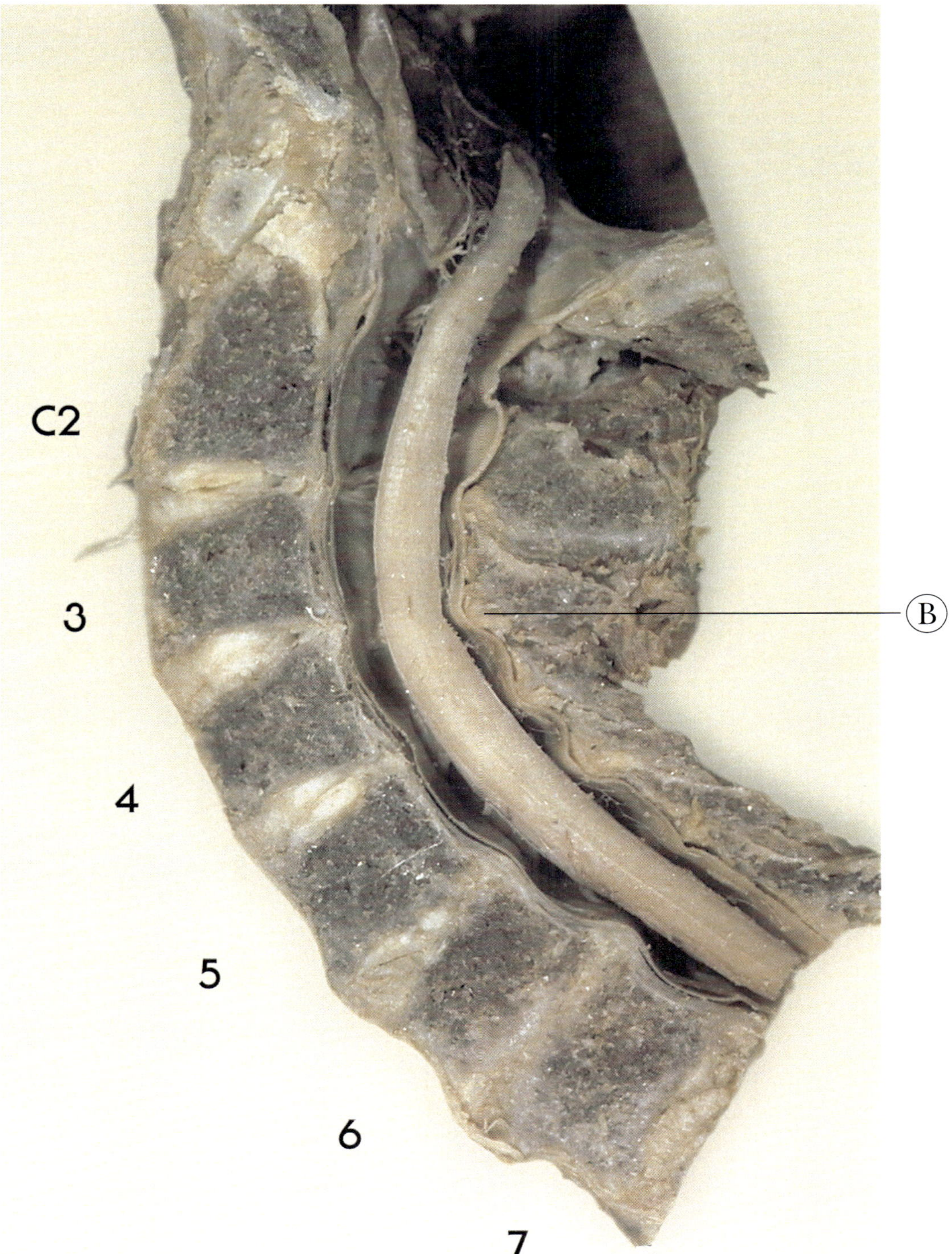

Plate 3-3 B

interspinous space-spinous contact can cause bony changes. This is secondary to the loss of the posterior disc height.

(A) Note; near fusion of posterior of vertebral bodies of C6 and C7 forming a permanent protrusion into the vertebral canal.

(B) Ligamentum flavum protrusion and cord contact at C3-C4 can be associated with loss of disc height, wedging and subluxation.

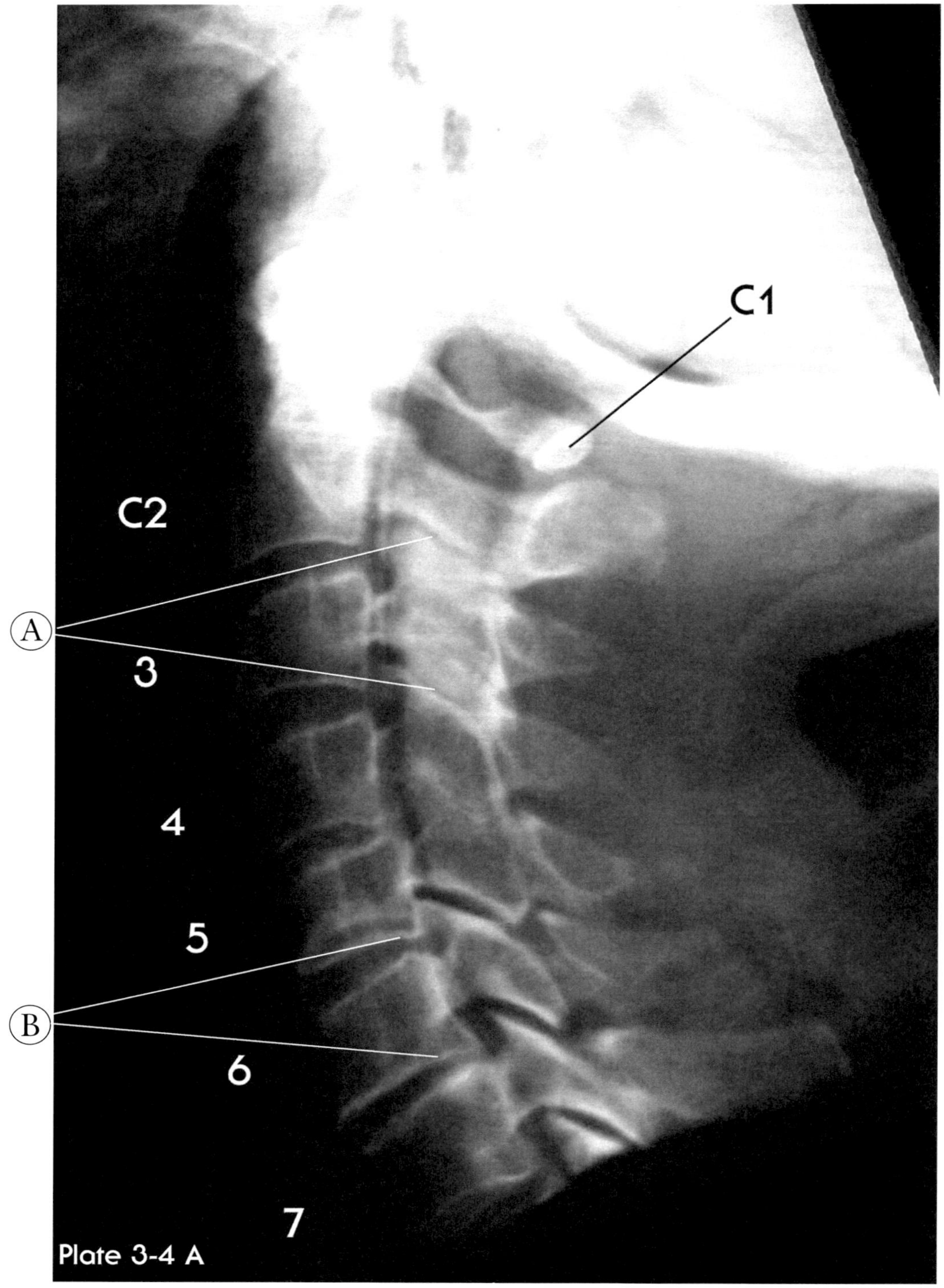

Plates 3-4 A & B

SUBLUXATIONS WITH LORDOTIC CERVICAL CURVE

The lordotic curve is maintained with C1 anterior to C2; C3 retro to C2 with disc tearing; C3-C4 looks all right with slight disc tearing; C4 is anterior to C5 (X-ray looks worse) disc tearing with some brown degeneration with loss of disc height; C6 slight retro to C5 with disc tearing and bulging anterior and posterior; C6 anterior to C7 with posterior spurring, disc tearing, and brown degeneration, posterior joint changes. The cerebellum and brain stem can be drawn down into the base of the occiput

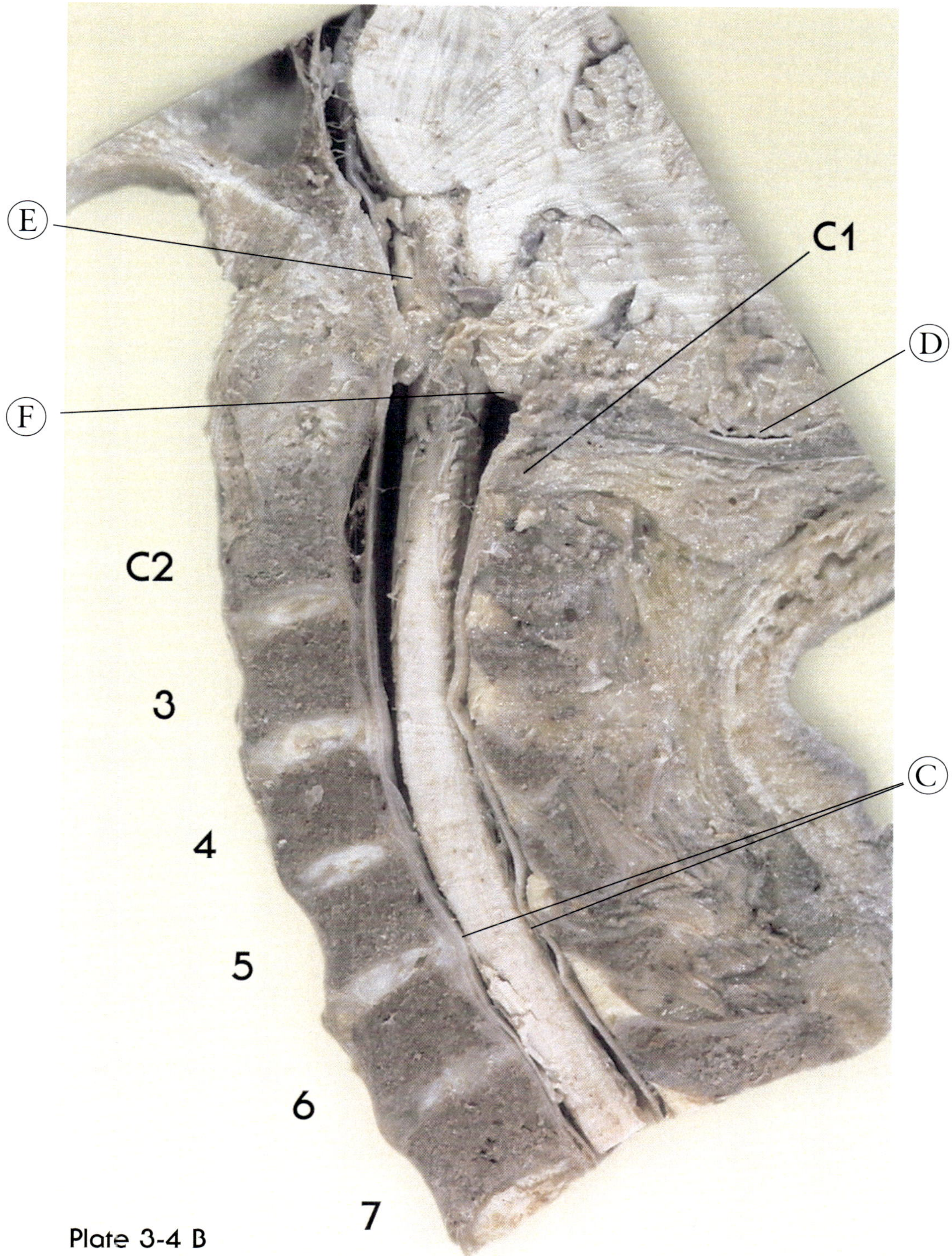

Plate 3-4 B

causing arterial compression and cerebellar invagination into the spinal canal.

(A) C2-C4 has little curve and loss of facet joint space.
(B) Inferior endplate widening is the hallmark of hyper loading the vertebral body and disc.
(C) Canal stenosis is the result of the widened endplates and bulging disc.
(D) Note cerebellar compression into occiput.
(E) Brain stem contact with the clivus.
(F) Cerebellum invaginating through the foramen magnum.

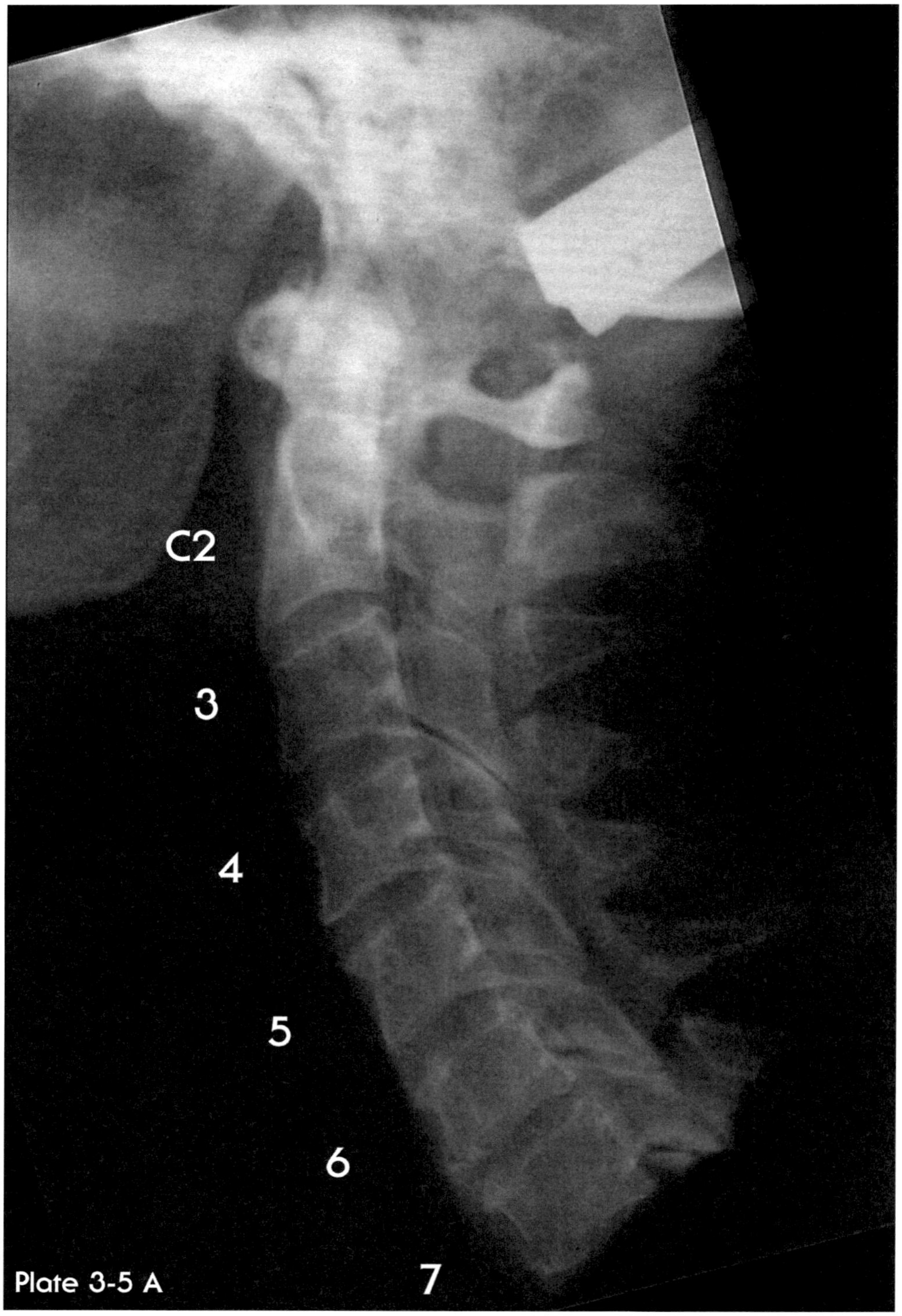

Plates 3-5 A & B

SUBLUXATIONS WITH LORDOTIC CERVICAL CURVE

Minor stairstepped retrolisthesis has occurred which developed posterior spurs and some disc bulging, but the normal lordotic curve has prevented major canal changes.

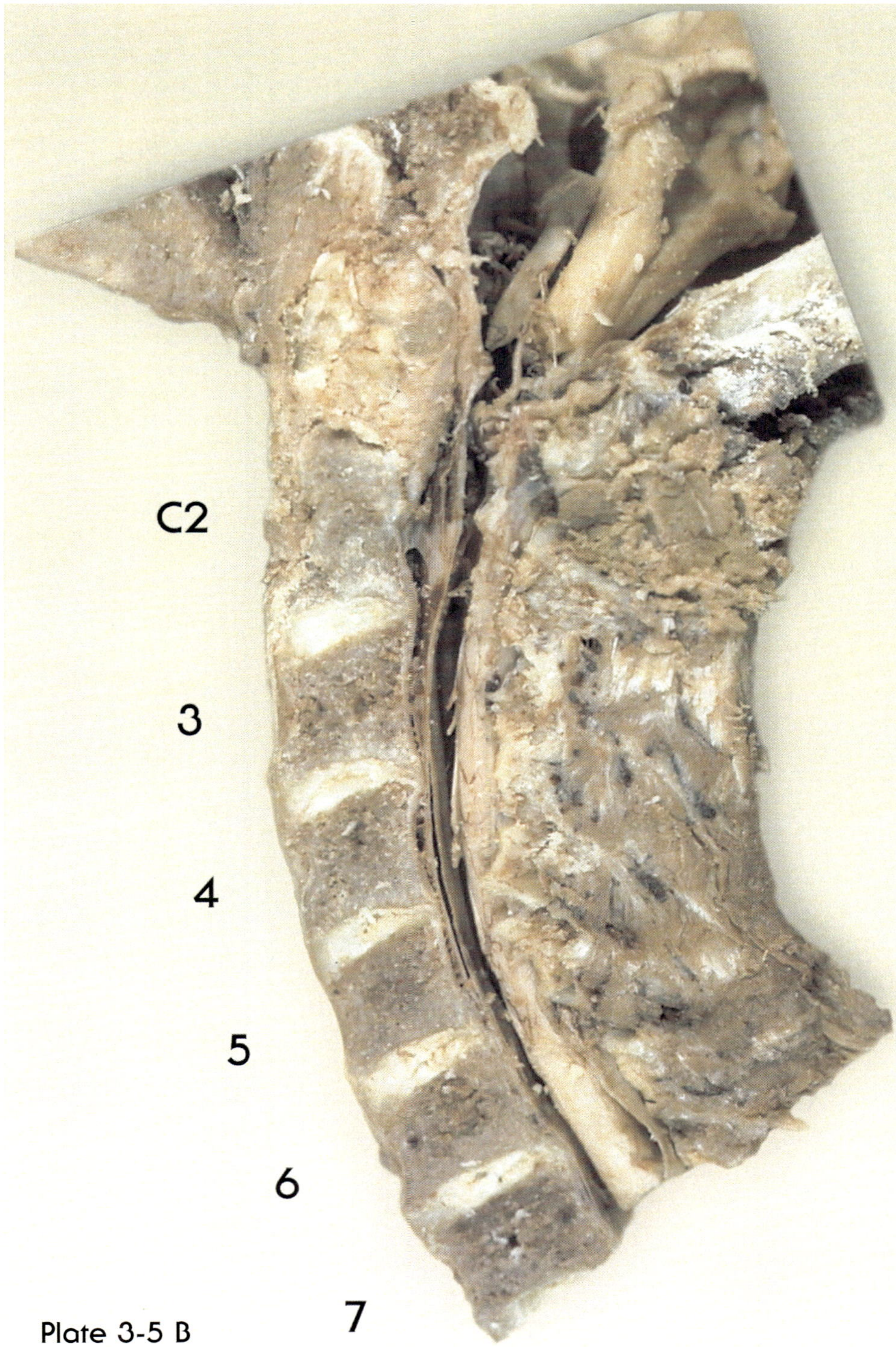

Plate 3-5 B

C3 is retro to C4, C4 to C5, C5 to C6 and C6 tc C7. Slight posterior bulging and loss of posterior disc height is visible between all segrr ents, and an anterior bulge can be seen at C6-C7. Deformation of the vertebral bodies indicates altered weight bearing beginning at C4.

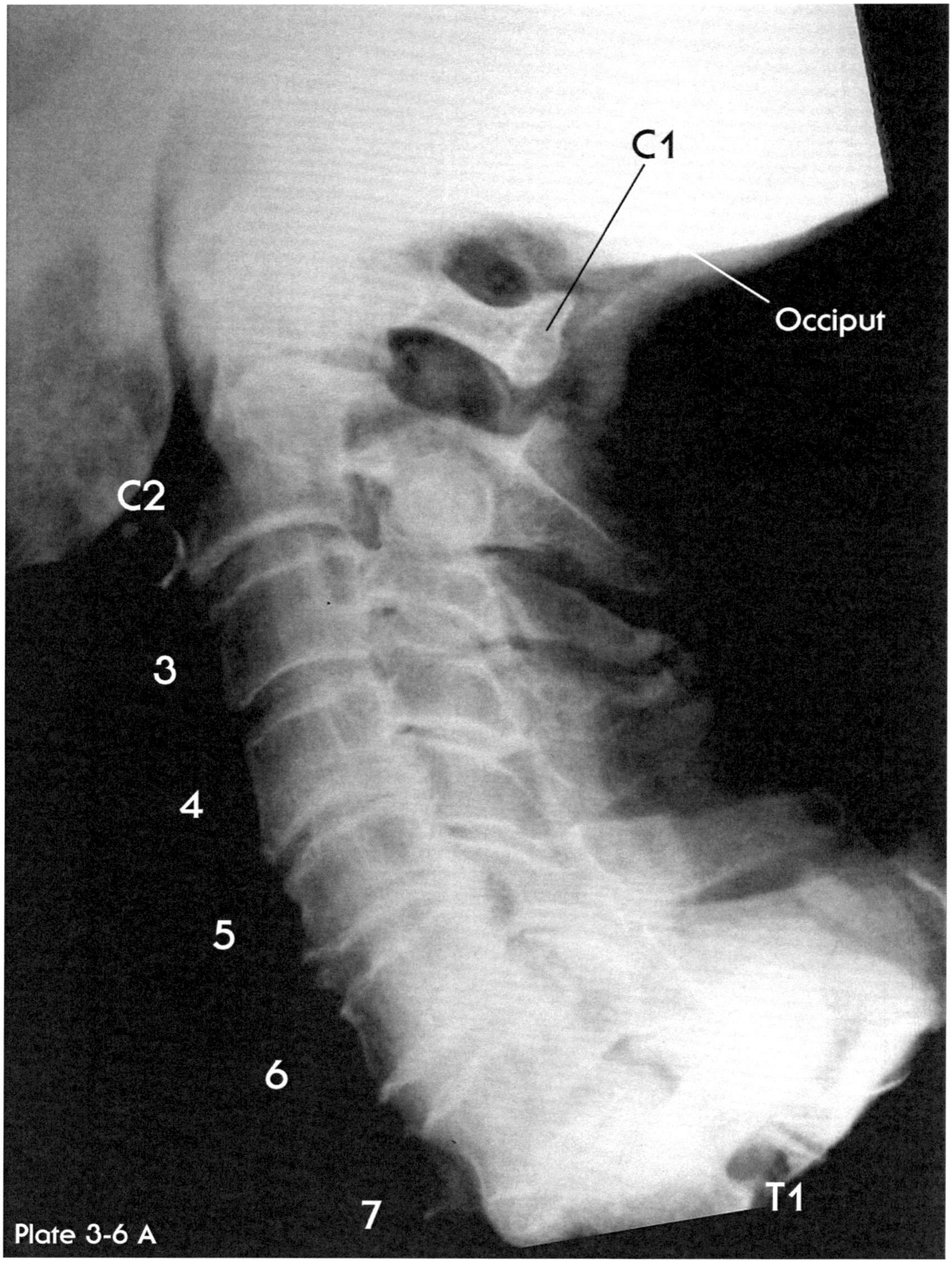

Plates 3-6 A & B

SUBLUXATIONS WITH LORDOTIC CERVICAL CURVE

This specimen shows relatively slight subluxations at every segment, with accompanying disc degeneration. C1 is anterior to the occiput and C2, C3 is retro to C2 and C4 (complete retrolisthesis). C4 is slightly retro to C5, and C6 is anterior to both C5 and C7 (complete anterolisthesis).

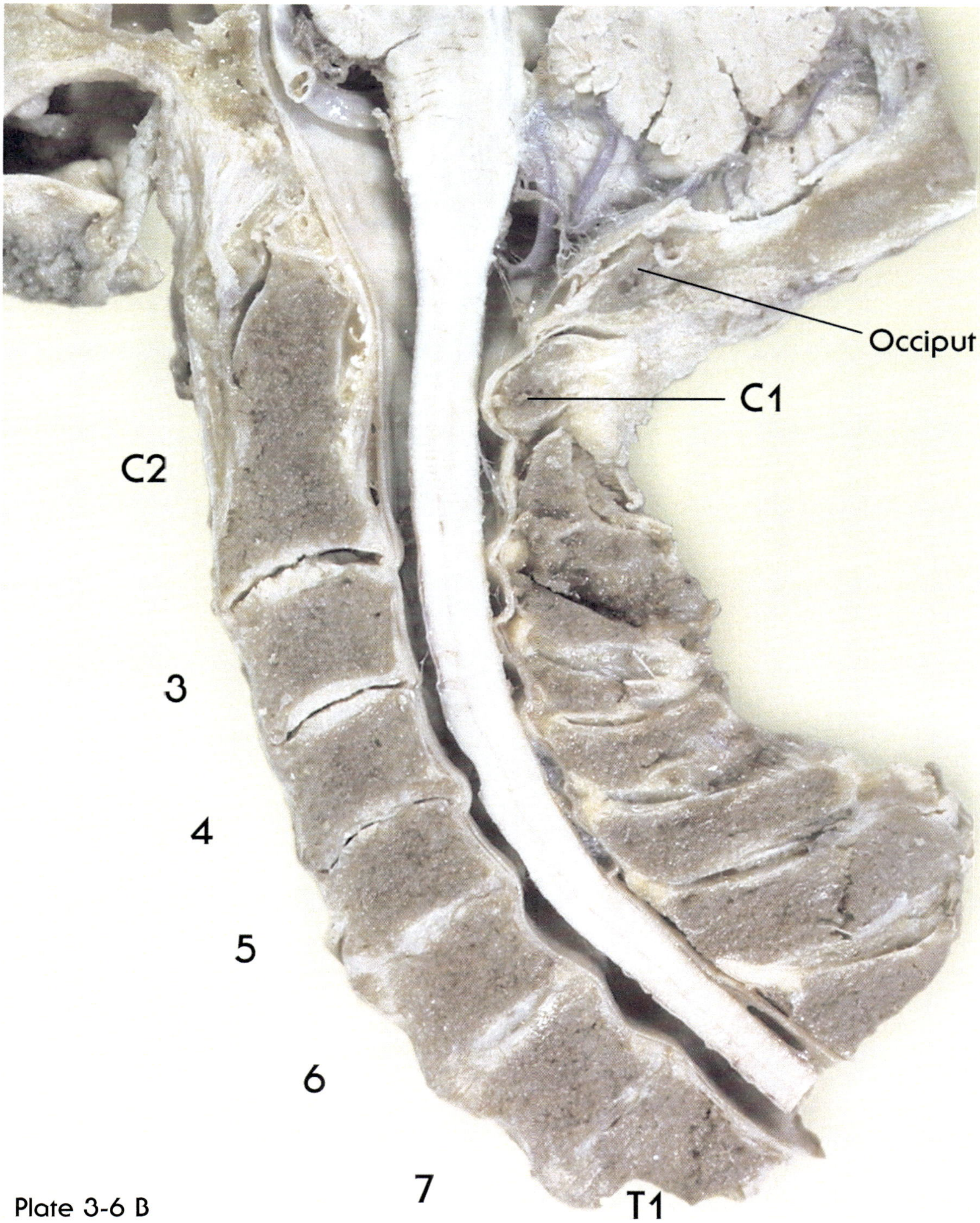

Plate 3-6 B

Note that the cervical lordotic curve has been maintained, indicating that the facets are still weight-bearing. Approximation of the spinous processes has occurred with loss of disc height and cavitation. Spurring has occurred in the lower segments, and the canal stenosis is minor. Encroachment on the spinal cord has occurred only at C4-C5 and perhaps slightly at C5-C6, and none of the segments have fused.
Anterior spurring is visible at C4-C5, C5-C6 and C6-C7, and a disc tear can be seen on the X-ray at C3-C4.
Note: Disc tears, even prominent ones (e.g. the disc between C2 and C3) may or may not show up on X-ray, however, they do appear on MRI's.

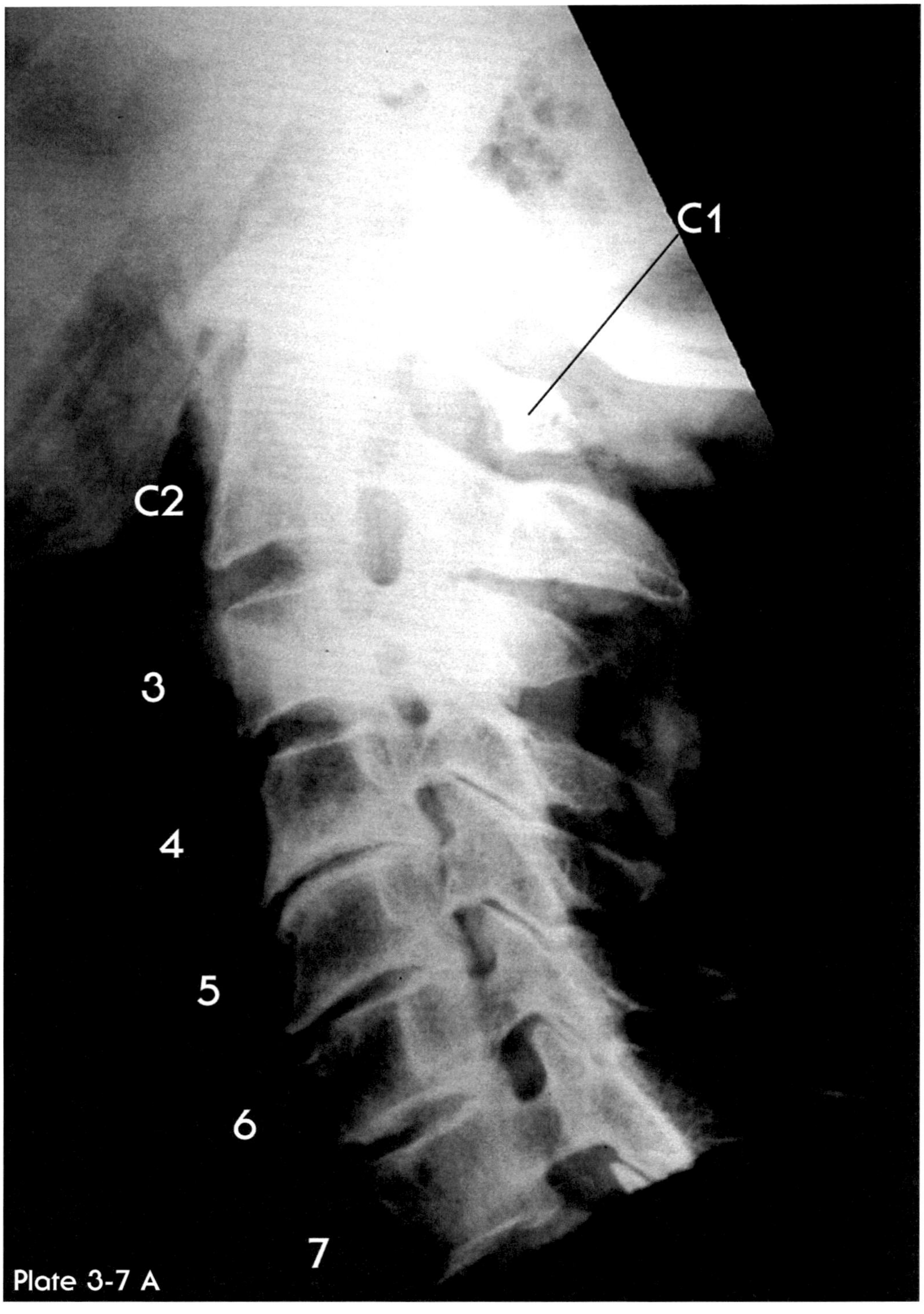

Plate 3-7 A

Plates 3-7 A & B

SUBLUXATIONS WITH LORDOTIC CERVICAL CURVE

This specimen has a moderate lordotic curve with significant disc degeneration and spurring at the subluxated segments. There is also cord contact from C3 to C5 with compression of the anterior cord at C4-5.

C1 is anterior; C4 is a complete retrolisthesis to C3 and C5; tearing of C3-C4 disc; but near fusion with spurring posterior and anterior; note tearing or fissure of C4-C5; C5 retro to C6 with

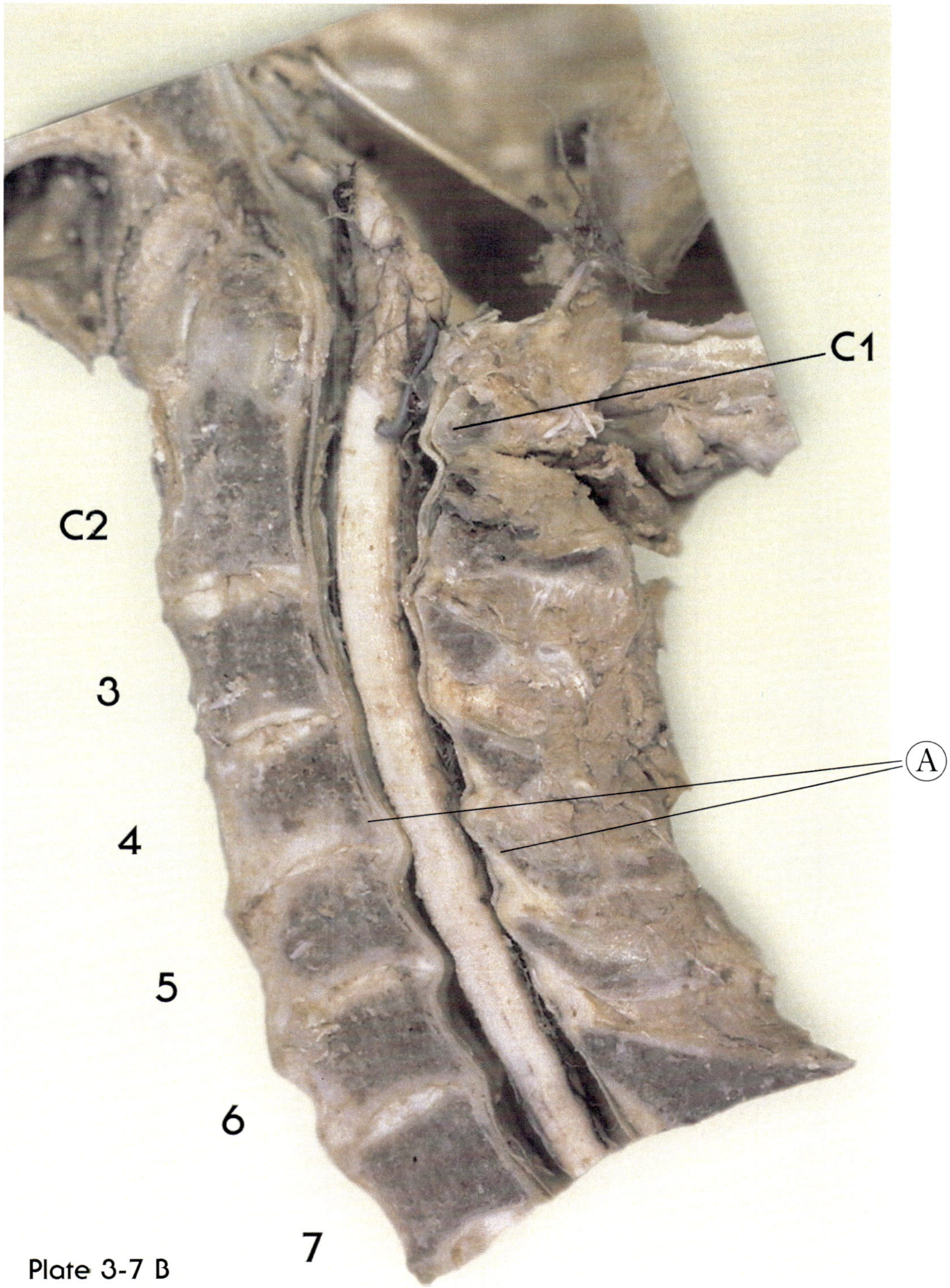

Plate 3-7 B

tearing and spurring; C6 retro to C7 with fusion of posterior C6-C7 tearing of disc without bulge of C7 superior endplate; moderate canal stenosis with C4-C5 disc bulge significant with flexion; also with C5-C6 slight significance with flexion.

(A) C4 posterior body retro to C3-C5 moves closer to lamina of C5, stenosis is worsened.

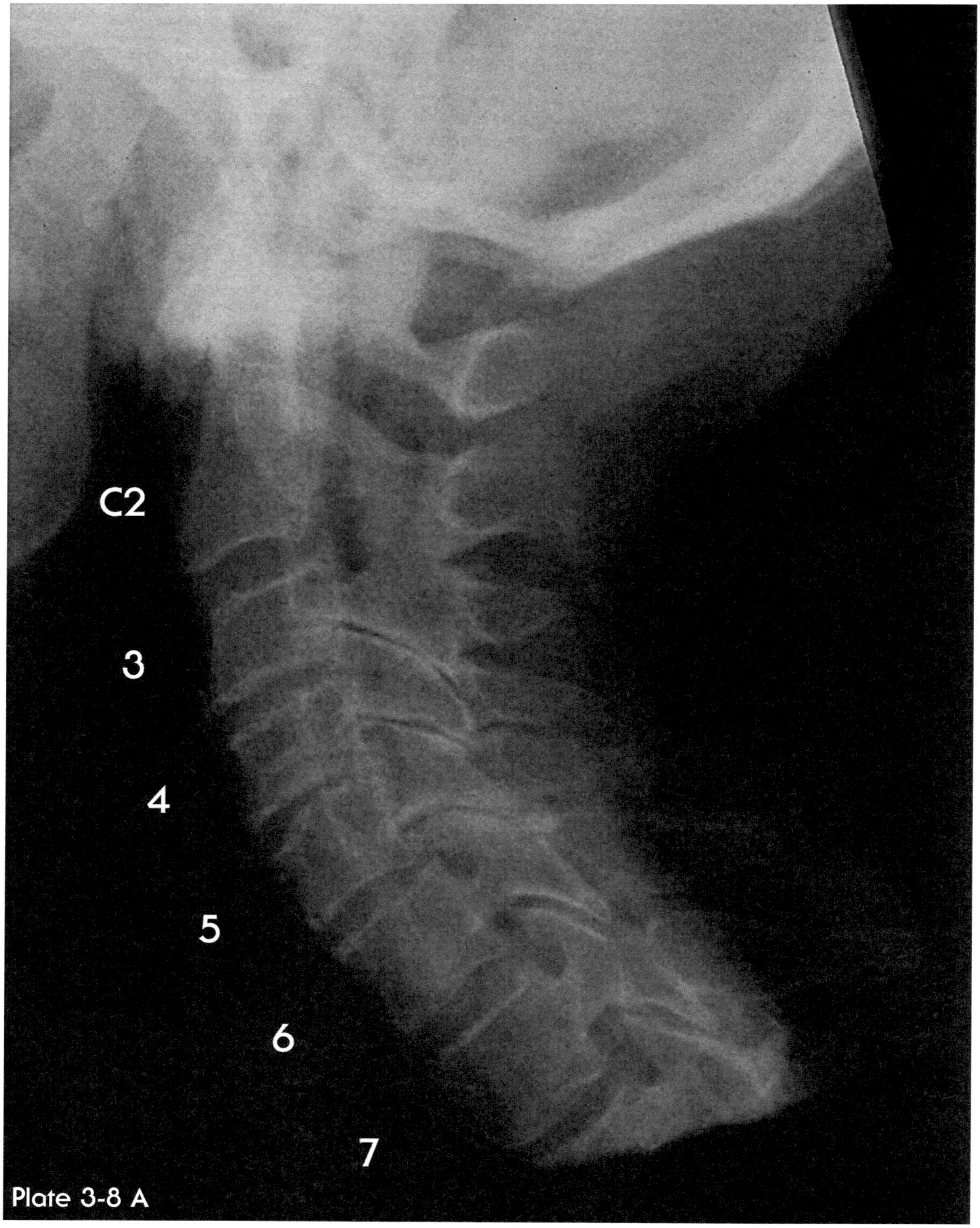

Plates 3-8 A & B

SUBLUXATIONS WITH LORDOTIC CERVICAL CURVE

Most commonly, injuries to the cervical spine occur at the C5-C6 and C6-C7 discs, which have the greatest capability for anteroposterior movement and which, being farthest from the head, are the most vulnerable to buckling. Occasionally, however, injuries specifically affect the mid-cervical vertebrae and discs.

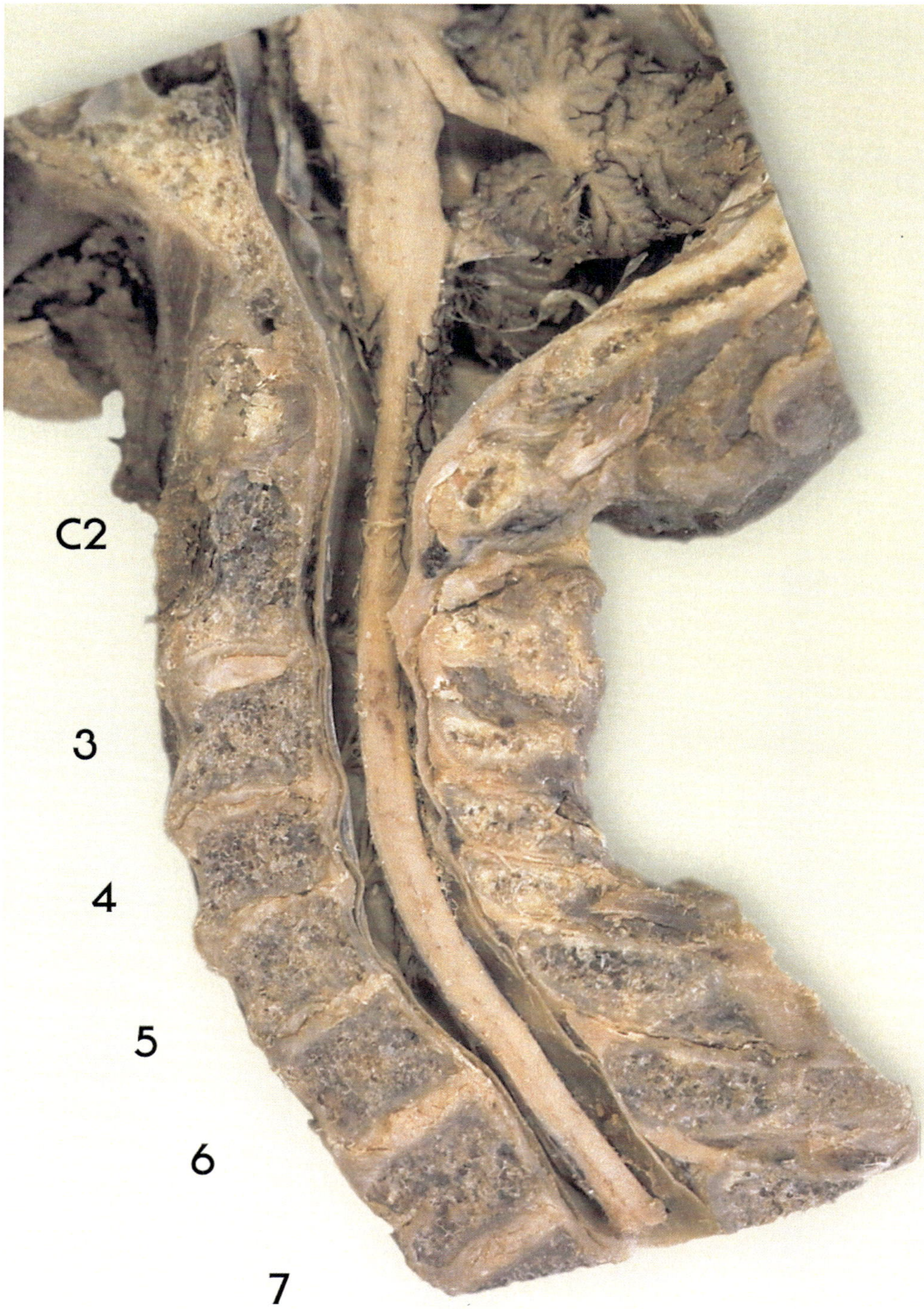

Plate 3-8 B

Almost all segments are subluxated; C3 is a complete retro (to C2 and C4), C4 is a complete antero (to C3 and C5), and C6 is completely retro (to C5 and C7). Disc tearing and bulging is evident throughout, and is most pronounced from C3-C4 through C5-C6, but because the lordotic curve has been maintained, stenosis of the vertebral canal is minor and the disc bulges do not impinge upon the spinal cord, although close at C6-7 disc. Spinous processes of C4-C6 have approximated because of disc height loss and the facets have been affected by the altered weight bearing.

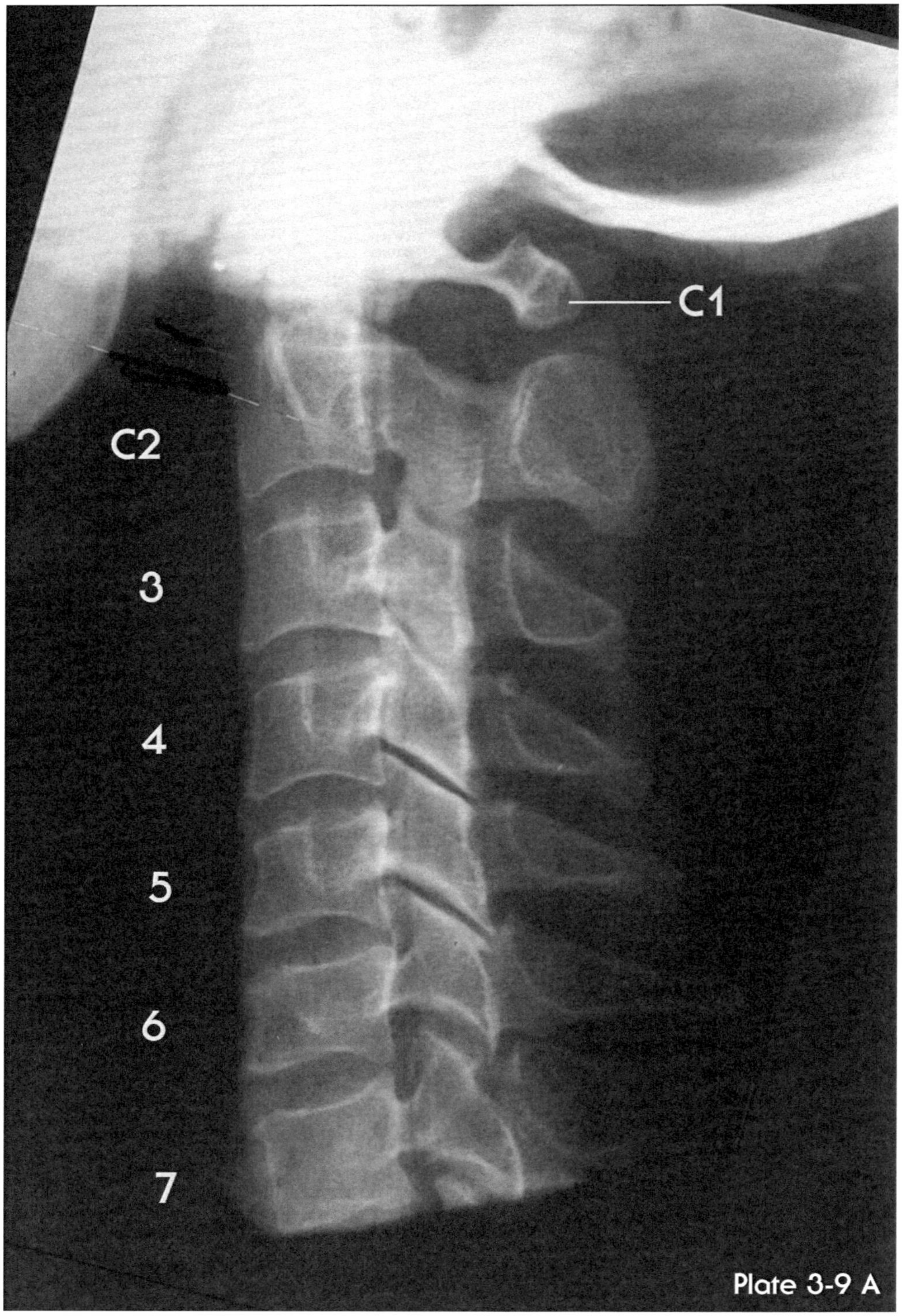

Plates 3-9 A & B
SUBLUXATIONS WITH LOSS OF LORDOTIC CURVE
Straight or military neck

This individual shows pronounced straightening of the neck as well as soft tissue and bony changes caused by altered weight bearing. C1 is anterior, C2 is anterior to C3, C3 is anterior to C4, C5 is retro to C6, and C6 is retro to C7.

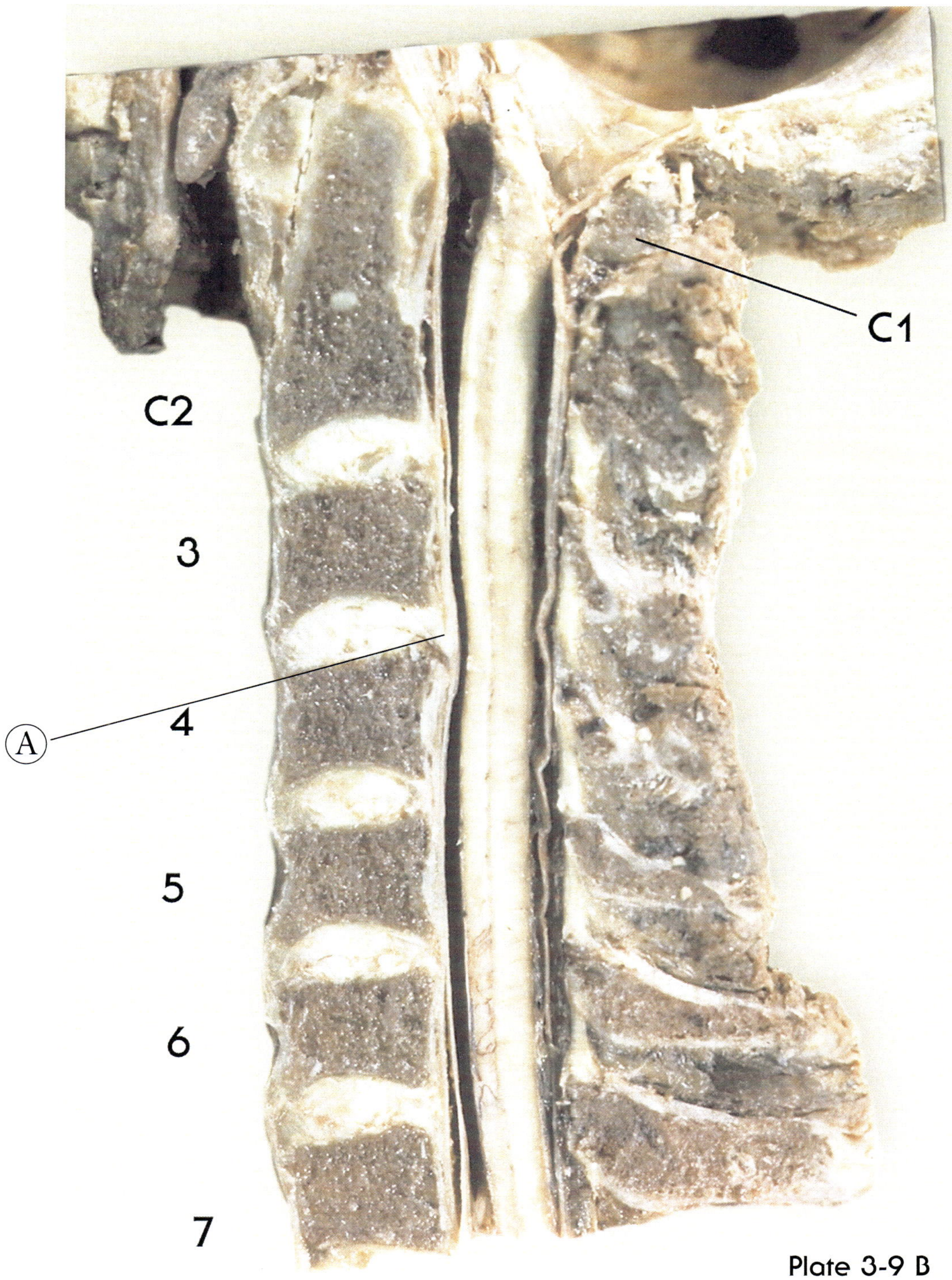

Plate 3-9 B

Total loss of the curve usually involves at least one or more retrolisthesis. Disc shearing and bulging occur from C3-C4 downward. Broadening of endplates is evident below C4, indicating increased weight bearing in the vertebral bodies. Anterior bulging and endplate deformation at C5-C6 and C6-C7 were probably traumatic in origin.

(A) Note that the relatively slight posterior disc bulge at C3-C4 impinges on the spinal cord.

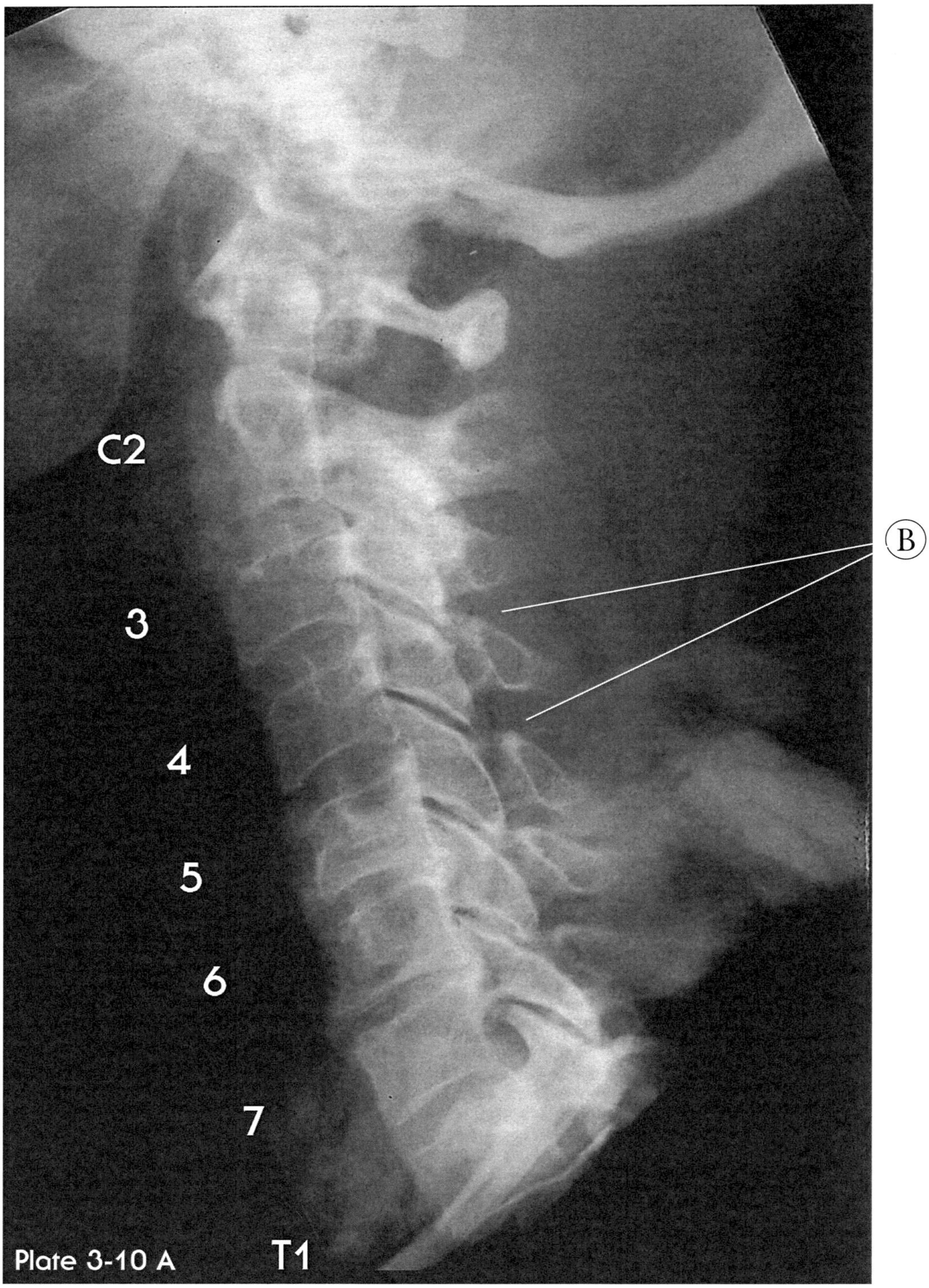

Plates 3-10 A & B
SUBLUXATIONS WITH LOSS OF LORDOTIC CURVE
Straight or military neck

This specimen shows a loss of cervical curve with a slight reversal from C4 through C6 with a retrolisthesis of C5. C2 is anterior to C3, C4 to C3, C5 is a complete retro (to C4 and C6), and C6 is retro to C7. Disc tearing (shear), spurring and loss of disc height can be seen indicating a long-standing forward alteration of weight bearing.

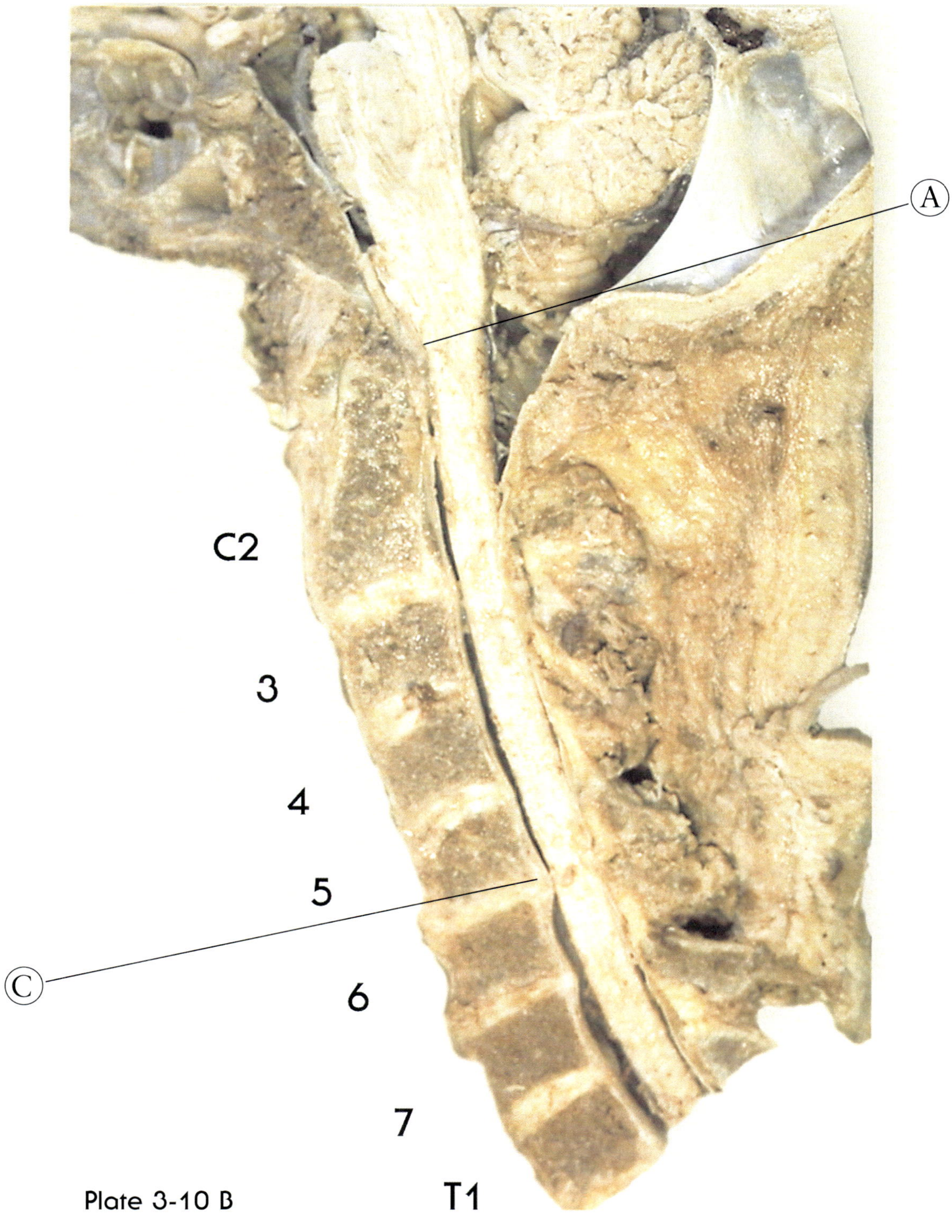

Plate 3-10 B

(A) Note that the pons and brainstem are tethered against the posterior surface of the dens and transverse ligament. Introduction of any flexion in the vertebral column will cause further tethering at this point.

(B) Increased interspinous distance indicates lengthening of the canal.

(C) Subluxation and endplate changes in this individual makes the posterior disc bulge at C5-C6 clinically significant. Advanced disc degeneration is evident at the most subluxated and structurally stressed part of the cervical spine.

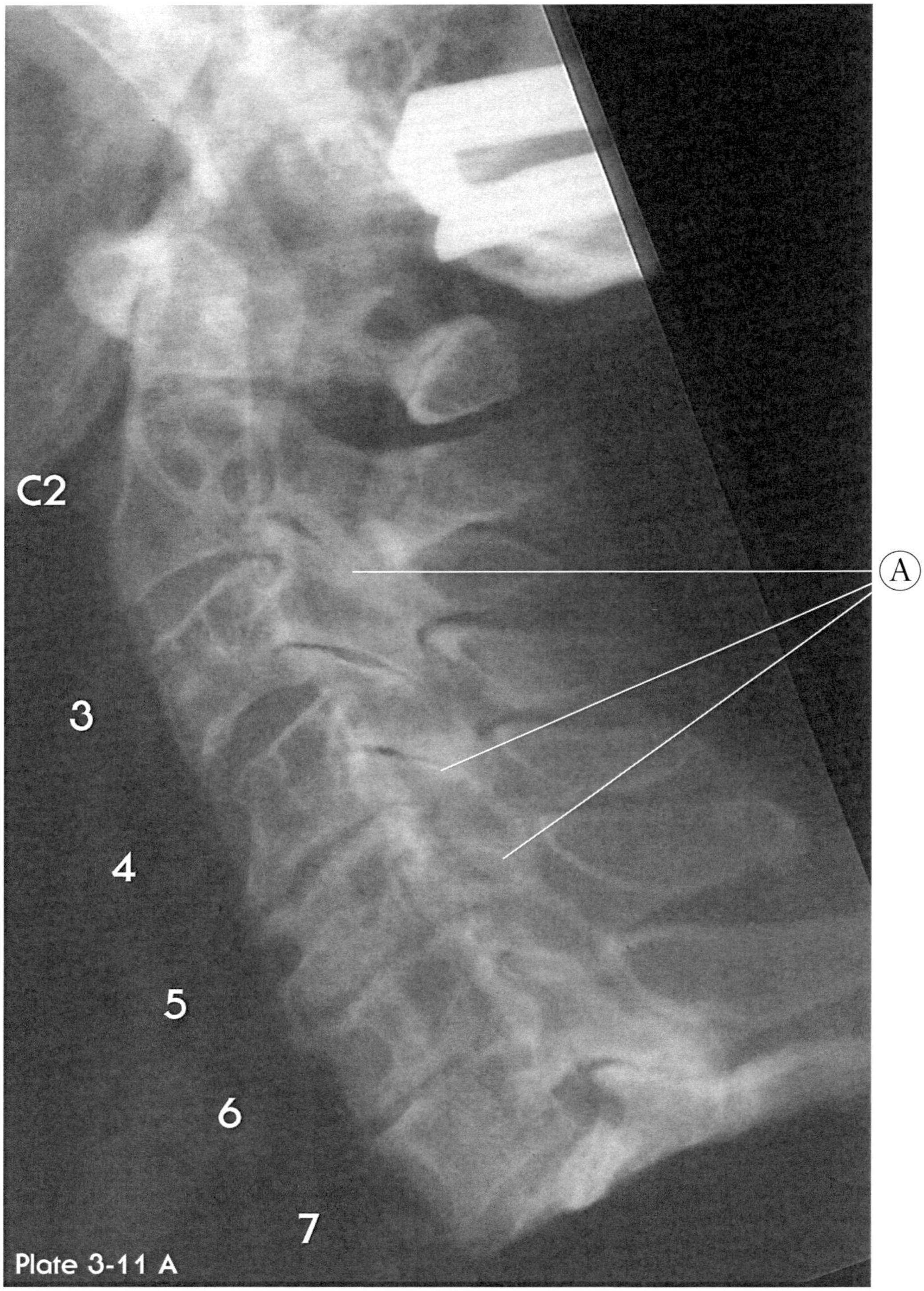

Plates 3-11 A & B
SUBLUXATIONS WITH LOSS OF LORDOTIC CURVE
Straight or military neck

Note the canal stenosis from chronic degenerative changes due to subluxation. C2 retro C3 with tearing and bulging of the disc, C3 anterior to C2 and C4; C4 retro to C3 with major vertebral body changes; C5 a complete retro to C4 and C6 with near fusion of C4-C5 and

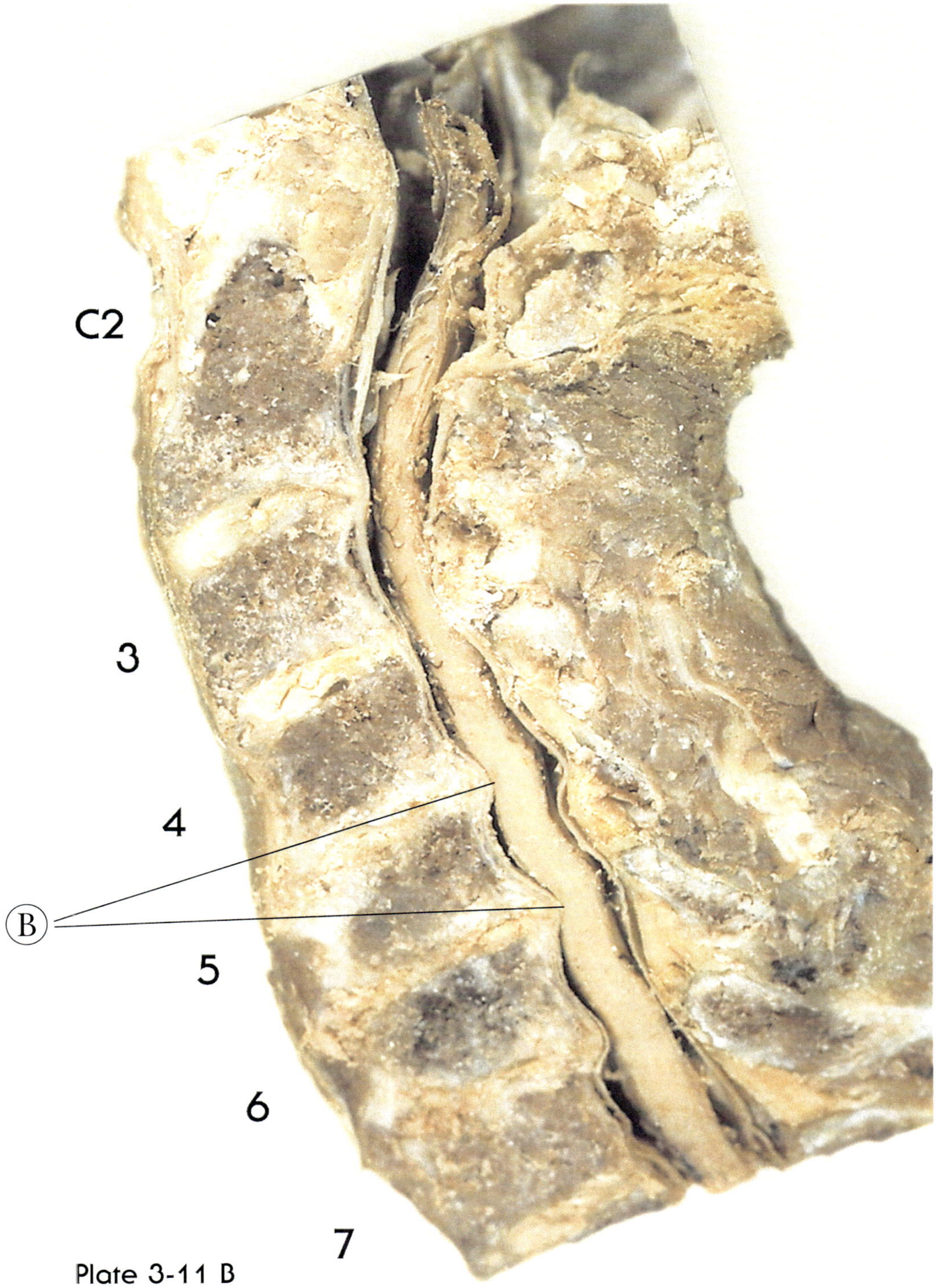

Plate 3-11 B

C5-C6 with posterior bone spurring and further stenosis; C6 retro to C7 with tearing near fusion. Note loss of posterior disc height C2-C3 with spinous contact and facet jamming and sclerosis. This can also be seen in all the facets due to loss of disc height and altered weight bearing of subluxation.

(A) Facet degeneration
(B) Cord-osteophyte contact.

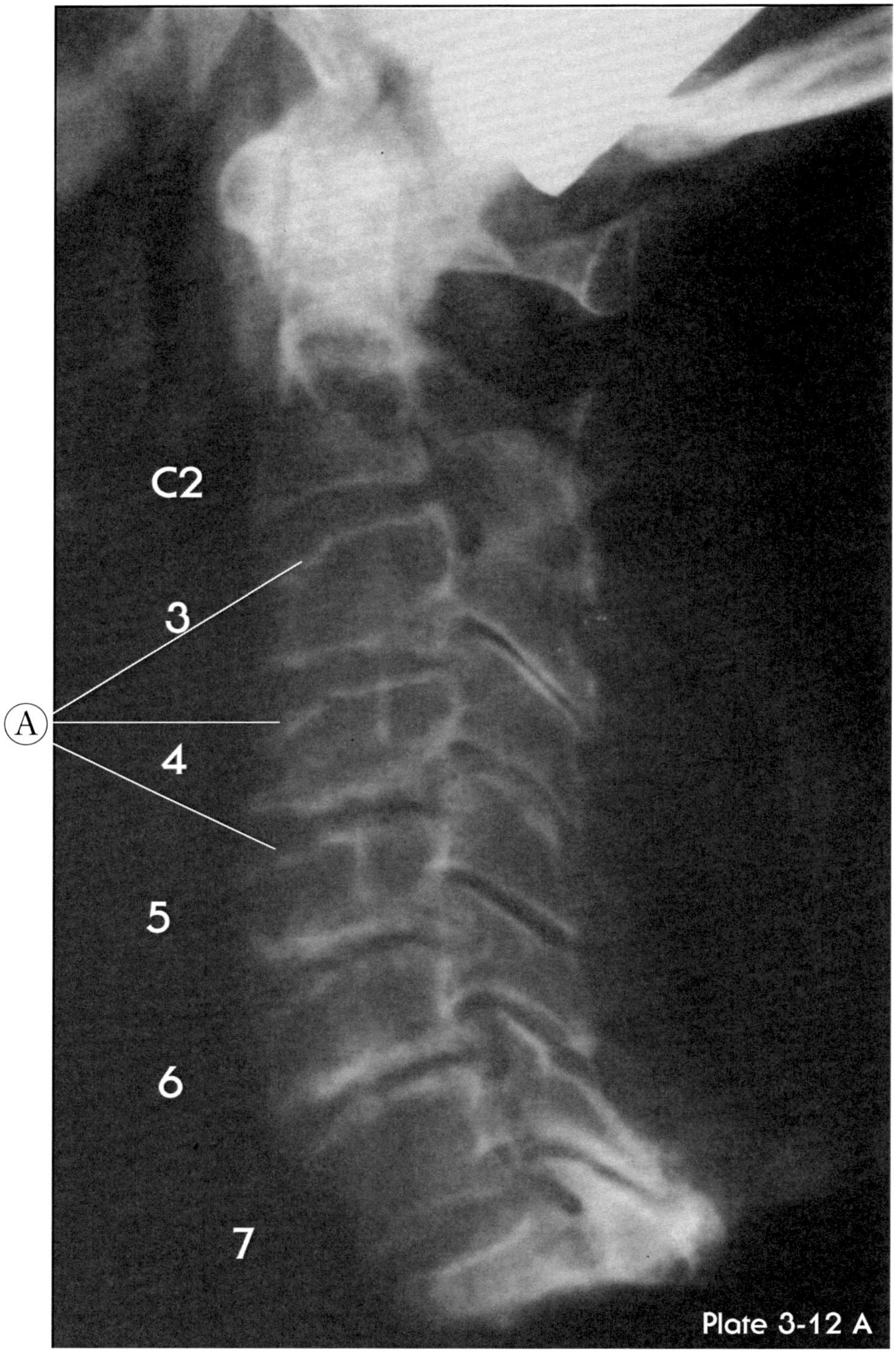

Plates 3-12 A & B

SUBLUXATIONS WITH REVERSED OR KYPHOTIC CURVE

Upper cervical subluxations

This view shows a reversal of the lordotic curve at C2-C3. Retro C3 to C2 with disc tearing and bulging; C4 is a complete retro to C3 and C5 with disc tearing, wedging, C6 is anterior to C5 with disc tearing and bulging and near fusion posteriorly.

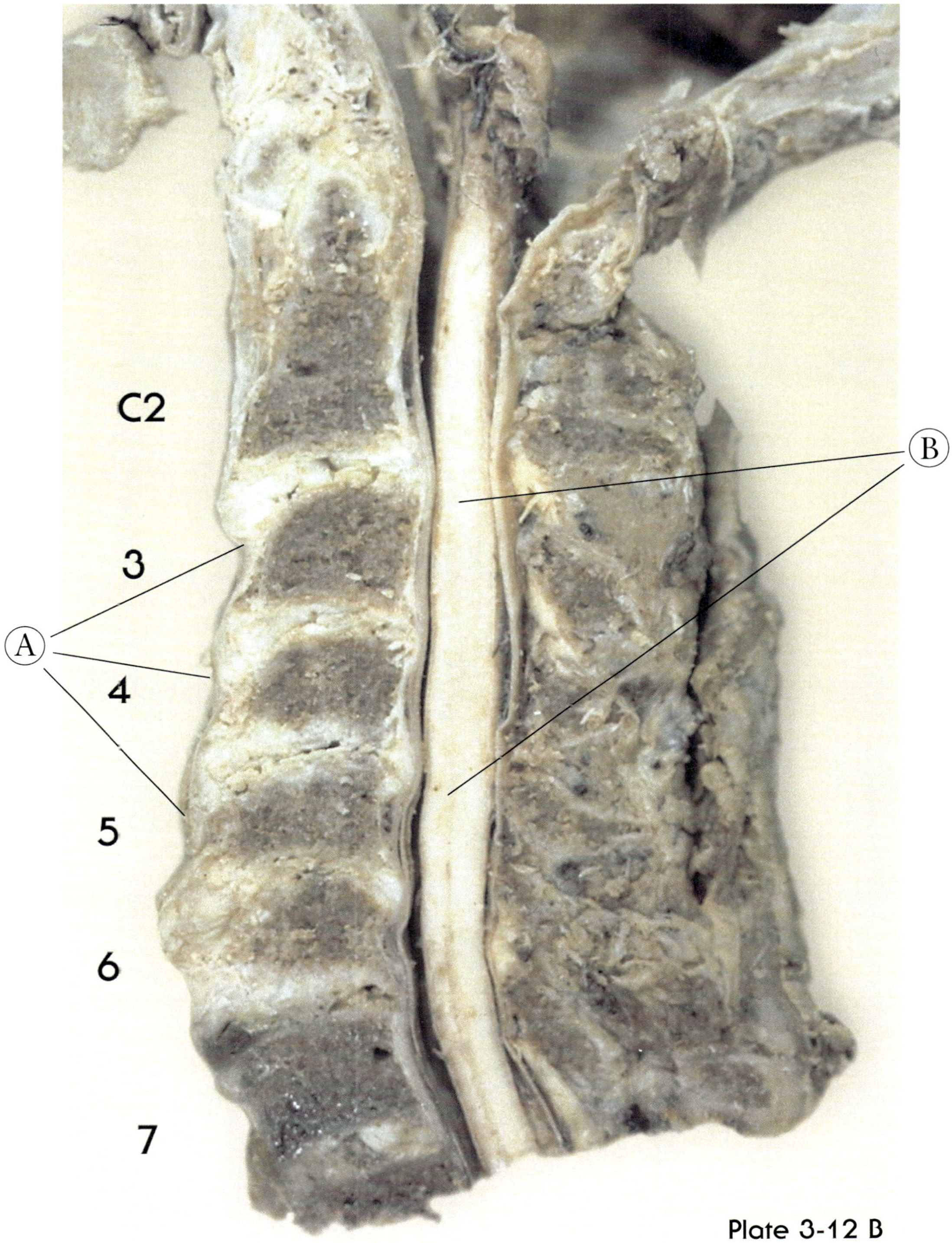

Plate 3-12 B

All discs are torn with anterior spurring and disc bulges posterior. Canal stenosis is due to the subluxations and the resulting alteration of soft and bony tissues.

(A) Small compression fractures of anterior and superior vertebral bodies C3-C5.

(B) Spinal cord and canal contact from C3-C5.

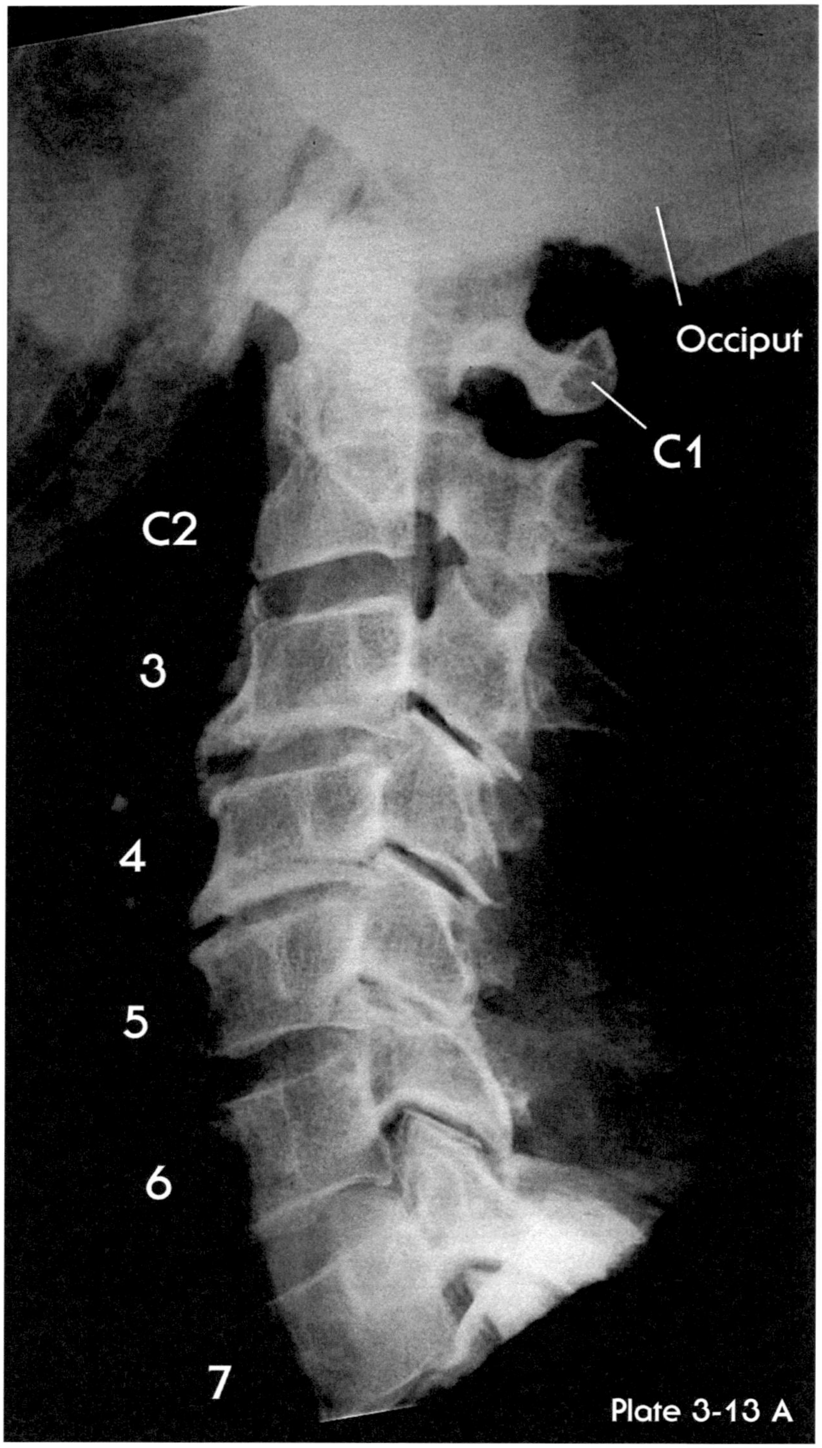

Plates 3-13 A & B

SUBLUXATIONS WITH REVERSED OR KYPHOTIC CURVE

Upper cervical subluxations

This specimen shows a reversal of the lordotic curve at C3 with stenosis of the vertebral canal at the subluxated segments, which makes the relatively minor disc bulges at C3-C4, C4-C5 and C5-C6 clinically significant.

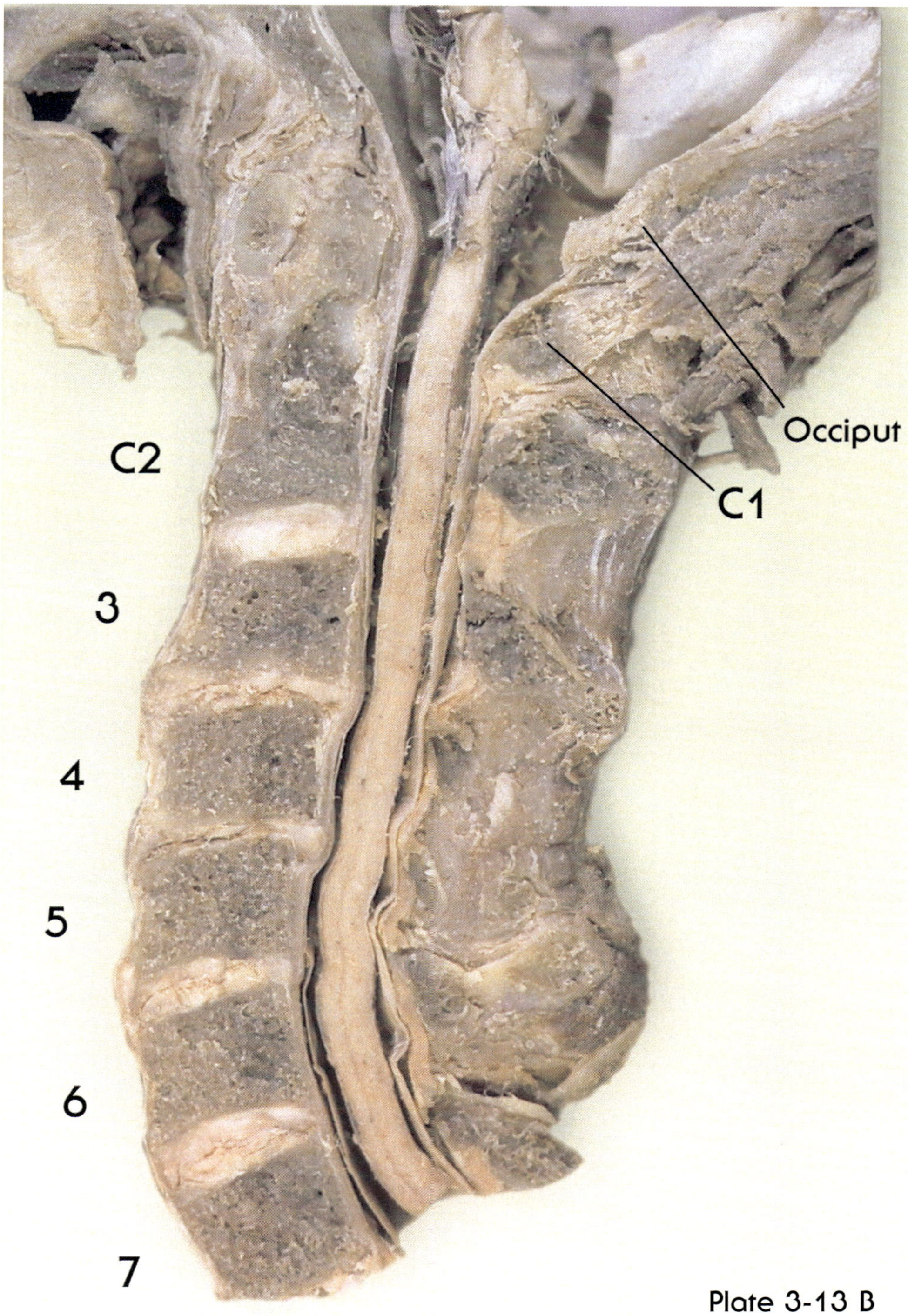

Plate 3-13 B

Gapping at the facets indicates that weight bearing has been transferred to the vertebral bodies in the mid cervical spine. The occiput appears to be posterior to C1. C2 is anterior to C3 and C3 is retro C4. Bulging and tearing of the C3-C4 disc have occurred. C5 is retro to C6, with a slight loss of disc height. A posterior disc bulge is visible at C5-C6 with cord contact. C6 and C7 are nearly aligned with normal canal shape and size. The subluxated vertebrae certainly have interfered with the central nervous system.

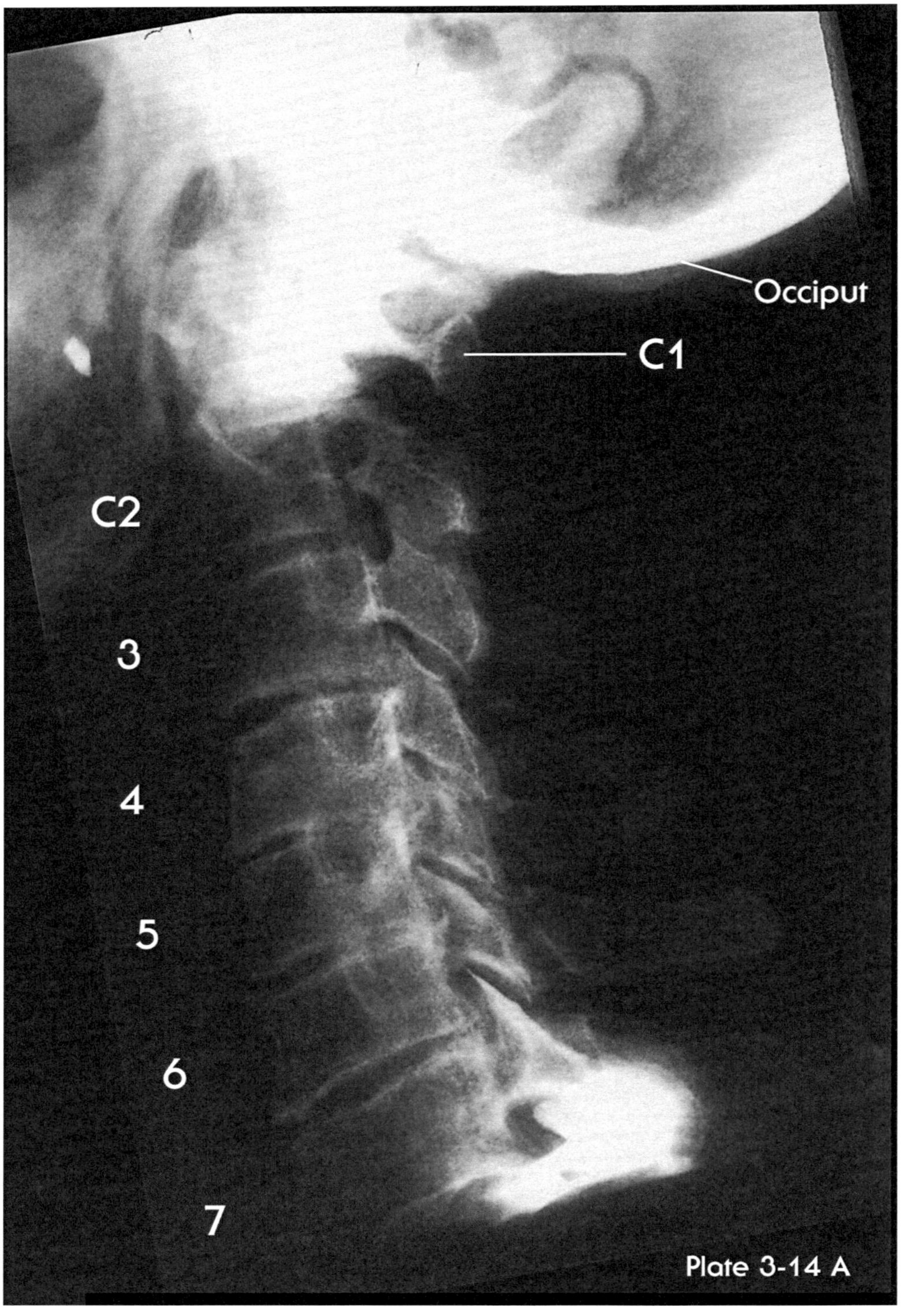

Plates 3-14 A & B

SUBLUXATIONS WITH REVERSED OR KYPHOTIC CURVE

Upper cervical subluxation

This individual suffered degeneration in all of his cervical discs due to subluxation of every segment. C1 superior on the dens and anterior to the posterior rim of the foramen magnum and the C2 spinous process contacting the dorsal surface of the spinal cord (see Plate B). C3 is a complete retrolisthesis with a reversal of the lordotic curve at this level..

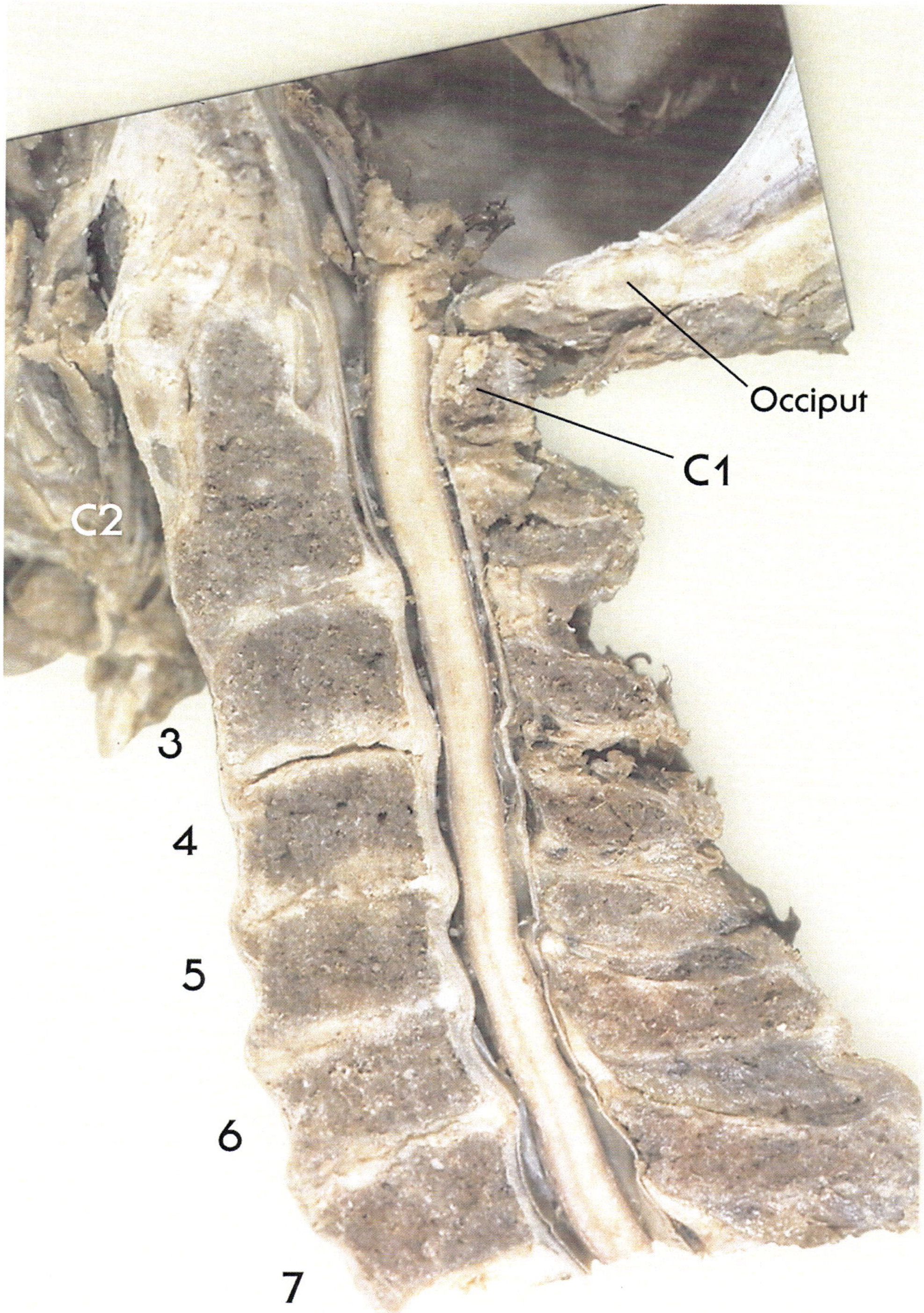

Plate 3-14 B

The degree of posterior bulging and spurring from the subluxations has resulted in acquired stenosis. The spinal cord is tractioned against the anterior wall of the vertebral canal, with contact on the cord. C3 is a complete retro to C2 and C4 with reduced disc height, tearing and posterior bulging, and with a cavitated disc at C3-C4. C4 is retro to C5 with spurring and partial fusion at C4-C5. C6 is retro to C5, and has partially fused with it posteriorly. C7 is retro to C6; the disc has collapsed, but fusion has not yet occurred. All of the discs are bulging posteriorly, and anterior bulging occurs from C3-C4 through C6-C7.

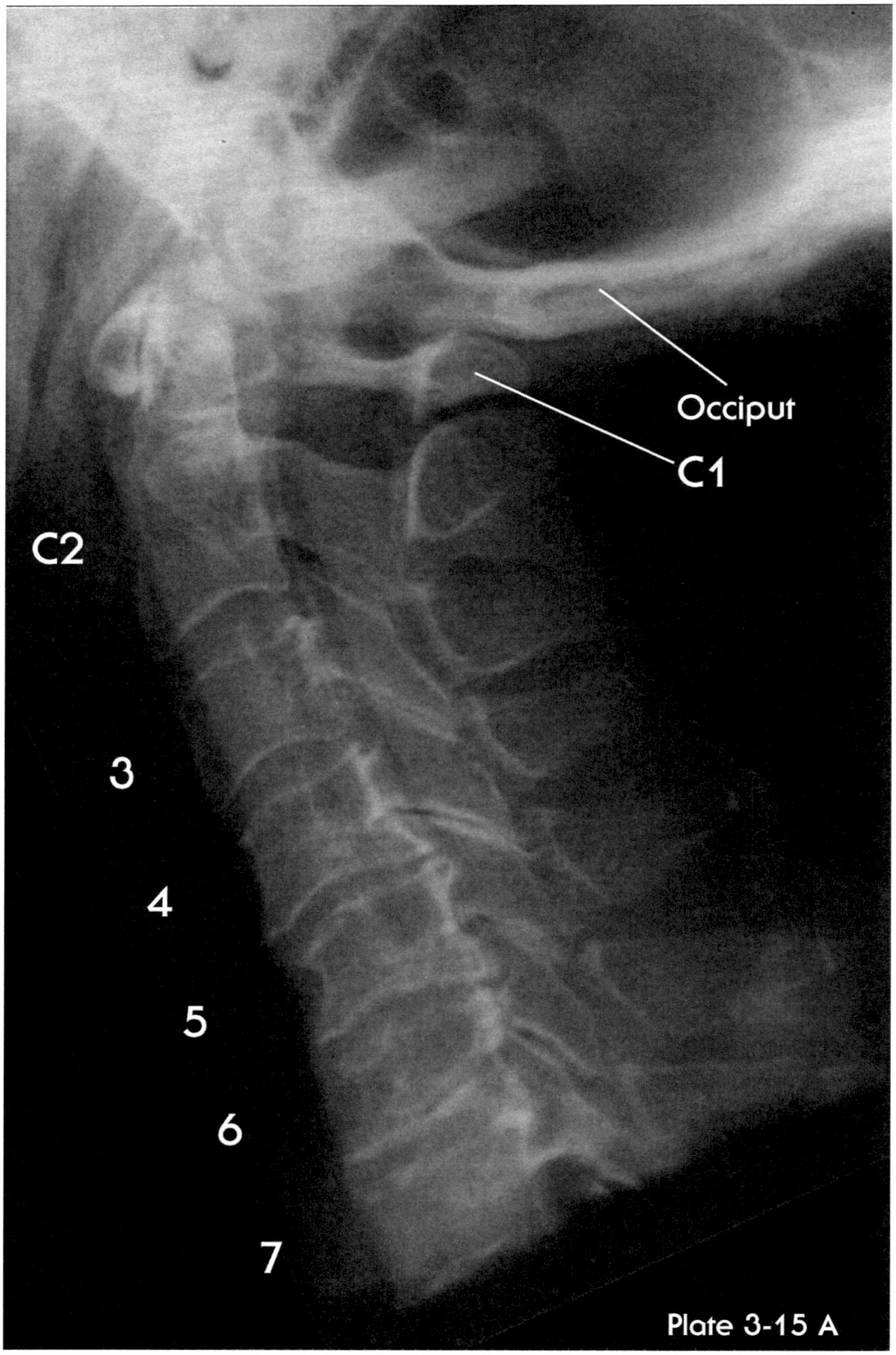

Plates 3-15 A & B
SUBLUXATIONS WITH REVERSED OR KYPHOTIC CURVE
Mid-cervical subluxations

Shown here is an interesting occiput C1/C2 relationship. The occiput is posterior to C1 and the posterior arch has become weight bearing. C2-C3 look good, with a good disc. C4 is retro to C3 with disc narrowing posterior and just a hint of anterior brown degeneration with significant endplate changes. C5 retro to C4 with disc tearing, necrosis, and moderately significant posterior spurring with cord impingement.

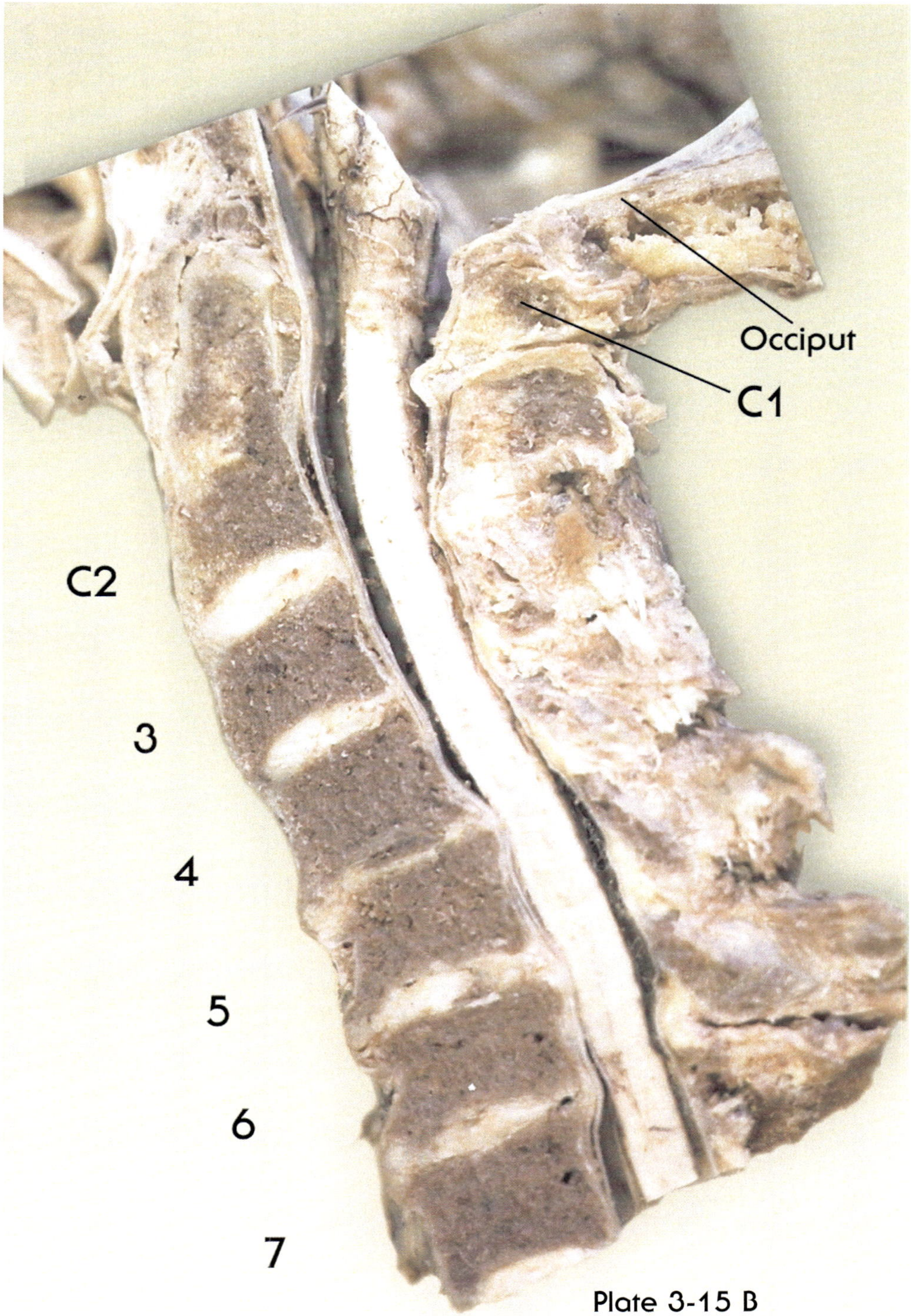

Plate 3-15 B

Note increased endplate thickness on the X-ray at C4-C5, which gives the appearance of a bulging disc in the specimen. C6 is a complete retrolisthesis to C5 and C7. Spinal cord contact and compromise from subluxation, posterior spurring and significant DJD with disc bulging of C5 & C6; C6-C7 looks significantly degenerated with minor bulge but near fusions - not seen on X-Ray.

Note facet jamming C3 to C6. Loss of disc height causes facet sclerosis and shortening of the canal.

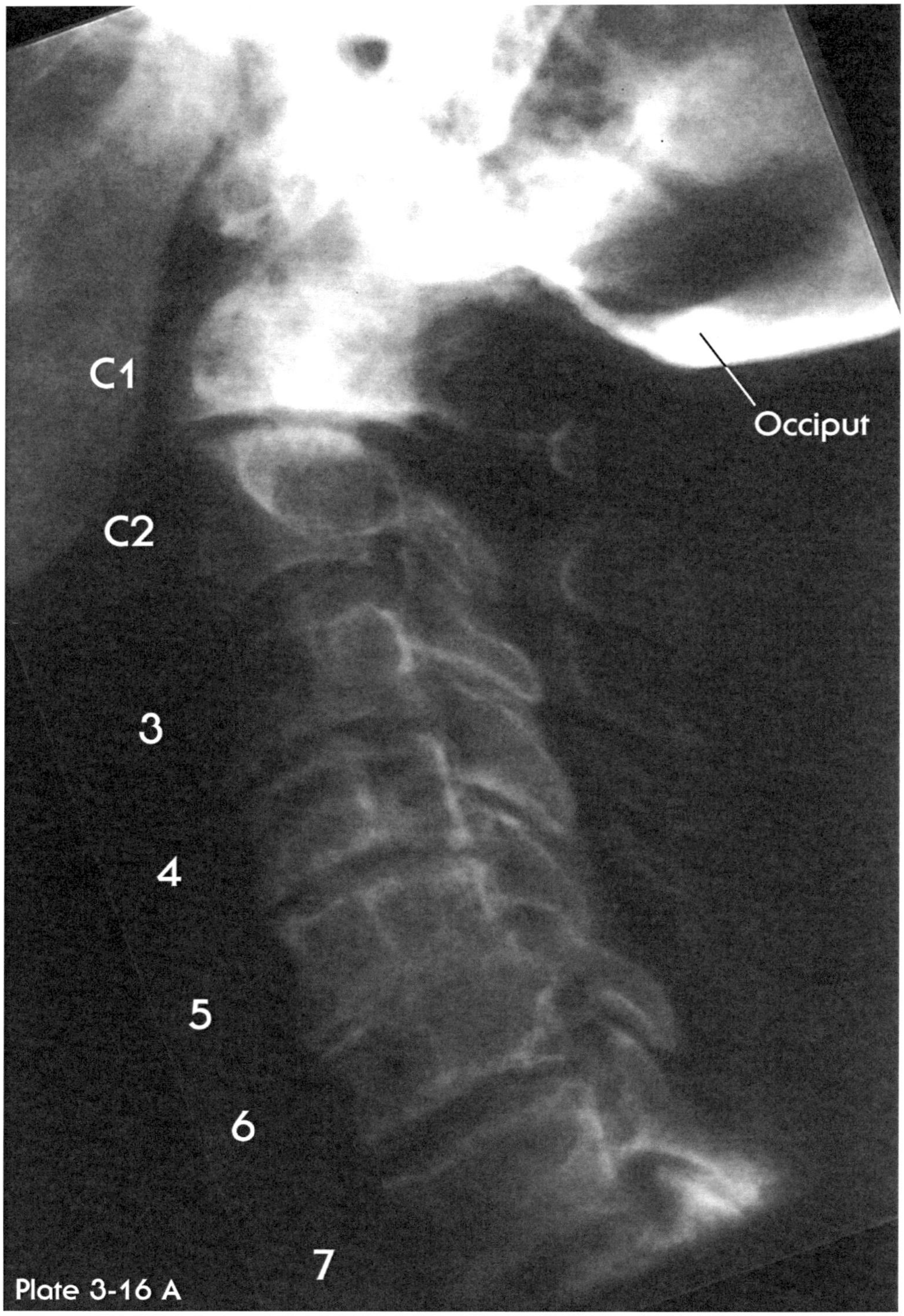

Plate 3-16 A

Plates 3-16 A & B

SUBLUXATIONS WITH REVERSED OR KYPHOTIC CURVE

Mid-cervical subluxations

The occiput is posterior to C1; C2 & C3 look aligned but facets show altered weight bearing; C4 retro to C3 and C5 retro to C4 with disc tearing of C3-C4 and C4-C5 with posterior spurs and loss of disc height; fusion of C5 and C6; C5 is anterior to C6 and C7

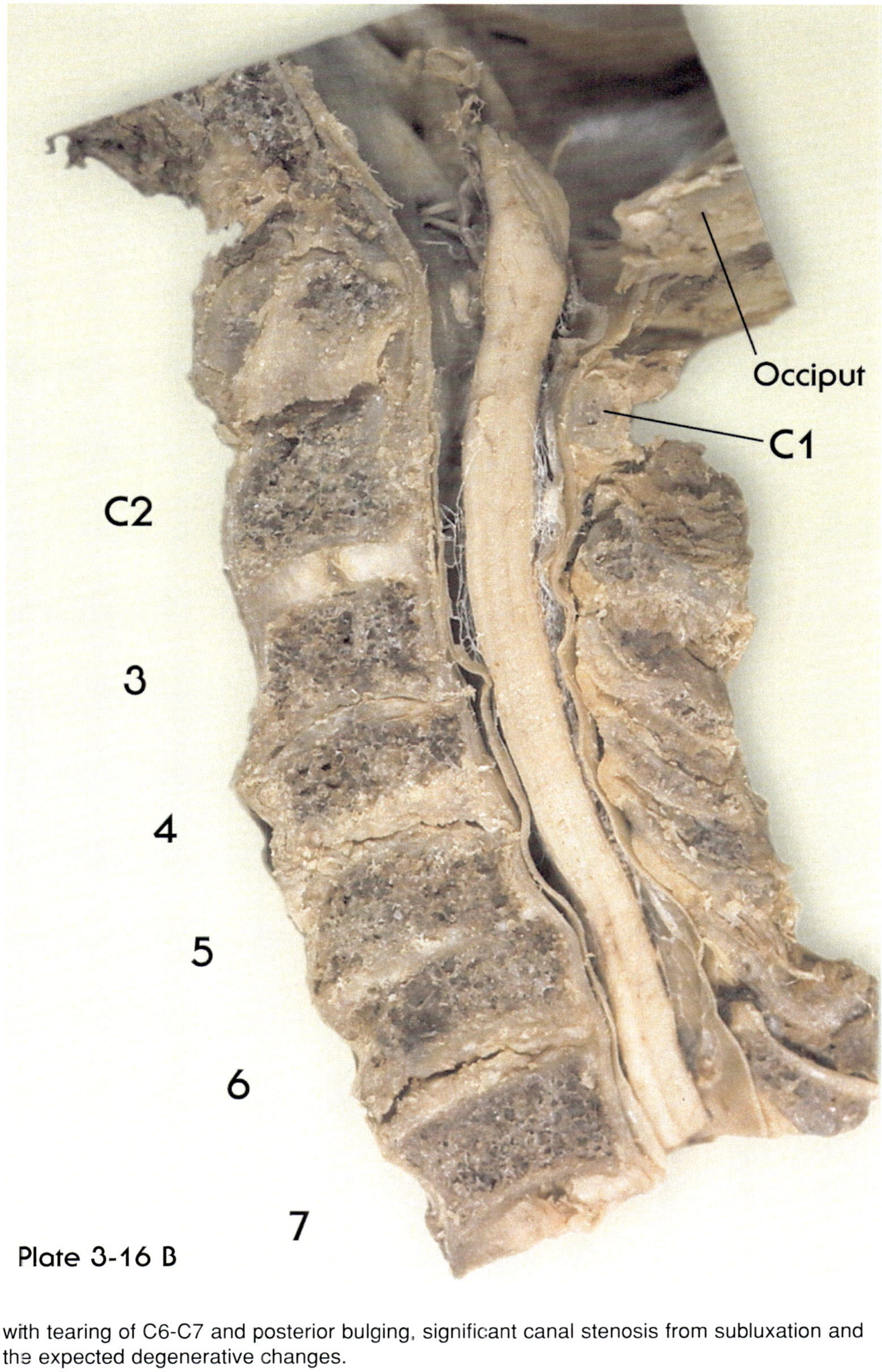

Plate 3-16 B

with tearing of C6-C7 and posterior bulging, significant canal stenosis from subluxation and the expected degenerative changes.
Note: vertebral body diameter of C4-C5 & C6 compare to C2 and C7; significant cord compression and canal stenosis at C6 and C7.

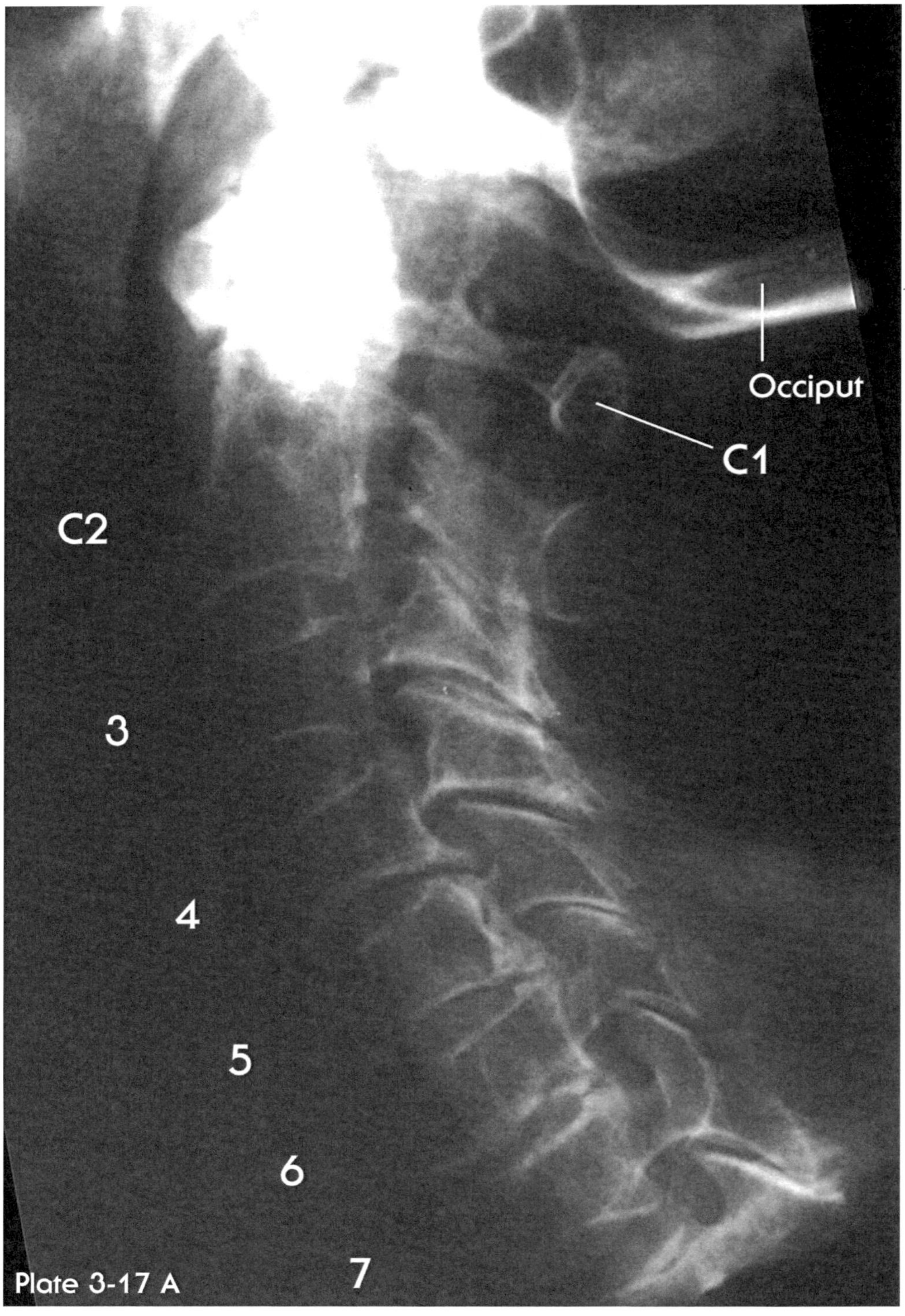

Plates 3-17 A & B
SUBLUXATIONS WITH REVERSED OR KYPHOTIC CURVE
Lower cervical subluxations

In this specimen there is a reversal of the curve at C6 but the lordotic curve in the upper cervical area is maintained and well-hydrated discs have persisted. Hypertrophy of the facets in this region indicates that they suffered altered weight-bearing function.

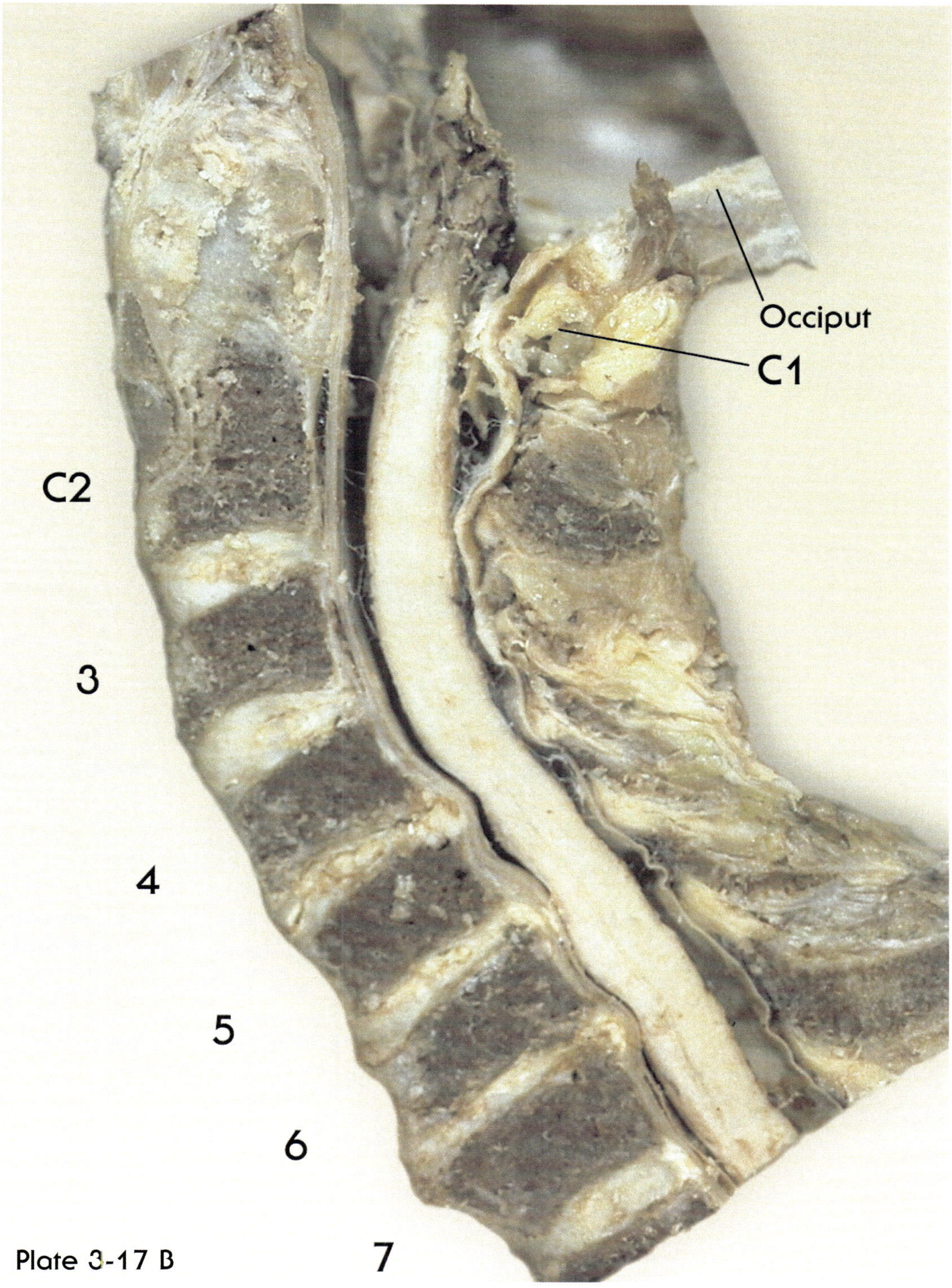

Plate 3-17 B

The occiput is posterior to C1 and C2, C3 is anterior to C4, C4 is anterior to C5, C5 is retro to C6 and C6 shows a retrolisthesis to C7. Bulging, spurring, loss of disc height and disc tearing have begun to develop at C4-C5 and C5-C6. Note canal stenosis and spinal cord impingement beginning at C4-C5. C6-C7 shows significant loss of disc height with bulging and spurring anteriorly and posteriorly. The whole disc appears to have collapsed (there is no visible line of shear). Note impingement on the spinal cord, which is tethered against the anterior surface of the vertebral canal at this level.

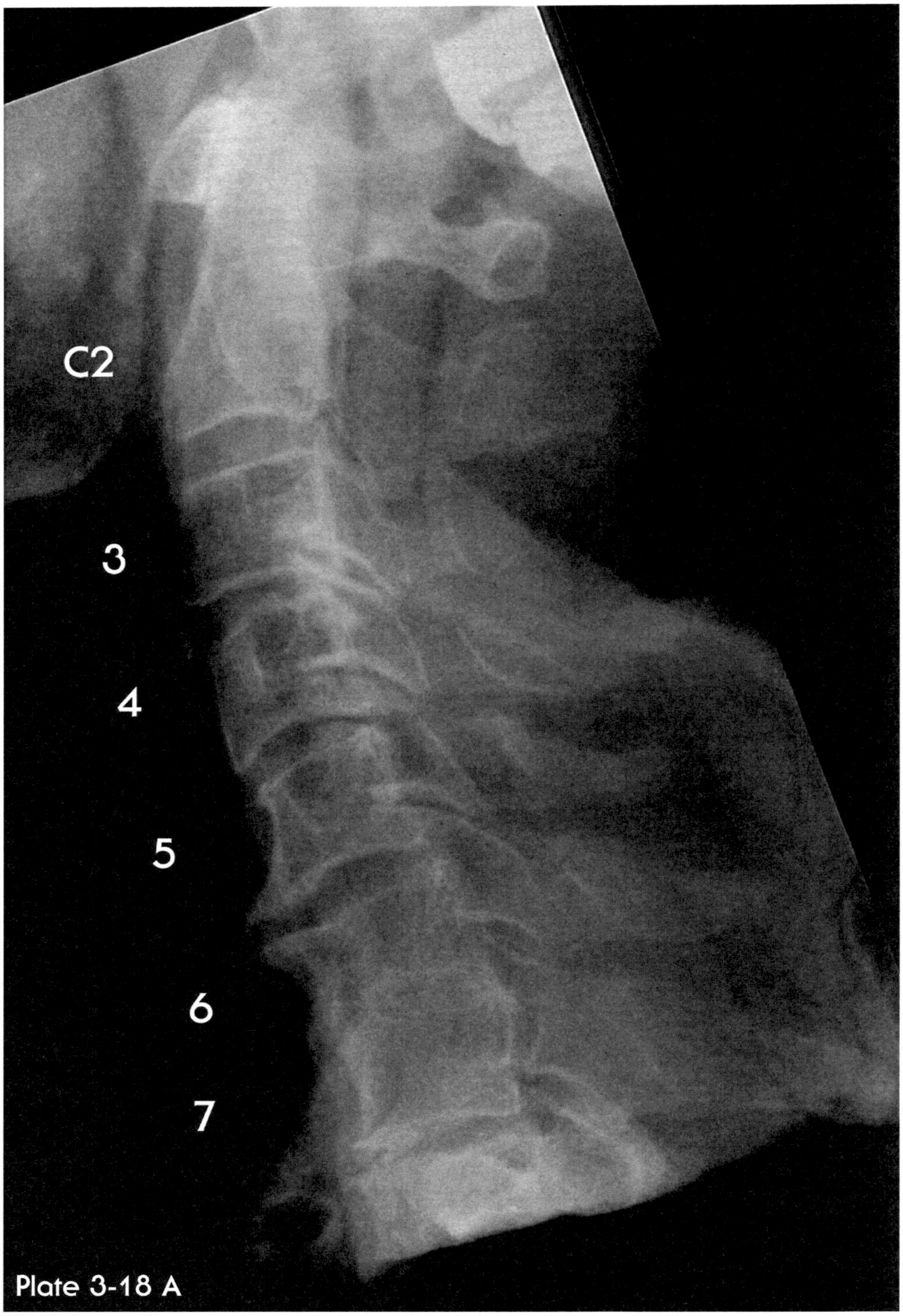

Plates 3-18 A & B
SUBLUXATION WITH REVERSED OR KYPHOTIC CURVE
Lower cervical subluxations

This specimen has a reversal of the lordotic curve at C6-C7 with significant cord compromise from C3-C7. The space behind cord at C5-C6 and compression of cord into anterior canal wall C5-C7 are due to tractioning. Moderate congenital stenosis. Note C2 and C7 canal size, these levels are near normal, while there is reduced canal diameter from C3-C6.

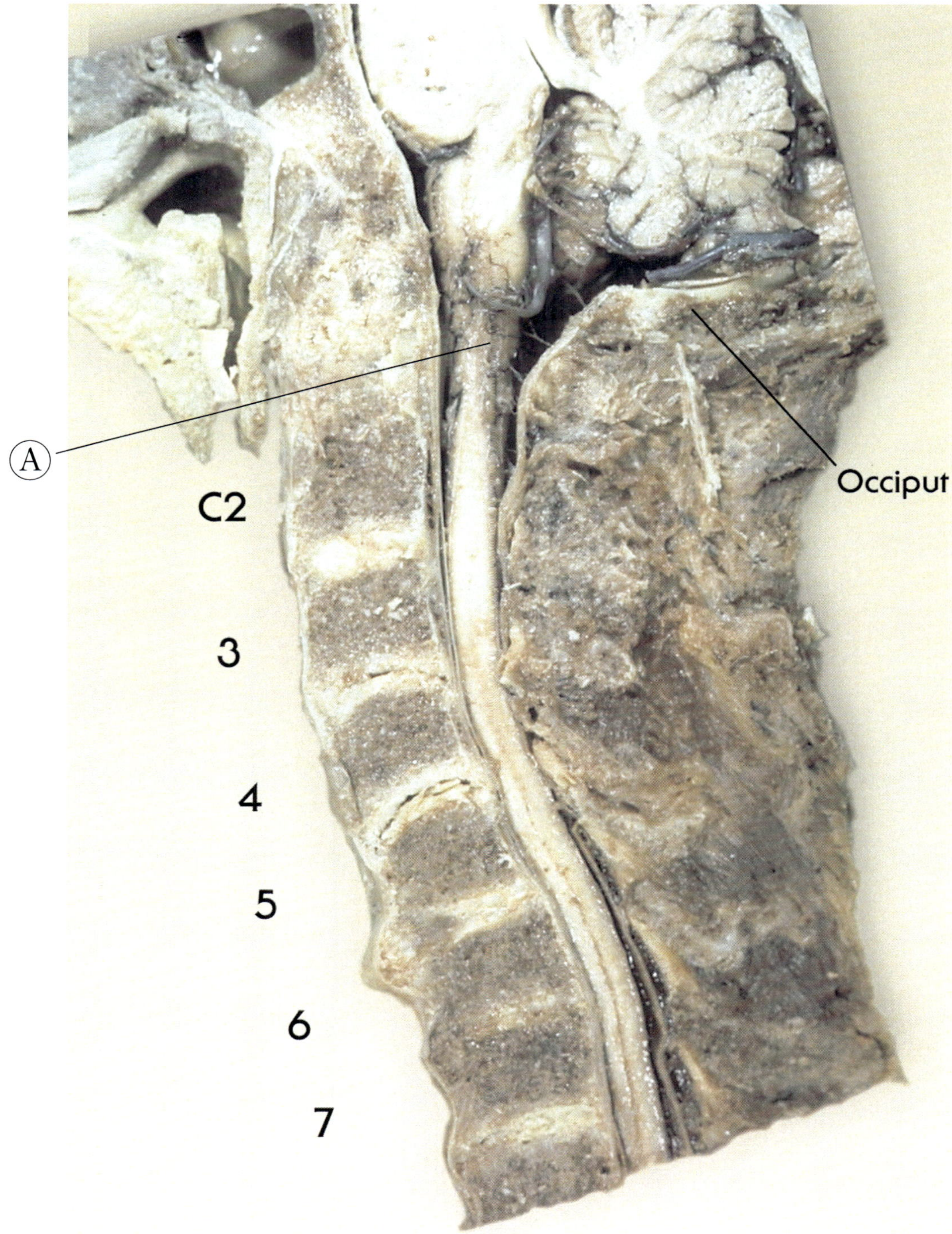

Plate 3-18 B

C2 is aligned with C3 with a healthy disc; C3 is stepped behind C4 - or C4 is anterior to C3 with disc tearing and bulging of C3-C4; C4 is retro to C5 with tearing and bulging; endplate changes are moderate; C5 is anterior to C6 (and C4); C5 has become a complete anterolisthesis; C6 is retro to C5 with significant endplate changes; note the necrotic (brown) tissue in C5C-6 disc, also the disc material all the way out between "spurs" of C5 and C6. C6-C7 fused with C7 retro to C6

Note reduced pontine flexure and the brainstem is well below occiput.

(A) Brainstem

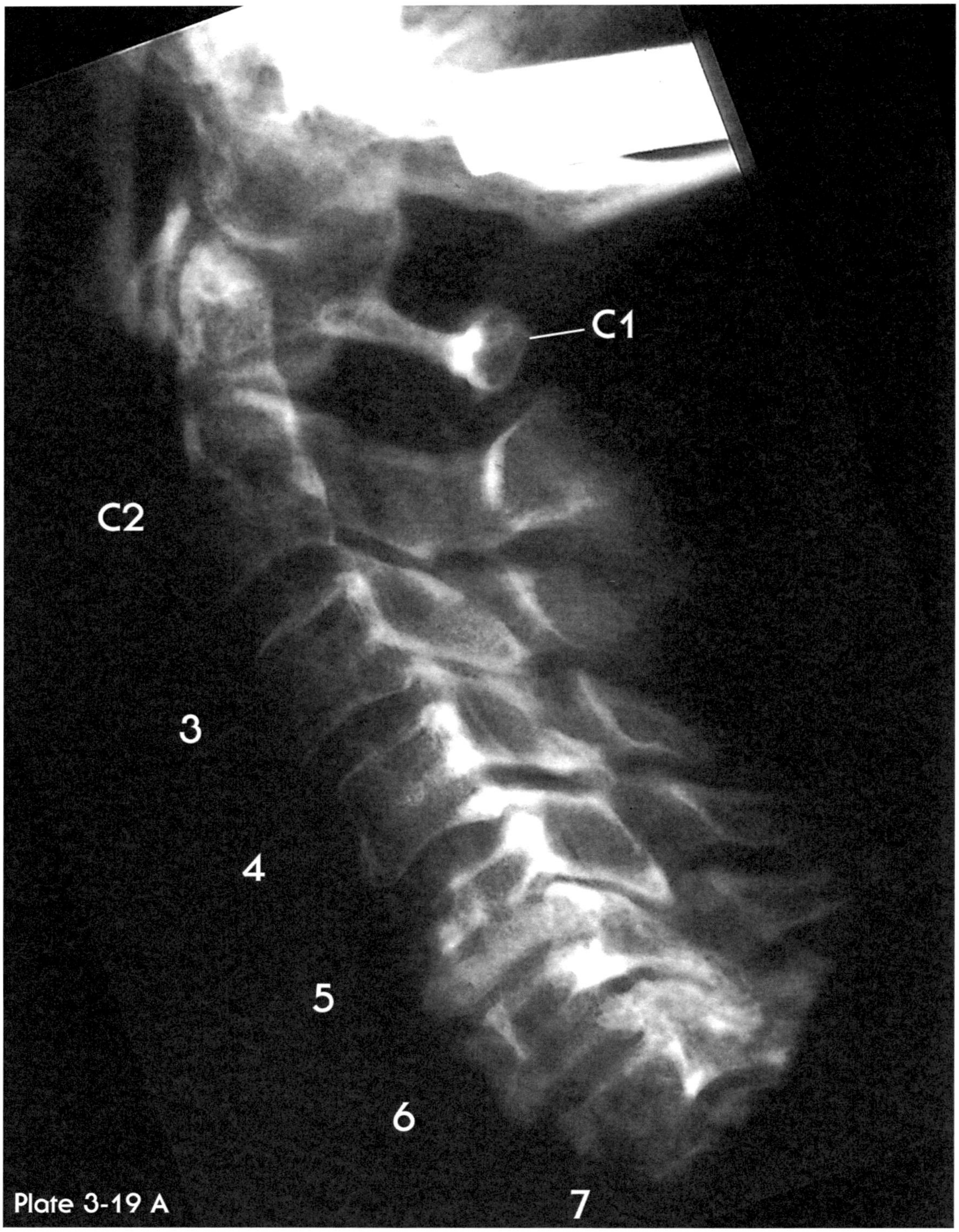

Plates 3-19 A & B

SUBLUXATIONS WITH REVERSED OR KYPHOTIC CURVE

Lower cervical subluxations

In this individual the C2-C3 disc is normal, but C4 is retro to C3 with a visible line of shear in the disc. C5 shows complete retrolisthesis (i.e. is retro both to C4 and C6), with a shear line and posterior spurring at the C4-C5 disc and complete fusion at C5-C6. C7 is retro to C6 with pronounced loss of disc height, disc shearing and posterior spurring.

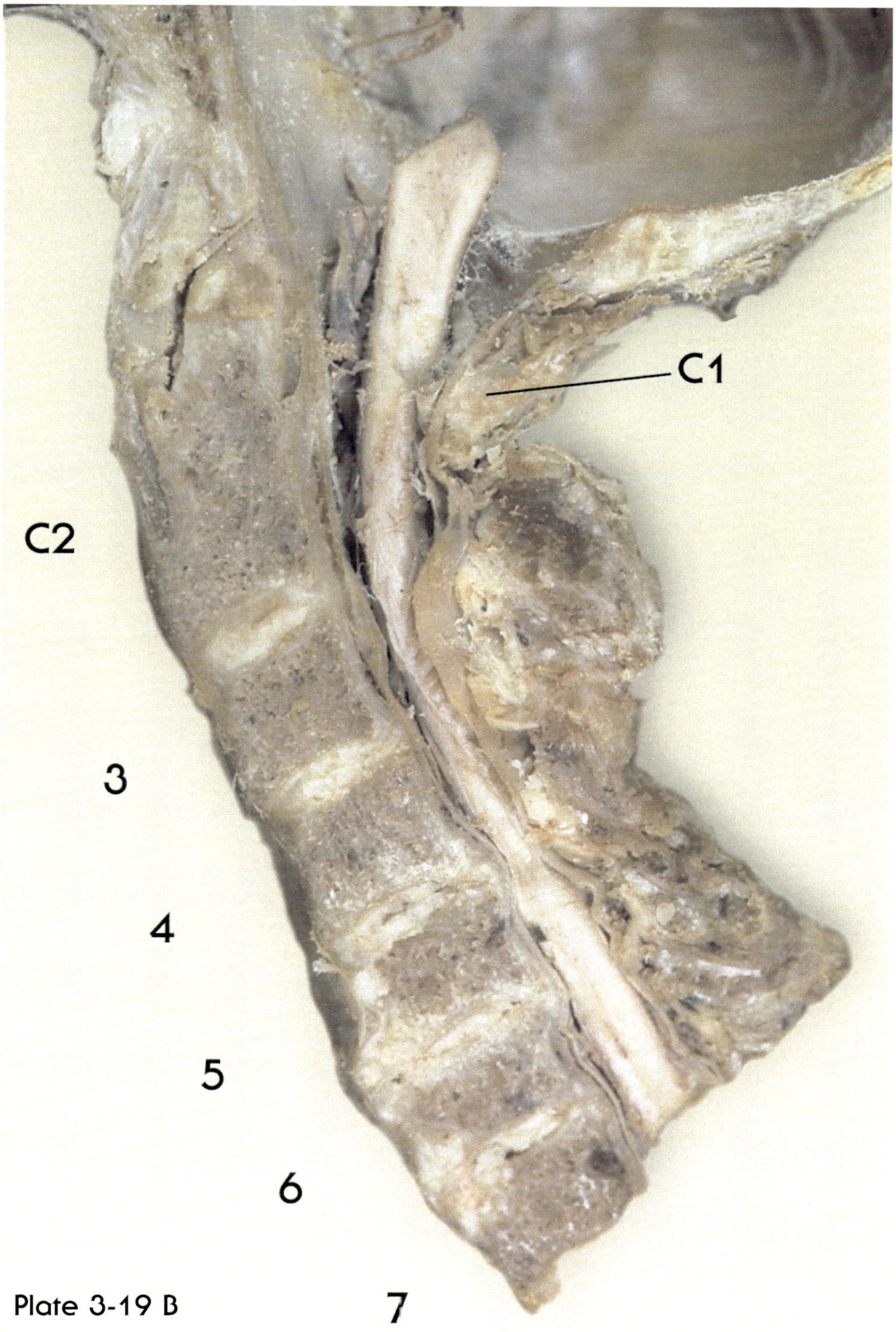

Plate 3-19 B

At the level of C2, the spinal cord rests in a spacious vertebral canal; however, at C4 through C7 the broadened endplates of the vertebral bodies have resulted in canal stenosis (narrowing) to the point where the spinal cord is actually compressed with clinical significance for the individual.

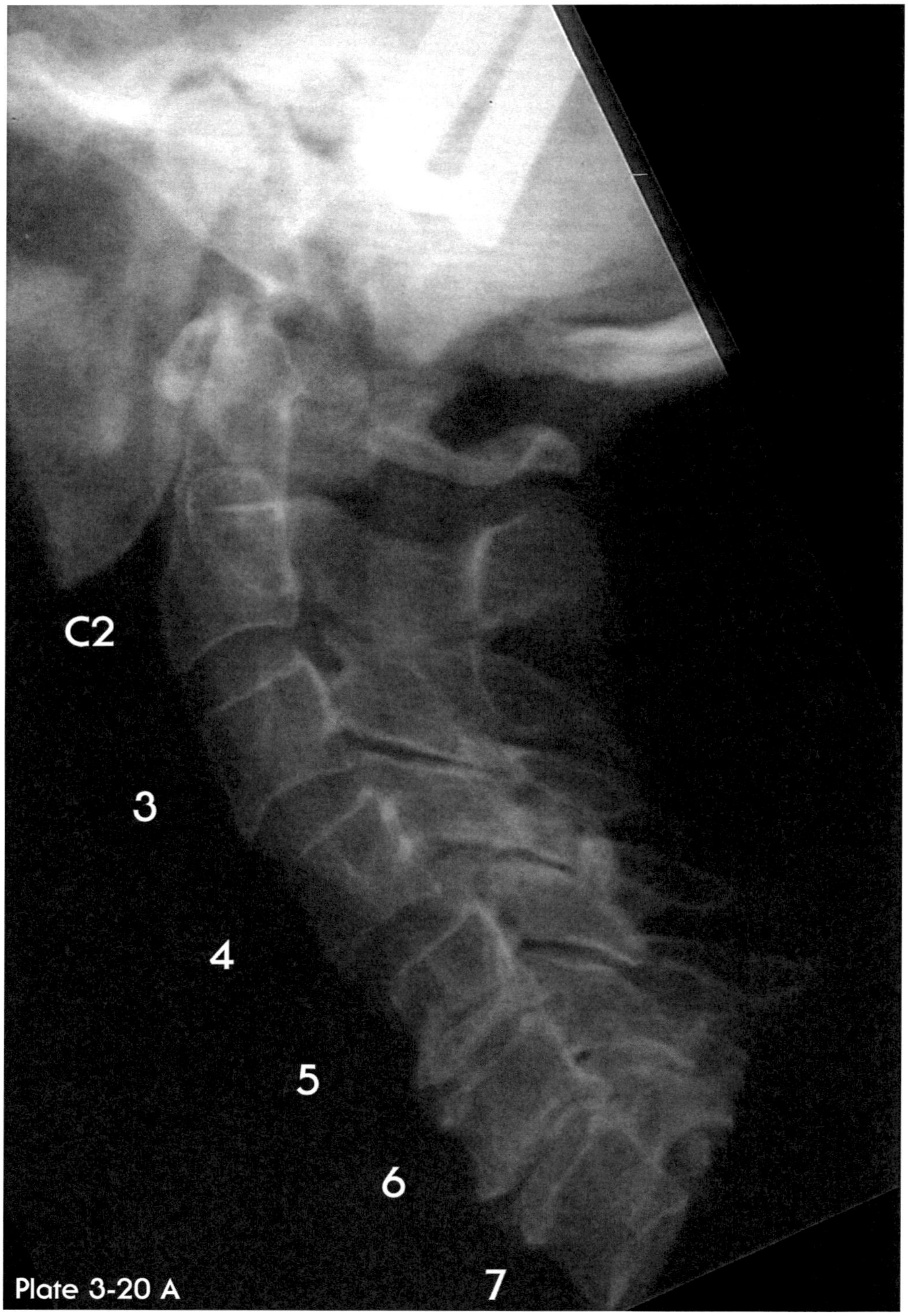

Plates 3-20 A & B

SUBLUXATIONS WITH REVERSED OR KYPHOTIC CURVE

Lower cervical subluxations

This person evidently sustained an injury which severely affected her lower cervical spine decades before her death, and a second, lesser trauma which altered her upper cervical spine shortly before her death. Note the almost normal lordotic curve from C1 through C4, with a dramatic straightening and reversal of the at the C5-C7 level. C3 shows a complete anterolisthesis (C2 and C4), and C4 is anterior to C5. However, the C2-C3 and C3-C4 discs

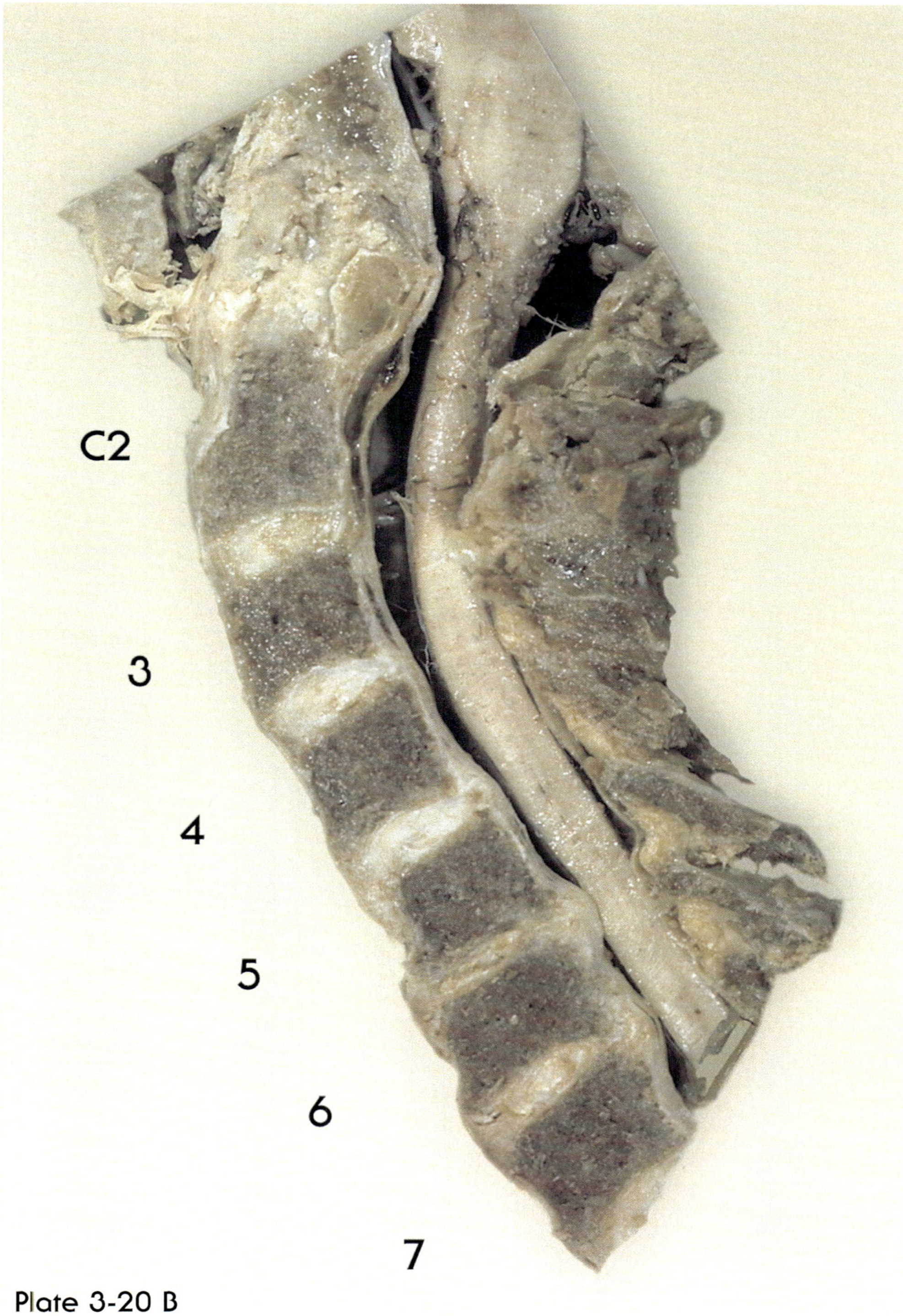

Plate 3-20 B

show only minimal degeneration. Despite slight disc bulging, the vertebral bodies have not yet begun to change shape. In the lower spine, C5 is completely retro (to C4 and C6) and C6 is completely antero (to C5 and C7). The C5-C6 disc has significant degeneration, showing dramatic loss of height, anterior and posterior bulging, and alteration of the shape of the vertebral bodies to accommodate altered weight bearing. The C6-C7 disc has sheared and bulged posteriorly, and has lost height posteriorly. The posterior bulge at C5-C6 is pressing into the spinal cord. The disc below it appears to be touching, but not yet deforming the cord.

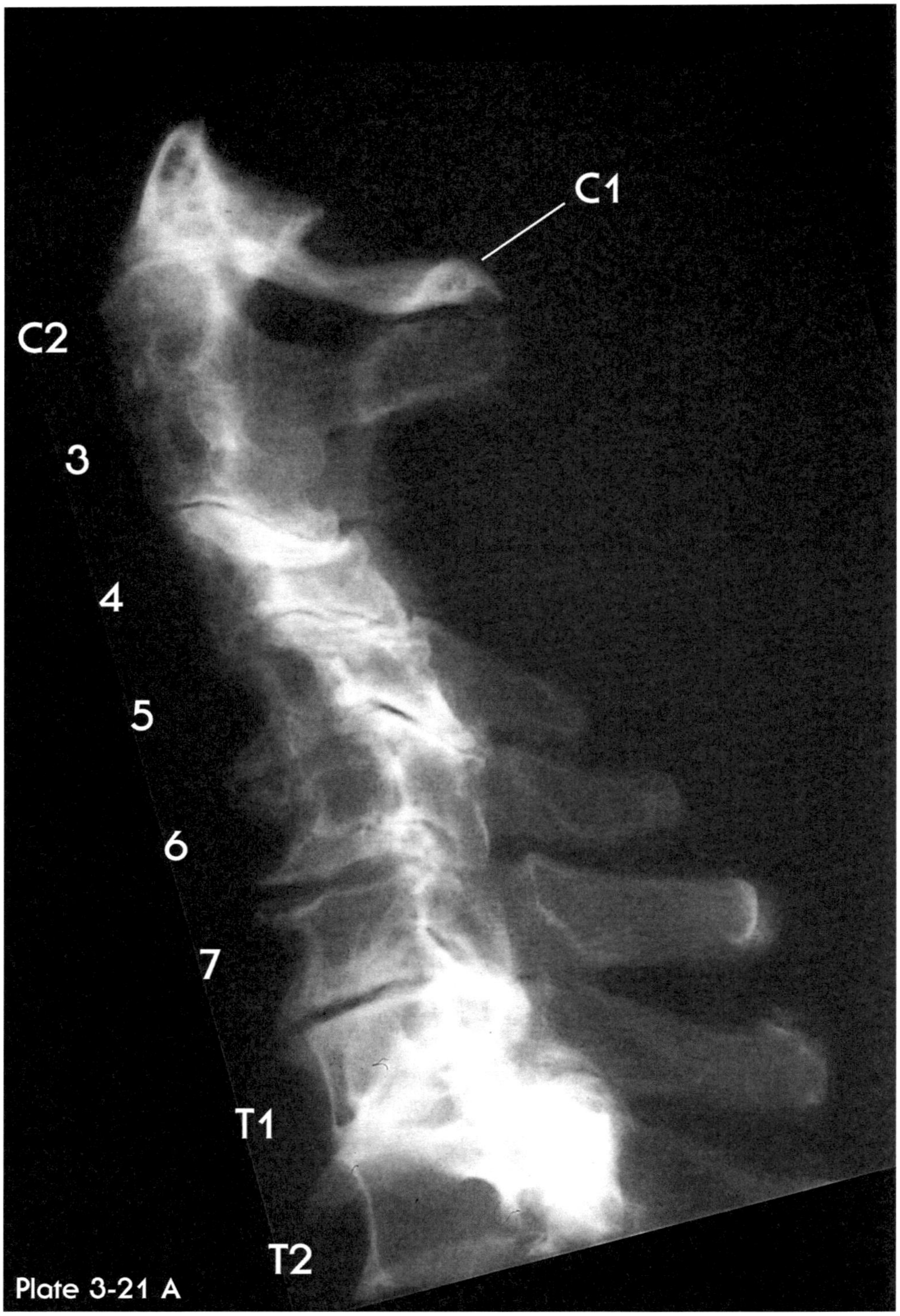

Plates 3-21 A & B

SUBLUXATIONS WITH REVERSED OR KYPHOTIC CURVE

Mid-cervical subluxations

In this specimen a reversal of the lordotic curve is present from C4 through C7. Canal stenosis has occurred, but the individual originally possessed a large vertebral canal as seen at the C2 and T2 levels. However, the cord is tethered against the anterior surface of the canal starting at C4. This is an extreme example of the spinal cord deforming to the shape of the spinal canal.

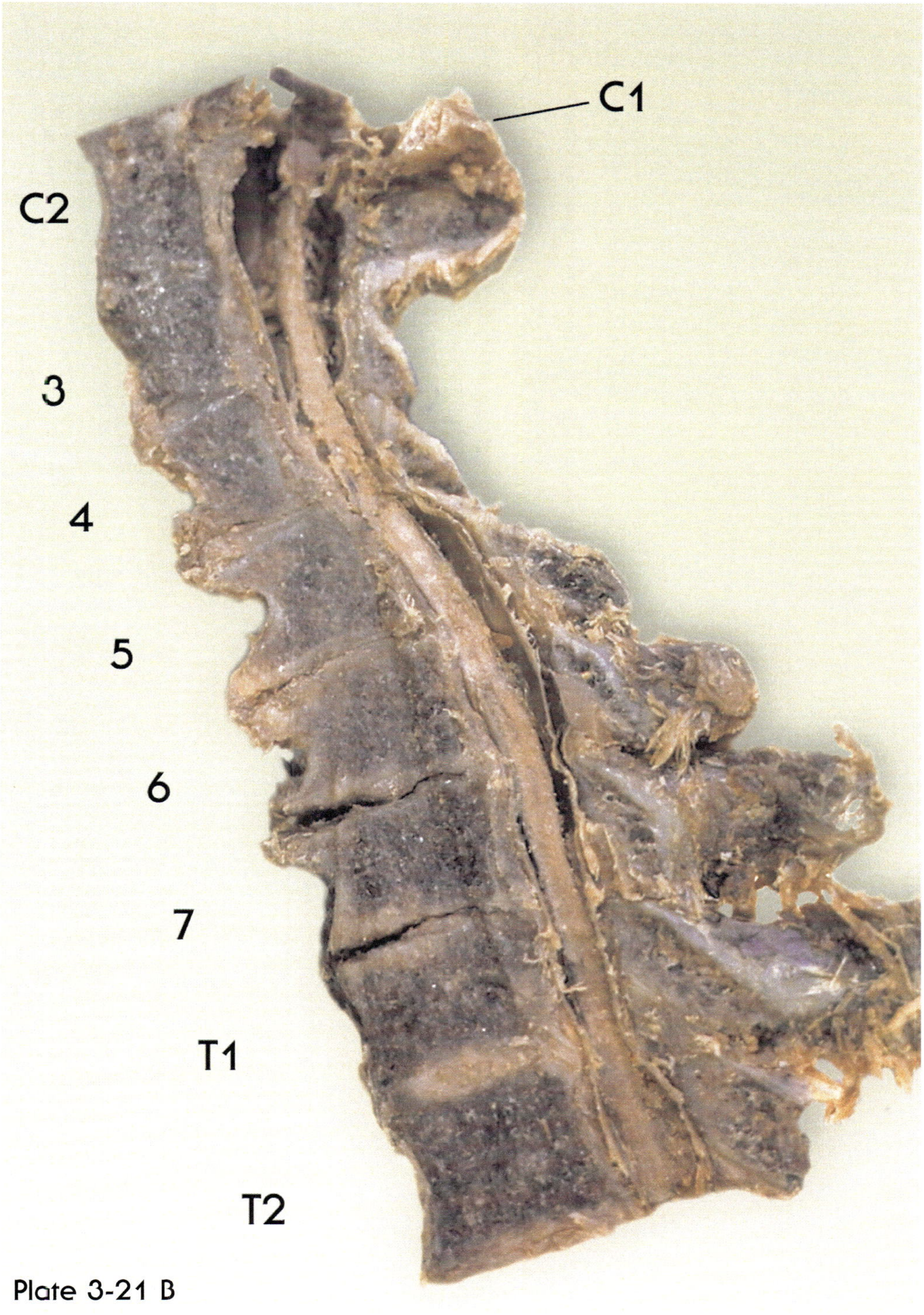

Plate 3-21 B

Note that a pseudo-joint has formed between the posterior arch of Atlas and the spinous process of C2. (The spinous processes of C3, C4 are missing because they were rotated out of the mid-saggital plane when the specimen was cut.) C3 is retro to C2, C4 is retro to C3. C5 is retro to C4, C6 is a complete retrolisthesis (to C5 and C7) and C7 is retro to T1. The C5-6, C6-7 and C7-T1 discs have completely degenerated, but the vertebrae have not yet fused. Anterior spurring is pronounced, but posterior spurring does not appear significant except at C6-7. Note that the T1-2 disc is not subluxated, and appears to be fully hydrated.

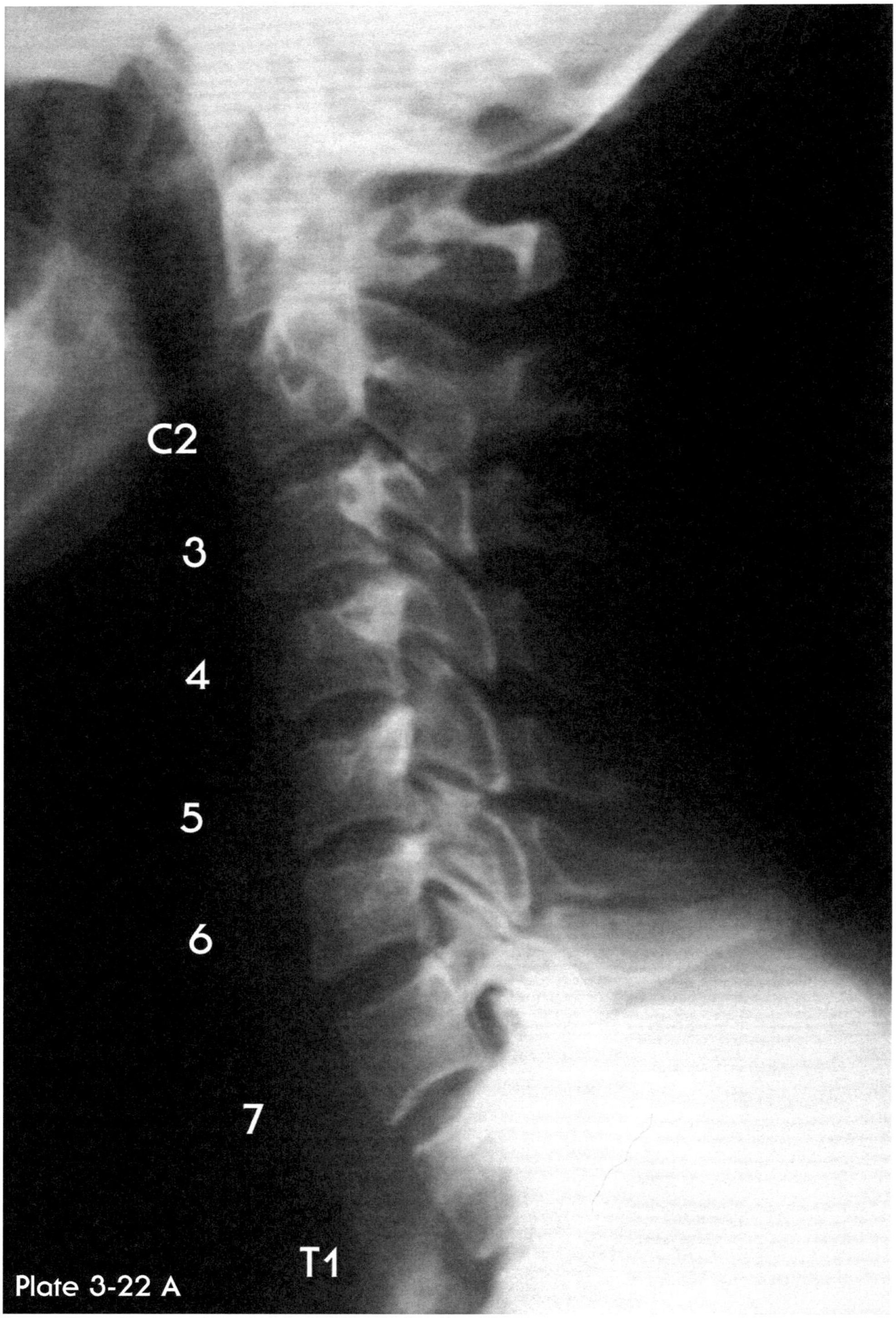

Plate 3-22 A

Plates 3-22 A & B

SUBLUXATION WITH REVERSED OR KYPHOTIC CURVE

An X-ray and MRI comparison.

This is a lateral cervical X-ray and mid-sagittal cervical MRI of the same person. This shows a reversed lordotic curve. There is a anterolisthesis of C2 to C3, C3 to C4 and C4 to C5, the latter pair form a posterior apex of the "kyphosis" or kyphotic curve.

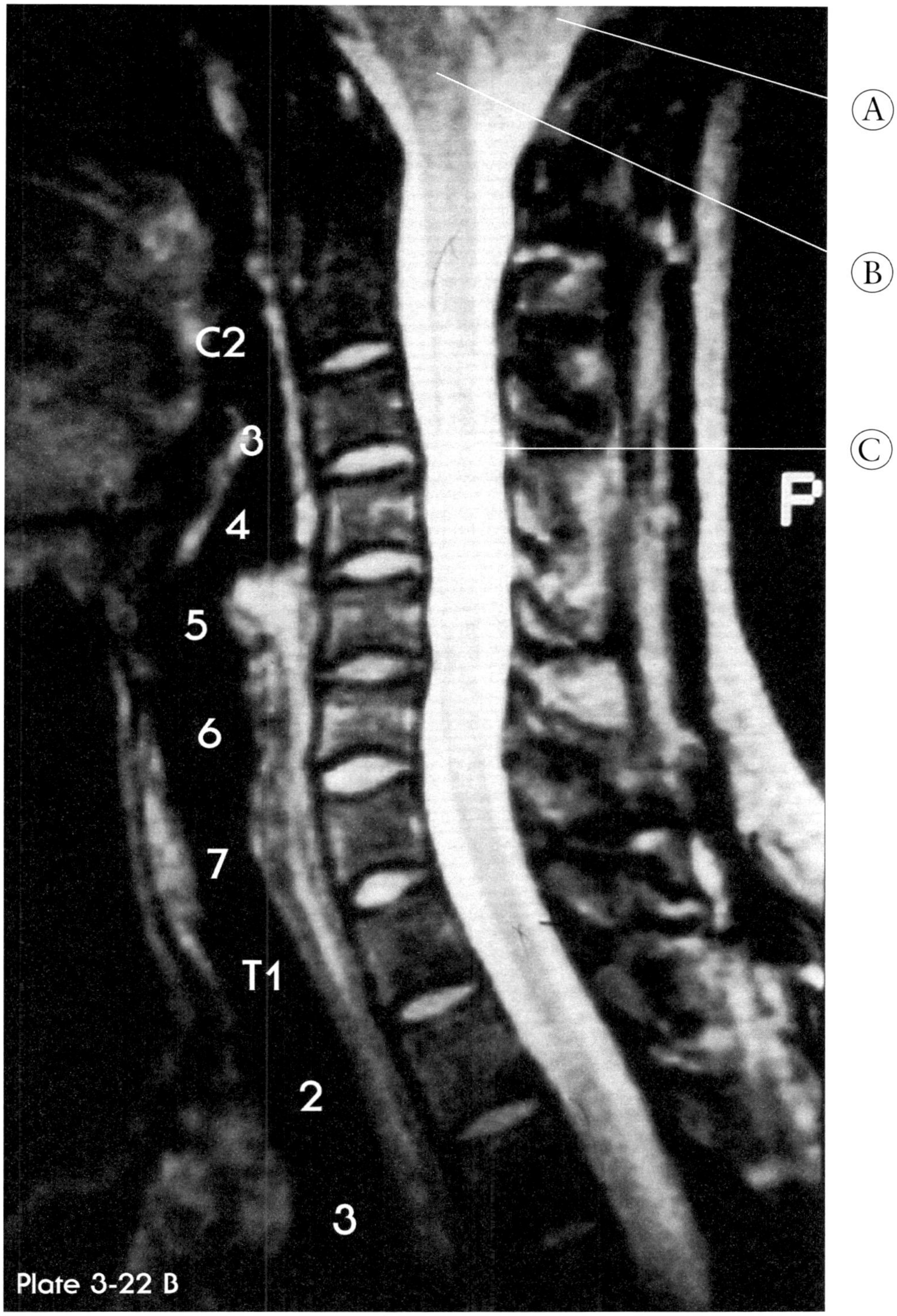

Note the brainstem and spinal cord have straightened and has close contact at the C5-C6 level and has direct contact at T3 and T4. The cerebellum has contact with the posterior inferior occiput in the neutral position. Cervical flexion and an increase in canal length will add to this deformity

(A) Cerebellum
(B) Brainstem
(C) Spinal cord.

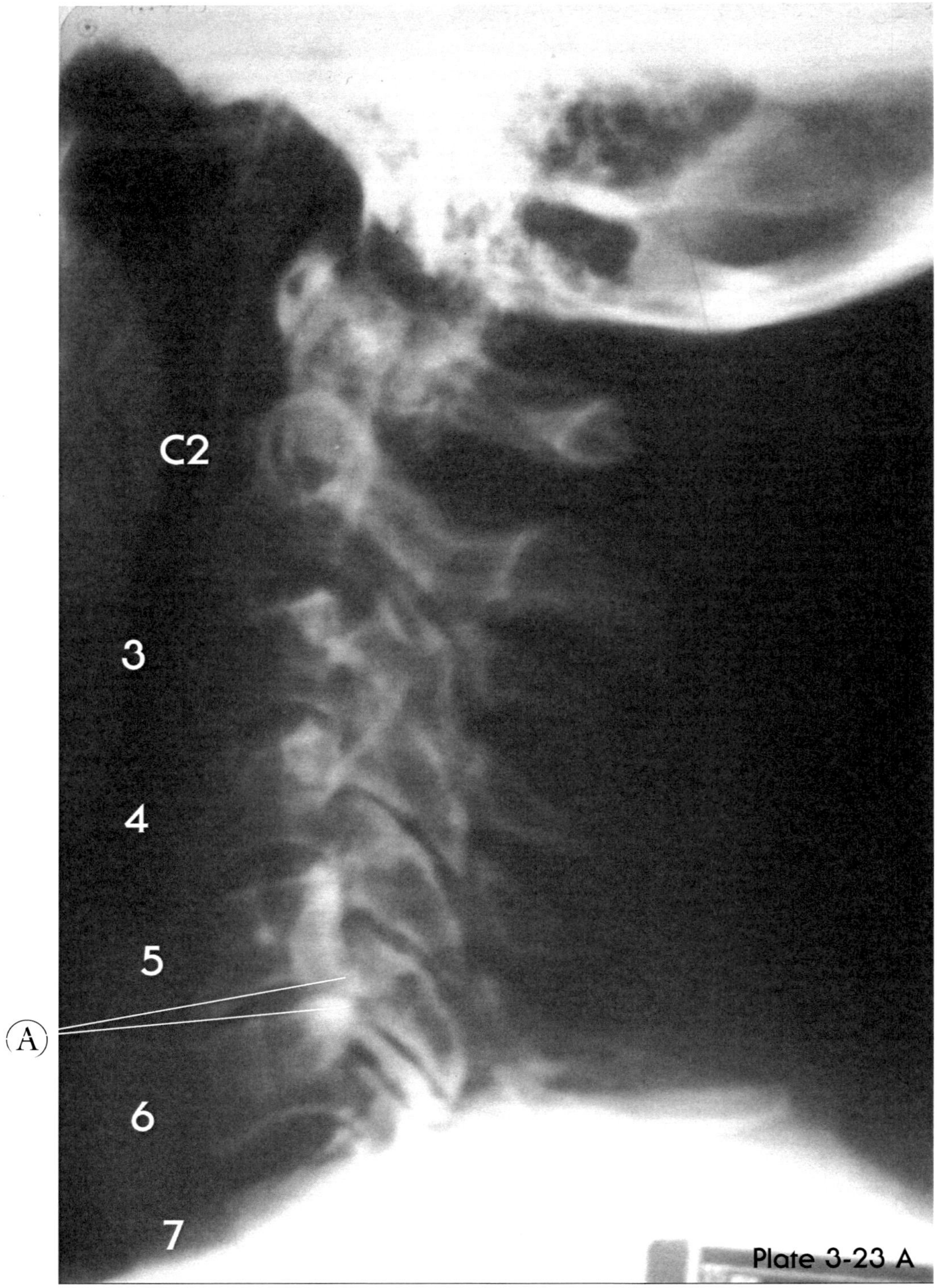

Plates 3-23 A & B
SUBLUXATION WITH REVERSED OR KYPHOTIC CURVE
An X-ray and MRI comparison.

This pair of images is the lateral cervical X-ray and MRI of the same person. The spinal cord is moved to the anterior portion of the canal. and has close contact with the C5-C6 osteophytes and disc. Ligamentum flavum at C6-C7 is bulging into the canal, partly from

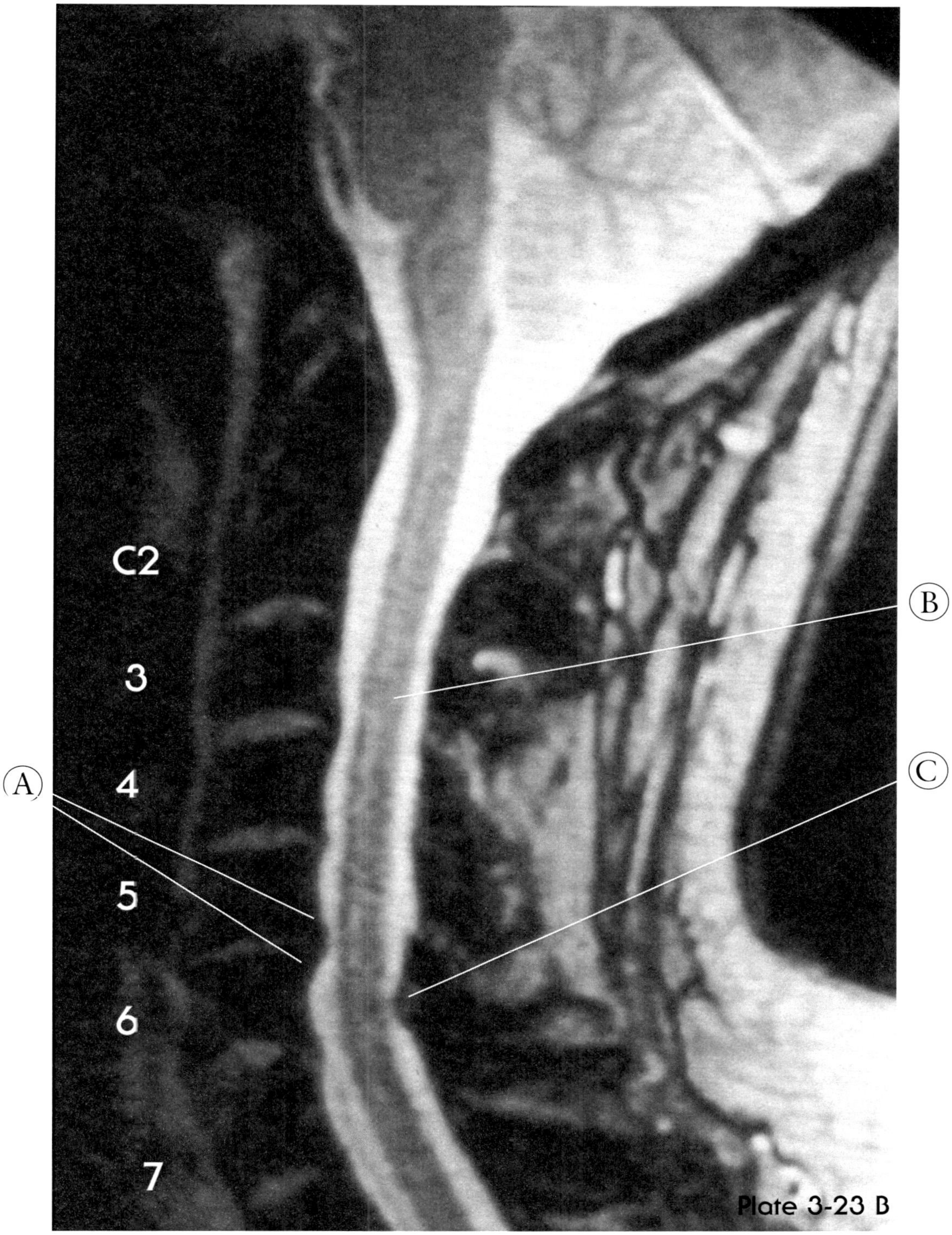

the loss of disc height and vertebral misalignment. The collective loss of disc height in the vertebral column can partly relieve cord tension by decreasing canal length.

(A) C5-C6 osteophytes
(B) Spinal cord
(C) Ligamentum flavum between C6 and C7.

CHAPTER FOUR

Subluxations Of The Thoracic Spine

Discussion

The way in which the ribs are attached in the thoracic region of the spine makes it significantly different from the cervical and lumbar regions. Each rib articulates with a transverse process to a set of demifacets on the same vertebra and to the adjacent superior vertebral body. The ribs between T2 and T10 also attach to the disc between demifacets, and have the appearance of three small joint complexes. These include two small synovial joints, and an intervening fibrous joint where it contacts the disc. In **Figure 4-1** the rib-disc articulation is seen at the T1-T2 disc. Subluxation can alter any or all of these articulations, just as it alters intervertebral discs and facets.

The combined effects of these complex rib articulations with the vertebrae and the extensive network of supporting ligaments and muscles, give the thoracic spine the quality of being a single functional unit. This is called the rib cage. The head, rib cage, and pelvis comprise the three masses of the axial skeleton. The connecting, and much more mobile, cervical and lumbar columns can buckle when these masses are displaced. The head can displace relative to the thoracic spine, and the thoracic spine can displace relative to the pelvis. Many different terms have been used to describe the events that generate common subluxation complexes. The primary subluxation complexes can occur in the thoracic spine itself as a result of various

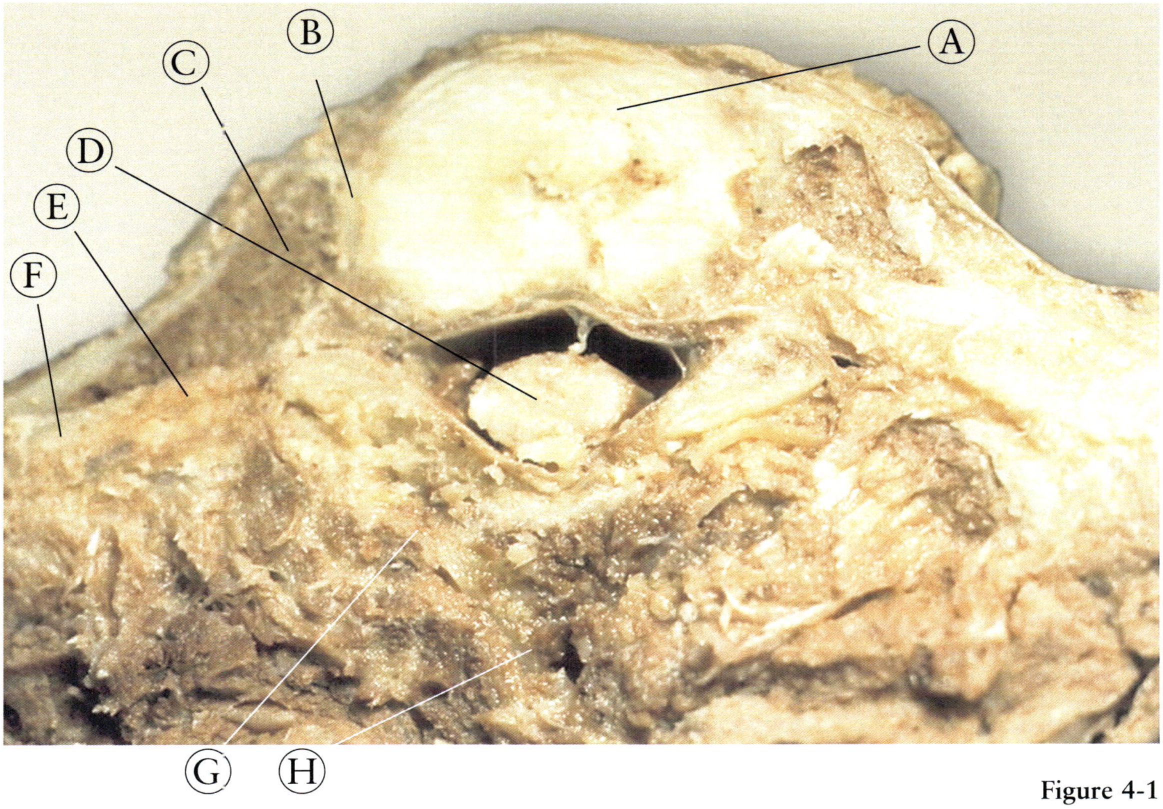

Figure 4-1

CROSS-SECTION OF THE VERTEBRAL COLUMN IN THE THORACIC REGION

This is an axial view of the second ribs articulating with the T1-2 disc. These are costo-vertebral joints.

(A) Disc
(B) Costo-vertebral joint
(C) Rib
(D) Spinal cord
(E) Costo-transverse joint
(F) Transverse process
(G) Lamina
(H) Spinous process

Illustration of thoracic spine with sympathetic chain, showing orientaton of Figure 4-2 and Figure 4-3.

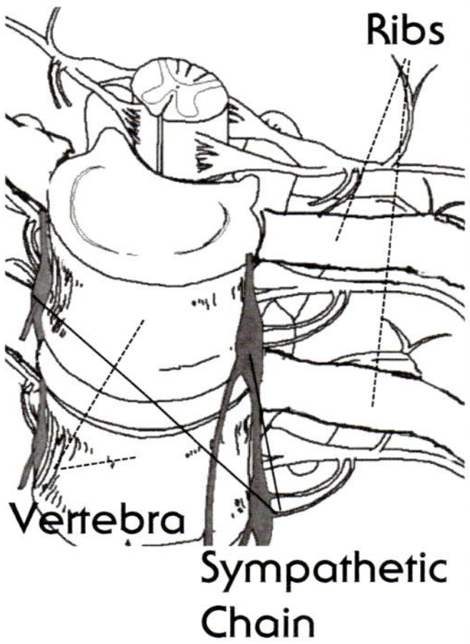

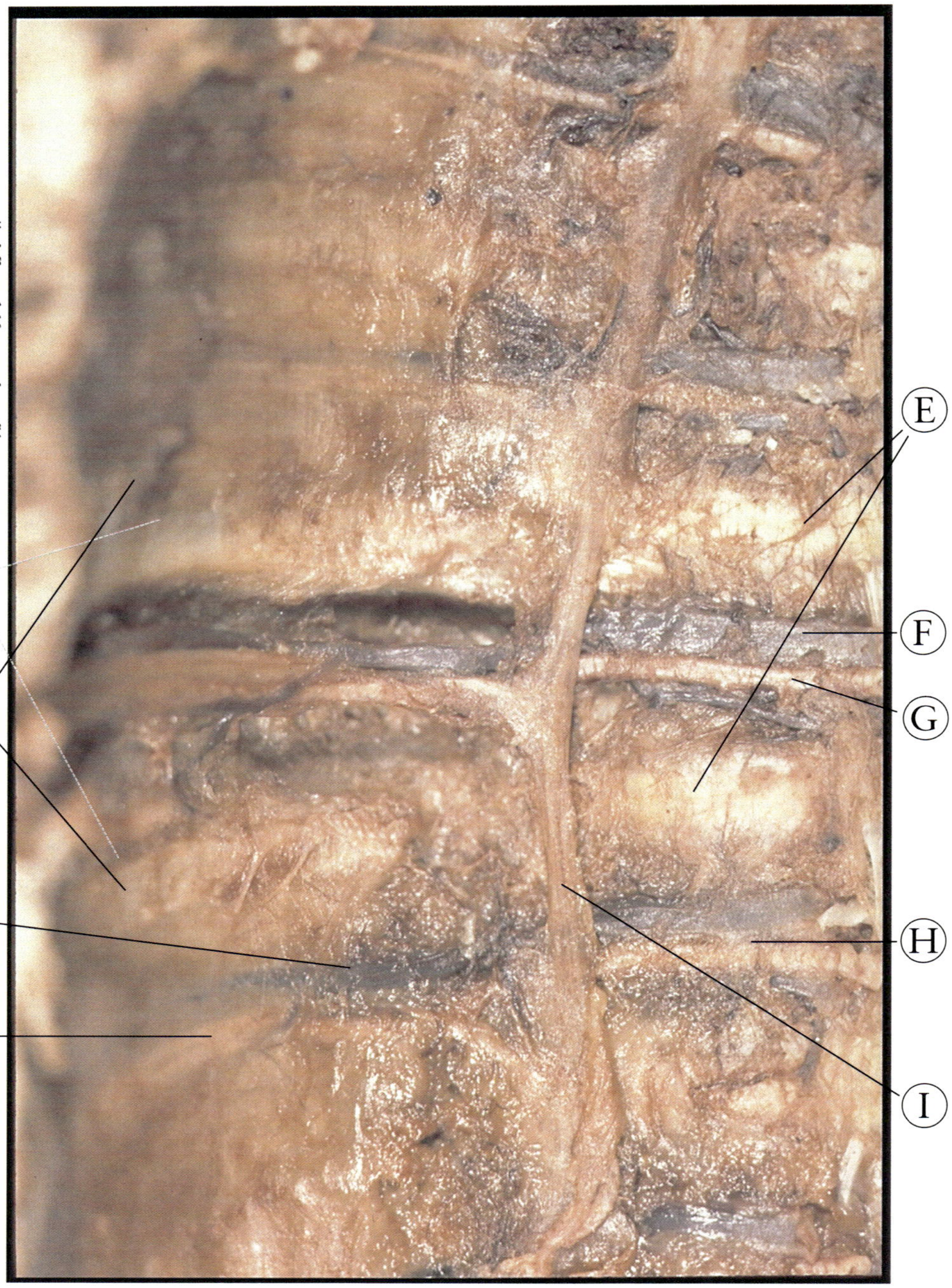

Figure 4-2
THORACIC SPINE ANTERIOR VIEW WITH SYMPATHETIC CHAIN AND RIB-SPINE RELATIONSHIP

Here is an anatomical proximity of the extra spinal nervous system to the costo-vertebral joints. The sympathetic chain can be immediately anterior to the costovertebral joints. Costo-vertebral subluxation and the resulting degenerative joint changes are concomitant with vertebral subluxation and the degenerative changes at those joints. Costo-vertebral subluxation and the sclerosis and inflammation can cause significant pathology to the autonomic nervous system.

(A) Endplates
(B) Discs
(C) Intersegmental twig arteries
(D) Anterior rami of nerve root
(E) Ribs
(F) Intercostal vein
(G) Intercostal nerve
(H) Intercostal artery.
(I) Sympathetic chain

traumas. Rib articulations with the spine are all posterior structures, and provide increased structural support in that area. The anterior aspect, comprised of the vertebral bodies and discs of the thoracic spine, is therefore more vulnerable to change than the posterior aspect, where anterolisthesis and retrolisthesis of the thoracic vertebrae occur, altering the shape of the vertebral canal. Even though I did not have the means to depict or study them in detail, I have to acknowledge the lateral listhesis and rotational subluxation complexes. More detailed anatomical studies in this area are needed. The vertebral canal is considered to be a posterior structure, but anterior changes of the thoracic spine can indeed effect the canal, ribs, and other posterior structures. More importantly, they can effect the neural contents, the spinal cord, and nerve roots. In the thoracic spine, there is an extra-spinal nervous system component to consider. The sympathetic chain in the thoracic spine is at or near the costo-vertebral joints, (**see Figure 4-2**). The integrity of the sympathetic chain is at risk when these joints are subluxated. Chronic degenerative changes have been observed to alter the nervous tissue of the sympathetic chain.[1,2] There can be a variation between individuals as to the location of the chain. In **Figure 4-2** the sympathetic chain is over the costo-vertebral joints and in **Figure 4-3** the chain is oriented over the costo-transverse joints.

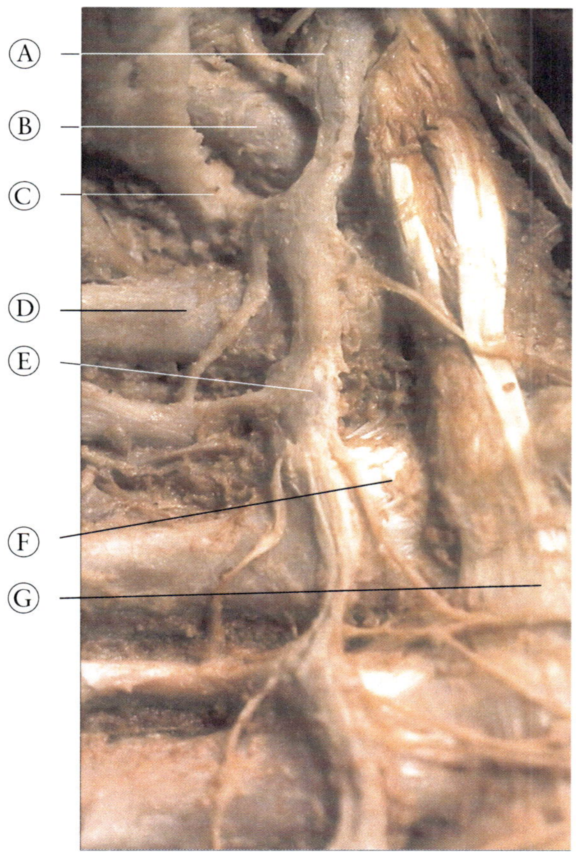

Figure 4-3

Anterior view of the upper thoracic spine.

(A) Inferior cervical sympathetic ganglion
(B) First rib
(C) First thoracic nerve root
(D) Second rib
(E) Sympathetic chain ganglion
(F) Costovertebral joint ligaments
(G) Anterior longitudinal ligament of the vertebral column

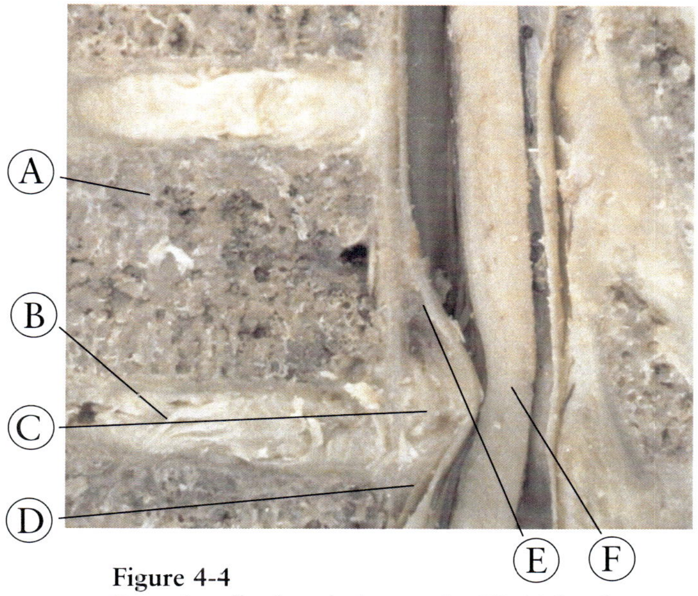

Figure 4-4

Posterior disc herniation at the T9-10 level.

The disc herniation has pushed the posterior longitudinal ligament and thecal sac into the spinal cord.

(A) Vertebral body
(B) Disc
(C) Herniation
(D) Posterior longitudinal ligament
(E) Thecal sac
(F) Spinal cord

One of the most common postural patterns in our society, is anterior weight bearing or displacement of the head anterior to the rib cage or shoulders, usually characterized by loss of the cervical curve. This has important implications for the thoracic spine. Over time, the weight of the head carried habitually in an anterior position can create a deforming force on the thoracic spine and cause increased kyphotic curvature. The condition appears gradually and becomes worse over a period of time, so the patient may not be aware of pain or discomfort, only an increasing perception of stiffness and lack of flexibility.

Vertebral bodies in the thoracic spine are compressed anteriorly more than posteriorly, making them wedge-shaped. The added posterior stability that the rib articulations and the network of ligaments provide to the transverse processes, canals, and pedicles may retard posterior crushing during certain kinds of trauma.

Posterior herniation of the thoracic discs does occur. **See Figure 4-4**, a T10 disc. It should be noted that the lower the thoracic disc herniation the lower the neurological involvement. Since the conus medularis ends at T12 or L1, the disc herniation at T11 could affect the neurons of the legs or even the bladder.

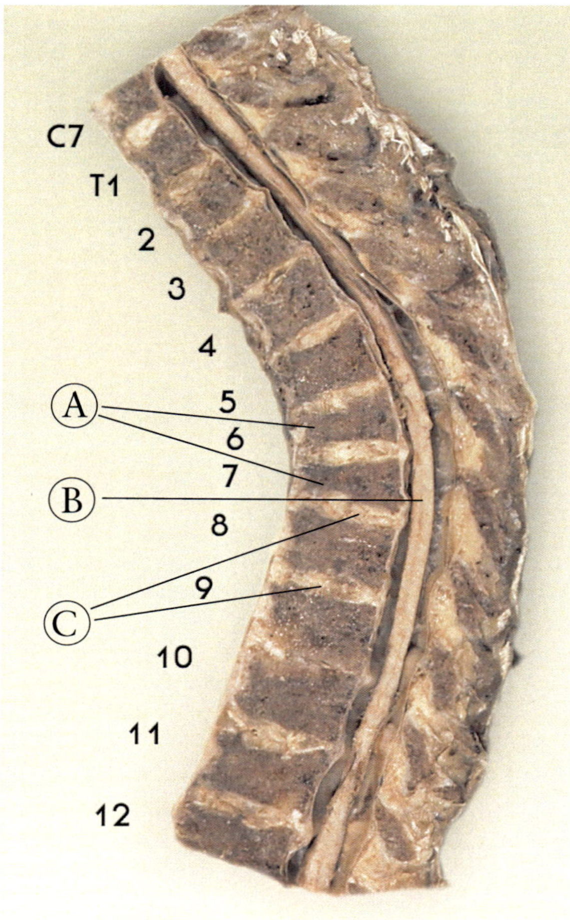

Figure 4-5
HYPERKYPHOSIS OF THE THORACIC SPINE.

The thoracic vertebrae 6 and 7 have compression fractures with more anterior height loss. The result is an anterior translation of the spinal cord to the anterior wall of the canal.
Note cord contact from T5 to T7.

(A) Compression fractures
(B) Spinal cord
(C) Discs.

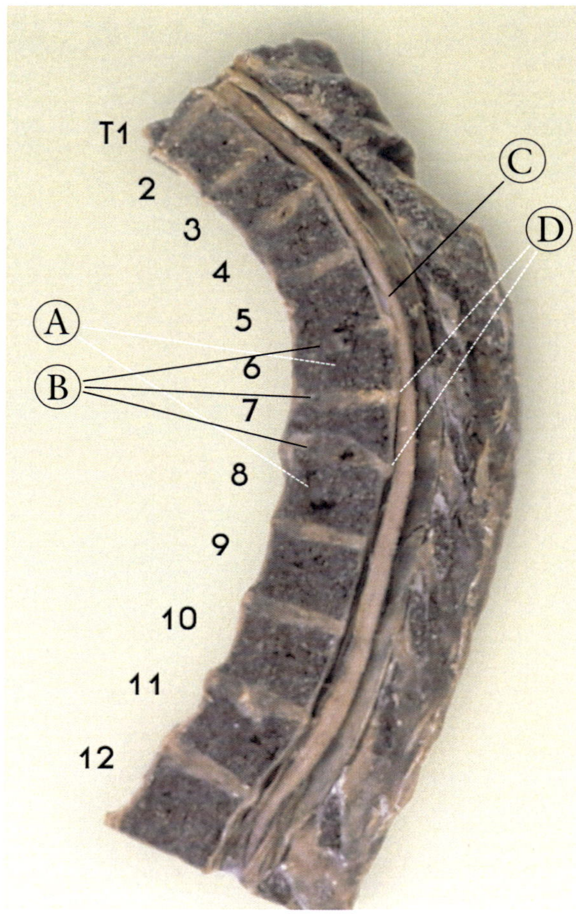

Figure 4-6
HYPERKYPHOSIS AS A RESULT OF OSTEOPOROSIS

Compression fractures of T6 and T7 have increased the kyphotic curvature. Note the spinal cord contact with the canal wall from T1 to T7 and small disc protrusions into the cord.

(A) Vertebrae
(B) Discs
(C) Spinal cord
(D) Disc protrusion

COMPRESSION FRACTURES

With traumatic or osteoporotic compression fractures, the thoracic kyphotic curvature increases (see **Figure 4-5**), pulling (tractioning) the spinal cord into the anterior portion of the canal and up against the vertebral bodies. Any structural defects such as osteophytes or disc bulges will exacerbate the clinical implications of this deforming compression fracture pattern. **Figure 4-6** shows how disc bulging and posterior spurs of thoracic vertebra 5, 6, and 7 have made impressions in the spinal cord.

The thoracic spinal cord gives rise to ventral nerve roots which are the motor and efferent (outgoing) nerve pathways for the viscera. The anterior spinal artery lies in close proximity, supplying blood to the neurons of the ventral horns where visceral and somatic motor neurons are found in close proximity. Hypoxia of this neural tissue and the exact clinical results are not known. The dramatic results by some chiropractors could be attributed to changing the vascular condition of the spinal cord. Further studies are recommended.

SUBARACHNOID ADHESIONS

Tractioning of the cord can lead to an inflammatory condition that results in fibrous adhesions inside and outside the thecal sac involving the cord and nerve roots. **Figure 4-7** shows the cord, (in the anterior compartment of the canal, indicating tethering) with nerve roots dropping down toward their intervertebral foramen. They are enmeshed in the dense, fibrous network that commonly results from chronic inflammation. This fibrous mass can trap nerve rootlets proximal to the nerve roots, so that certain positions and actions could create more severe inflammation and tractioning. Further, the increase in kyphosis leads to an overall increase in canal length and length of the cord itself, and can affect the entire middle portion of the thoracic spinal cord.

Over a period of time, in the absence of compression, tethering results causing a decrease of neural conductivity. Studies show that an initial period of irritation and increase in sensitivity and conductivity of the nervous tissue is followed by a drop in conductivity that results in a loss of all impulses.[3,4,5,6] This must correlate with loss of visceral and motor function. This is a significant factor in the chronic, debilitating postural changes that afflict many people in Western society.

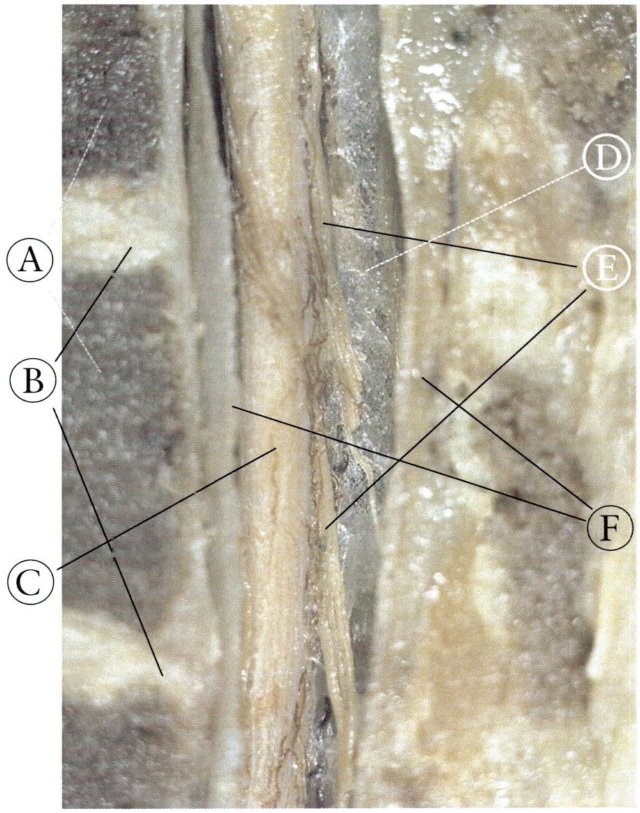

Figure 4-7
SUBARACHNOID ADHESIONS.
Adhesions in the subarachnoid space are common when the spinal cord is tethered
Note the nerve rootlets in the adhesions.
(A) Vertebral bodies
(B) Discs
(C) Spinal cord
(D) Subarachnoid adhesions
(E) Nerve rootlets
(F) Thecal sac.

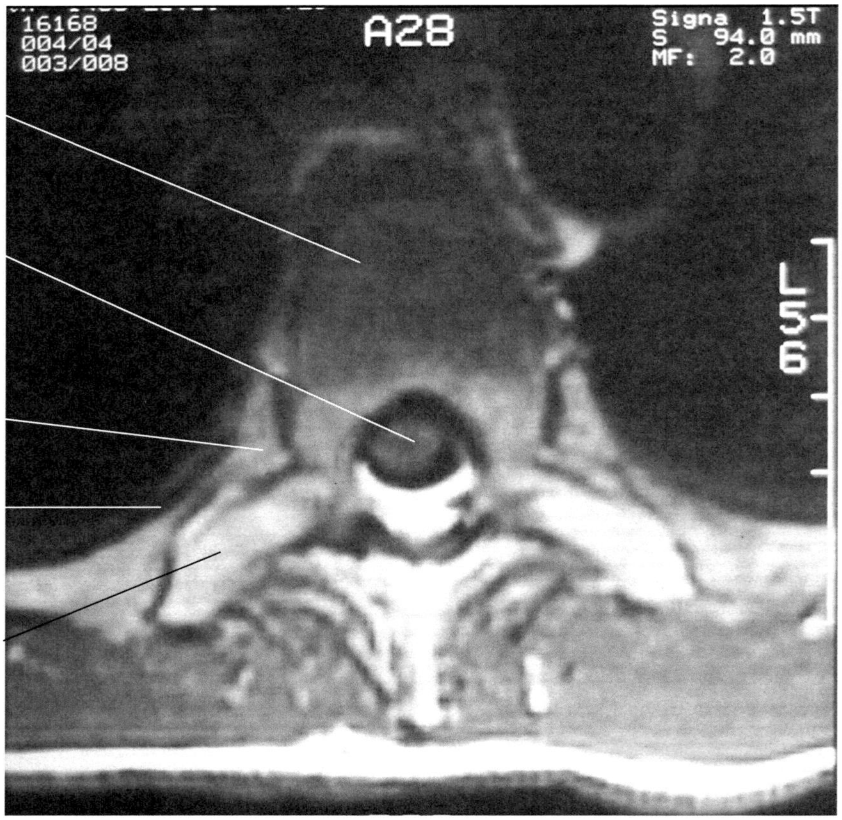

(A)
(B)
(C)
(D)
(E)

Figure 4-8
Thoracic Spine: MRI Axial View of Tethered Spinal Cord

(A) Vertebral body
(B) Spinal cord
(C) Rib head
(D) Neck of rib
(E) Transverse process.

Note the spinal cord-canal contact even in the recumbent position, giving the patient relief. Because of gravity, these studies indicate spinal cord pre-tension in the neutral position. The relaxed spinal cord should be in the posterior or bottom part of the canal. Adverse physiological tension will result in flexed positions.

Rib Cage Subluxations

The ribs are subject to deforming events in the normal course of human activity. The rib cage is a flexible structure, regularly deforming with breathing, coughing, sneezing and moving with normal twisting and bending. Rib subluxation can be very painful to completely silent. It can manifest itself as mild stiffness of the neck and shoulders, or cause nerve and vascular entrapment that is disabling. Many studies suggest that the degree of symptoms and the appearance of degeneration in the cervical spine, are unrelated, since they have shown that patients can be both pain-free with significant degenerative changes on imaging, or in severe pain, even though having apparently normal imaging findings. Most studies of the cervical spine and neck pain do not include evaluation of the rib cage for injury. Rib cage distress will cause a neuromuscular guarding reflex that will tighten all the "voluntary muscles" that attach to the ribs. This includes the scalene muscles, splenius capitis and the other muscles that attach the head to the thorax, the shoulder muscles and even involves the rotator cuff muscles of the shoulder girdle including levator scapulae. This rigidity of all these muscles is required by the central nervous system to hold everything together. I also use the term "subluxation" to describe displacement of these rib-vertebral joint complexes. The body's response to an insult to a "vital cavity" is to prevent an "impending luxation," which would be fatal if this occurred to the rib cage. The volume and shape of the chest cannot vary or change past a certain point without failing. This would be fatal. A collapsed lung would result from the luxation of the ribs.

In **Figure 4-1** we see the ribs and the relationship to the vertebra. The joints that the ribs have with a spine are spinal joints. These joint capsules have the same nerve supply as the facet joints and are as highly innervated. In **Figures 4-9** and **4-10** specimen dissections show the displaced ribs. Illustration of **Figure 4-11** shows the displacement pattern. This is a global event for the rib with a displacement over the whole course of the rib and involves the costosternal joints and the intercostal muscles. The distress will be easily palpable, especially in the axilla. In **Figure 4-8** we see the MRI of the normal alignment of the ribs to the vertebral body and transverse processes. In **Figures 4-12** and **4-13** we see the MRI studies with rib subluxations.

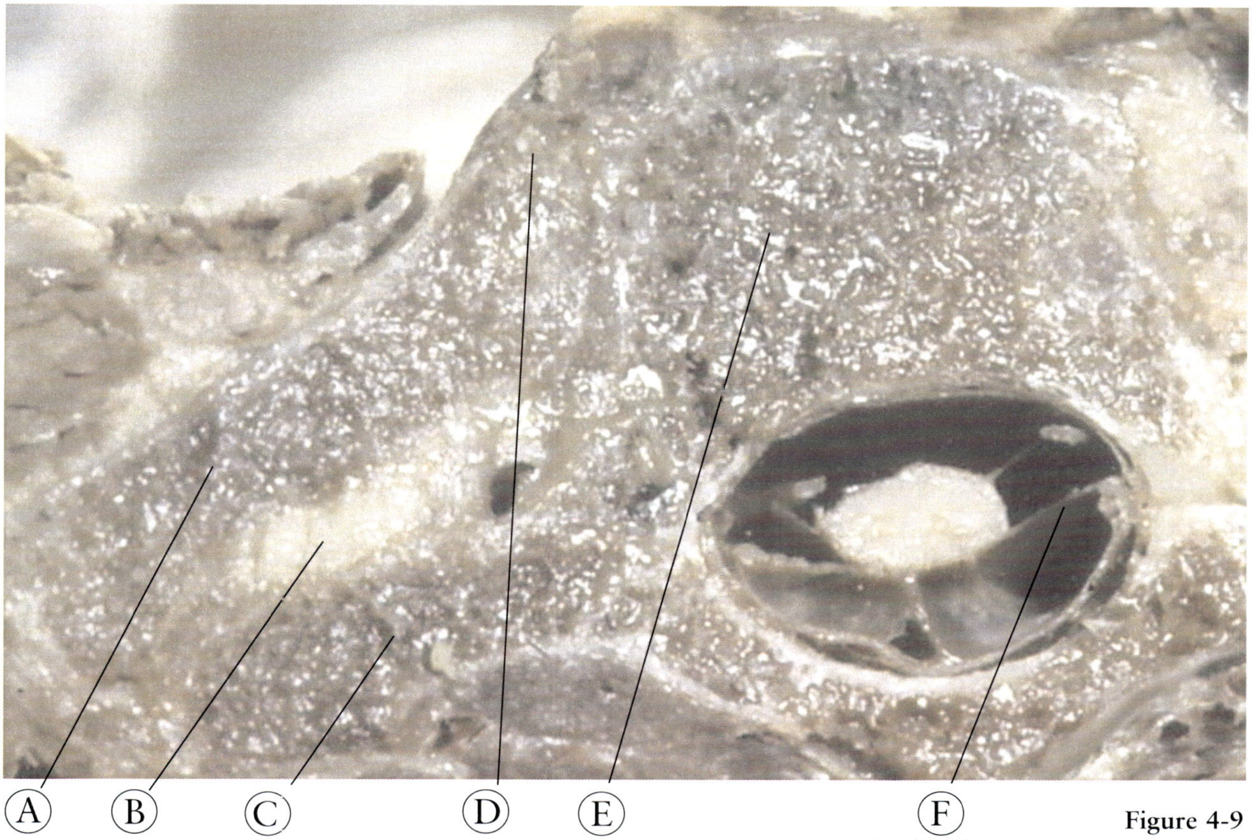

Figure 4-9
Costo-vertebral and Costo-transverse Joints

(A) Rib neck
(B) Gap
(C) Transverse process
(D) Rib head
(E) Vertebral body
(F) Dentate ligament

The X-ray appearance is subtle and the need of physical examination is essential for the definitive diagnosis. **Figure 4-14** is the normal AP view of the upper thoracic spine. Note the overlap of the ribs over the transverse processes and the proximity of the rib heads to the spine. **Figure 4-15** shows the loss of that relationship. This patient, a quadriplegic, had upper extremity function return with adjusting the rib cage. **Figure 4-16** shows a similar pattern of subluxation of the ribs, this patient had constant shoulder and neck pain following spinal fusion of C4-6. **Figure 4-17** is the illustration of that displacement that would explain that X-ray appearance. The prevalence of motor vehicle accidents in the population makes this subluxation pattern of the ribs very common.

Injury to the chest and the costovertebral and costotransverse joints can possibly irritate the sympathetic chain, due to their proximity to each other (**see Figure 4-3**). Chest wall pain has been associated with panic attacks.[7,8] Anxiety disorders and hypertension plague our society and we attack the nervous system with pharmacology. This would imply the nervous system is the problem with these disorders.

The plain X-ray AP views that are taken of the cervical spine usually include the top of the thoracic spine and it's joints with the first few ribs. In **Figure 4-14** the normal alignment of the ribs and thoracic spine are seen. Note the slight overlap of the transverse processes and the neck of the ribs and the proximity of the rib heads with the vertebral bodies. **Figures 4-15** and **4-16** are AP X-ray studies of two individuals whose cervical injuries needed surgical intervention. Note the lack of overlap of the rib necks and the transverse processes and the gap the rib heads have with the vertebral bodies. Both had significant post surgical problems that were reversed with realignment of the ribs. **Figure 4-17** is an illustration of the rib subluxation pattern common with motor vehicle accidents. This subluxation pattern will also be palpable at the costosternal joints and axilla. These type of injuries need to be evaluated by physical examination and correlated with the findings on the imaging.

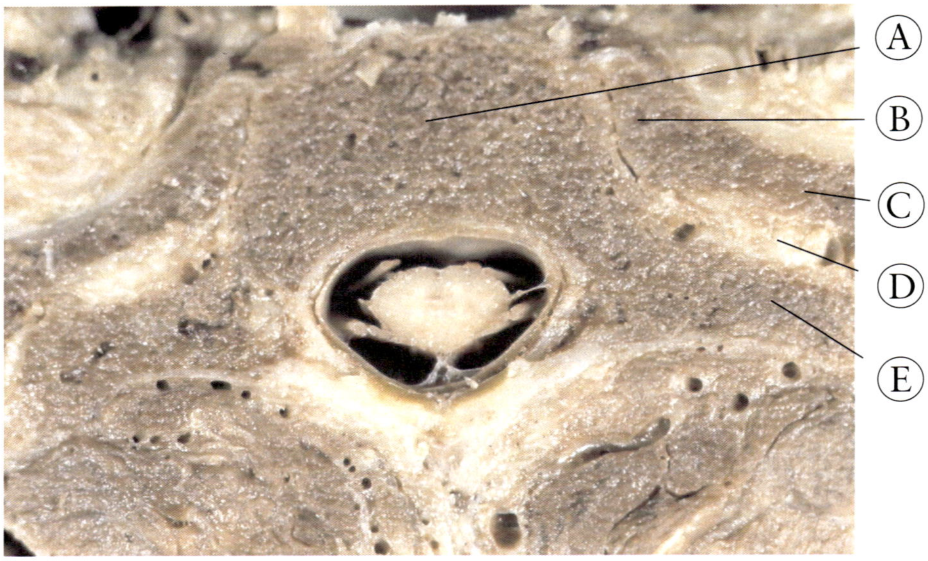

Figure 4-10
Rib Subluxation seen in Specimen

(A) Vertebral body
(B) Head of rib
(C) Neck of rib
(D) Gap
(E) Transverse process

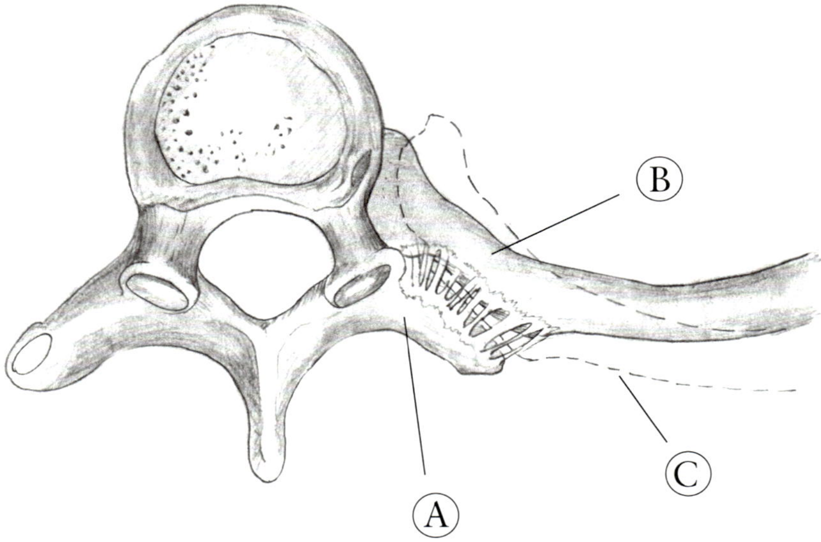

Figure 4-11
Illustration of Rib Subluxation

(A) Transverse process
(B) Neck of rib
(C) Dotted line indicates subluxed rib

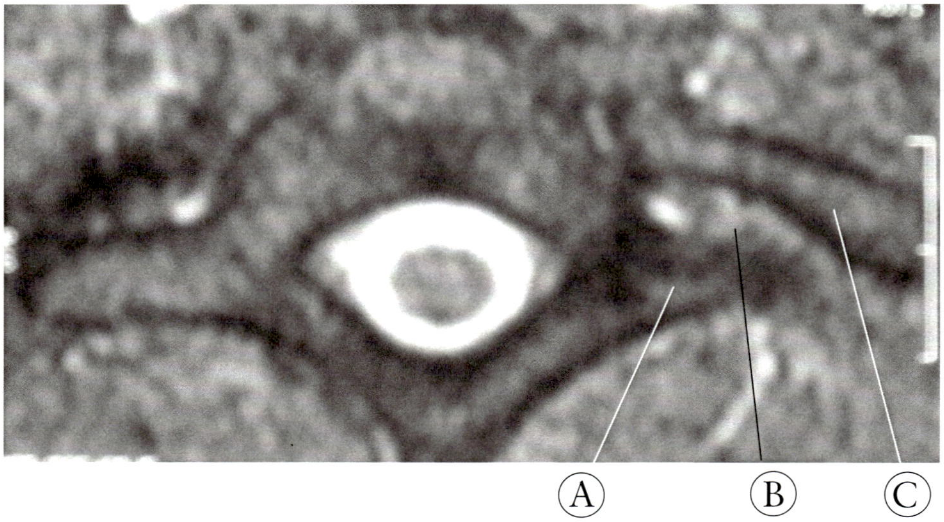

Figure 4-12
MRI View of Rib Subluxation

(A) Transverse process
(B) Gap
(C) Neck of rib

This patient had debilitating hand pain for 18 months. The brachial and axillary plexuses attach to the ribs. Realigning the ribs allowed her to return to work within 2 weeks.

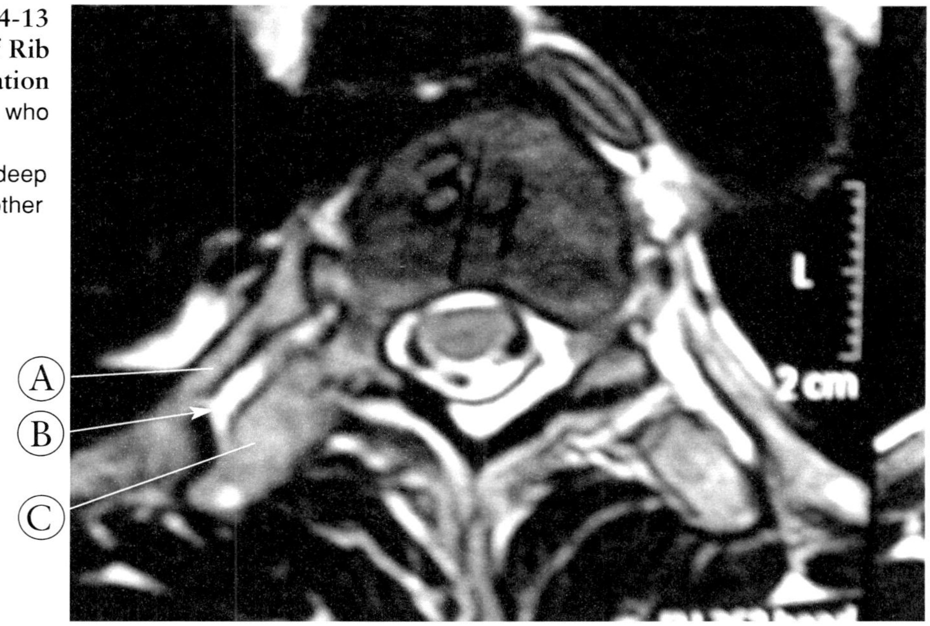

Figure 4-13
MRI View of Rib Subluxation
This is an MRI of patient who has pain with breathing, diaphragm spasms and deep mid back pain. He is another victim of motor vehicle accident.

(A) Neck of rib
(B) Gap
(C) Transverse process

This pattern of change can often include distress of the sympathetic chain. The distress of the central nervous system from deformation of the central canal would also include autonomic dysfunction. This would be a very gradual and insidious onset of symptoms, decades after the traumatic event. Anatomical studies have shown that the sympathetic nerves stretched by osteophytes have lost the histological appearance of nervous tissue, they are fiber and incapable of conductivity.[9] This an example of persistent deformation altering the histology of tissue.

If there is a history of rib fracture, or surgical procedures to the chest then all assumptions should be suspended and a thorough rib by rib evaluation should take place. The most common rib joint injuries are presented here. Any patient has the right to their own unique injury pattern.

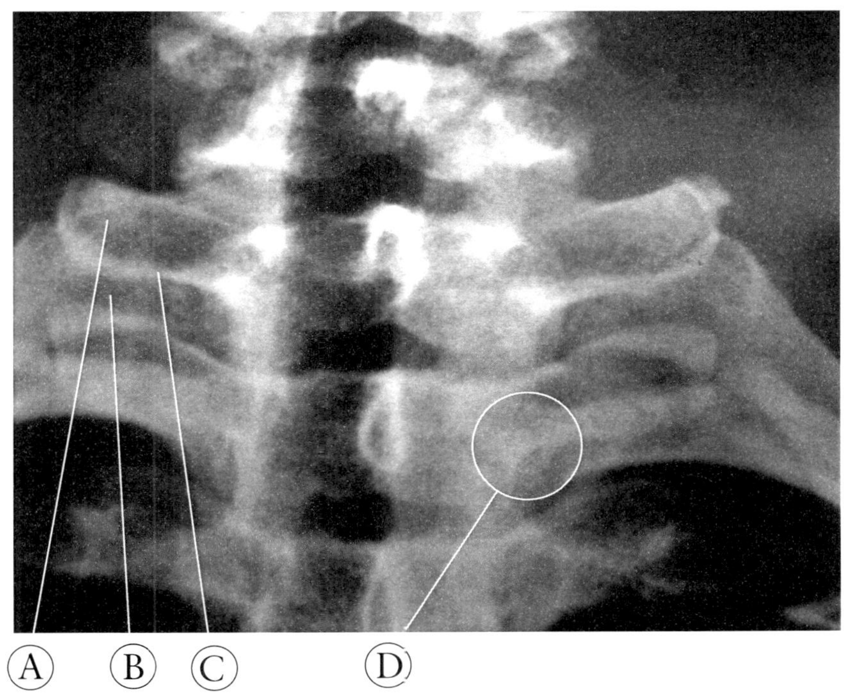

Figure 4-14
Anterior to posterior X-ray of a normal upper thoracic spine.

Note overlapping of the ribs and transverse processes and the closeness of the rib heads to the spine.

(A) Transverse process
(B) Head of rib
(C) Overlap of rib and transverse process
(D) Note: no gap

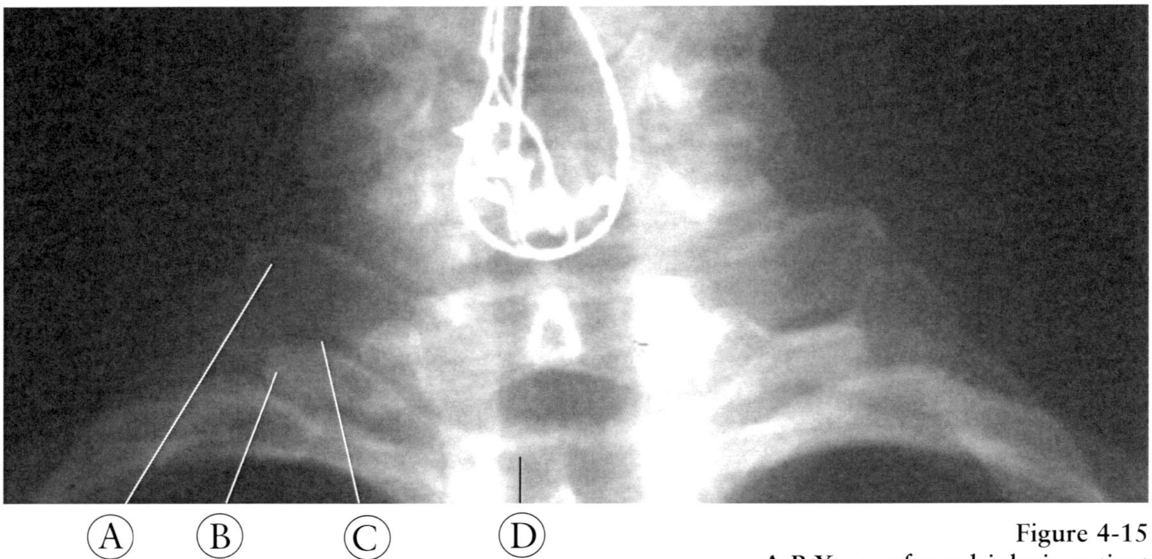

Figure 4-15
A-P X-ray of quadriplegic patient

(A) Transverse process
(B) Neck of rib
(C) Gap
(D) Vertebral body

This patient was a quadripelegic at the time this film was taken. Note the significant subluxation of the ribs. The axial and brachial plexuses attach to the ribs. The displacement of the ribs away from the spine traction these neurological structures interfering with their conductivity. Chiropractic adjustment of the ribs restored arm and shoulder function.

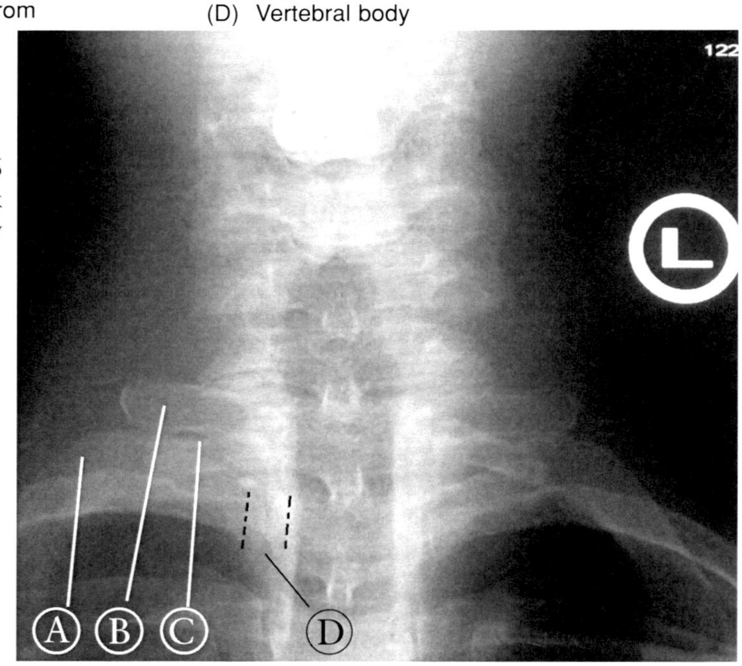

Figure 4-16
A-P X-ray of patient with persistent neck and shoulder pain following surgery

(A) Neck of rib
(B) Transverse process
(C) Gap
(D) Gap

This patient was suffering from significant neck and shoulder pain and limited motion post surgery. Note the significant rib displacement from the vertebra. The subluxations of the ribs will cause the scalene muscles, pectoralis muscles and serratus anterior muscles to be rigid and tense. The patient has restricted motion and painful symptoms with activity. Significant relief was experienced with chiropractic adjusting of the ribs.

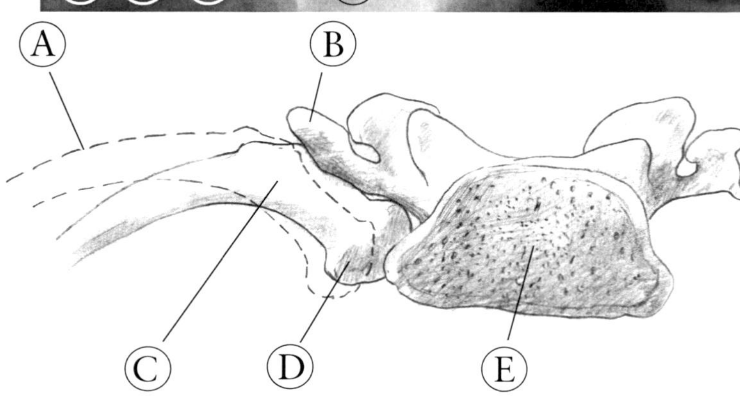

Figure 4-17
Illustration of typical rib subluxation

(A) Dotted line indicates subluxation of rib
(B) Transverse process
(C) Neck of rib
(D) Head of rib
(E) Vertebral body

ANTERIOR WEIGHT BEARING

Anterior weight bearing is a very common condition, and is a by-product of our postural habits. What Western society considers normal posture is, from the human body's point of view, not normal at all. We sit in chairs, get in and out of cars, sit in cars, and spend hours reading, studying, or staring at a computer screen with our heads inclined forward, cantilevered into space. Evolutionarily speaking, these are not "normal" human activities. They are recently acquired, and often mandatory postural situations that are having profound effects on our spines.

In most people, sitting increases the curvature of the thoracic spine because most desk or computer work, and even watching TV, causes the head to go forward relative to the thoracic spine, thus reducing cervical curvature and increasing thoracic kyphosis. This causes long-term malpositioning and tethering of the spinal cord, which can be associated with visceral problems, primarily cardiovascular.

Loss of ligament and joint integrity causes soft tissue changes. These have been given different names, i.e. non-marginal osteophytes, spondylosis, but all represent the same degenerative process. The result is altered weight bearing leading to altered bone. There are many different mechanisms of injury and ways to lose normal weight bearing. The severity increases with time. The degree of subluxation and chronic neurological distress due to overall postural changes are producing significant health conditions. Duration and magnitude of the distress on the nervous system are the major factors.

Figure 4-18
Anterior view of the mid-thoracic spine.

(A) Sympathetic chain ganglion
(B) Ribs
(C) Intercostal nerves
(D) Anterolateral osteophytes of the vertebral column

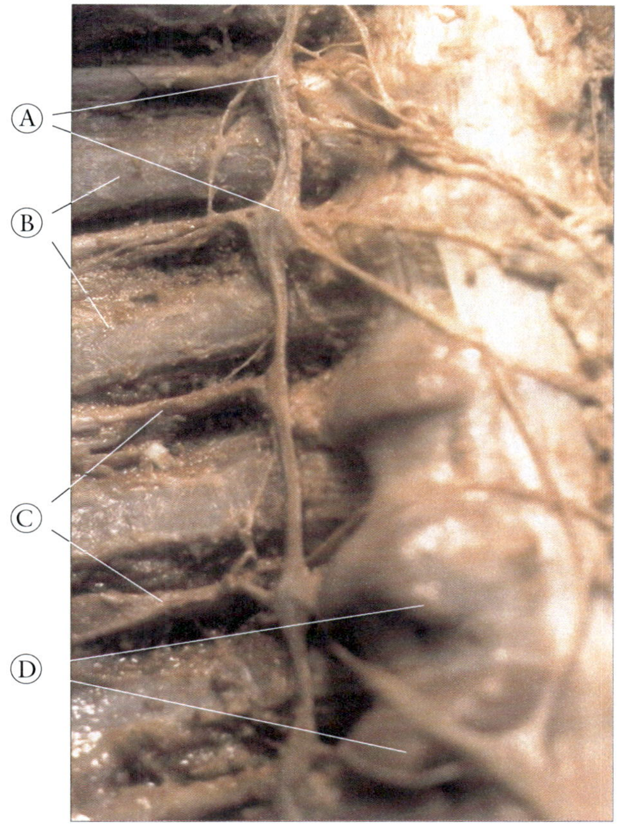

CHAPTER FOUR — EXPANDED TABLE OF CONTENTS

Atlas of Subluxations of the Thoracic Spine

SECTION I:

Subluxations with a normal thoracic curve (1 pair)

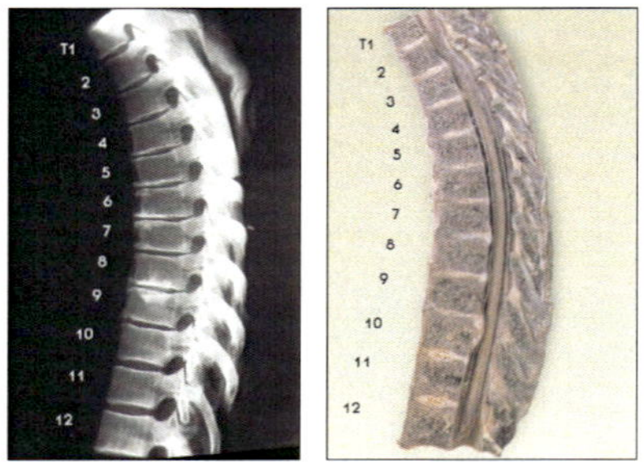

Plates 4-1 A&B
SUBLUXATIONS WITH A NORMAL KYPHOTIC CURVE
This shows the thoracic spine with minor compression fractures and multiple disc herniation.

SECTION II:

Subluxations with a reversed upper curve (3 pairs)

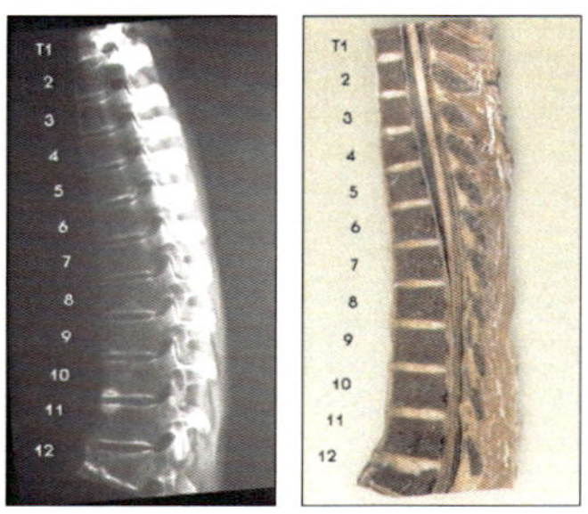

Plates 4-2 A & B
REVERSED UPPER THORACIC CURVE
Anterolisthesis: Upper Thoracics

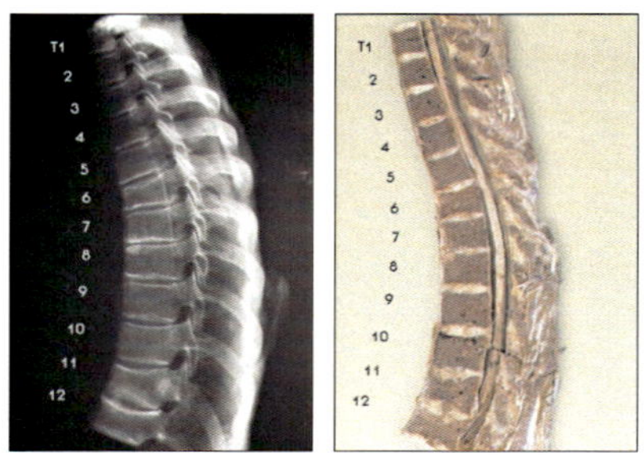

Plates 4-3 A & B
REVERSED UPPER THORACIC CURVE
Thoracic Anterolisthesis: Upper Thoracic

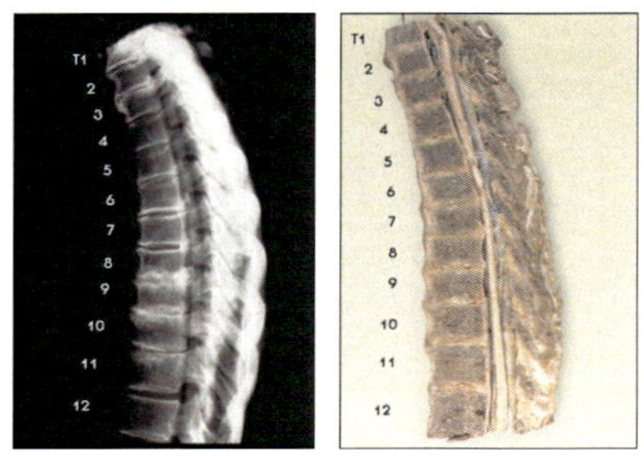

Plates 4-4 A & B
REVERSED UPPER THORACIC CURVE
Thoracic Spine: Anterolisthesis: Upper Thoracic

SECTION III:

Subluxations with a reversed lower curve (3 pairs)

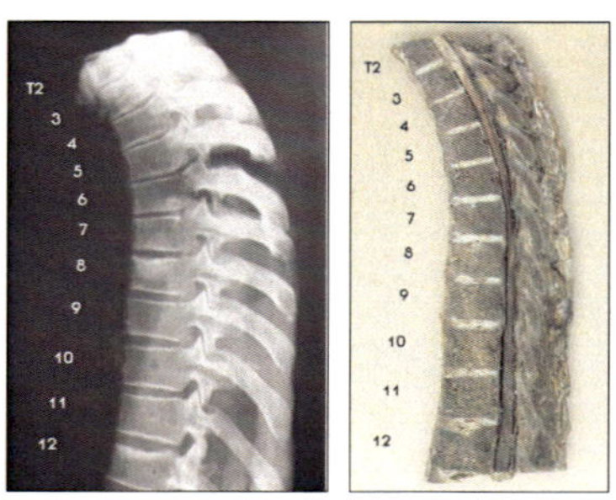

Plates 4-4 A & B
REVERSED LOWER THORACIC CURVE (T7-11)
Thoracic Spine : Anterolisthesis Lower Thoracics

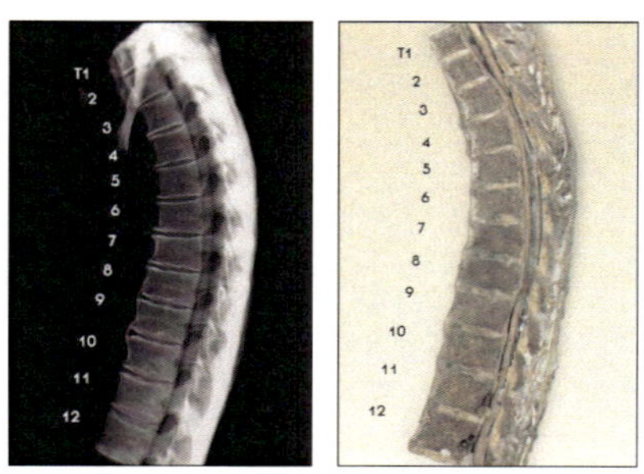

Plates 4-6 A & B
REVERSED LOWER THORACIC CURVE
Thoracic Spine: Anterolisthesis of Lower Thoracics

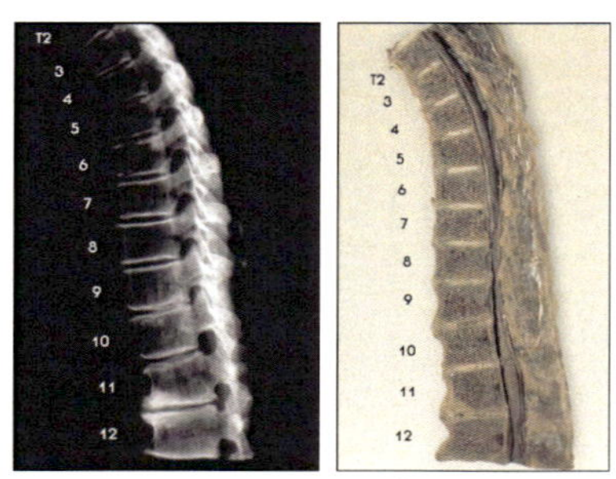

Plates 4-7 A & B
REVERSED LOWER THORACIC CURVE

CHAPTER FOUR — EXPANDED TABLE OF CONTENTS

Atlas of Subluxations of the Thoracic Spine

SECTION IV:

Subluxations with anterolisthesis of the upper and lower thoracic vertebrae (3 pairs)

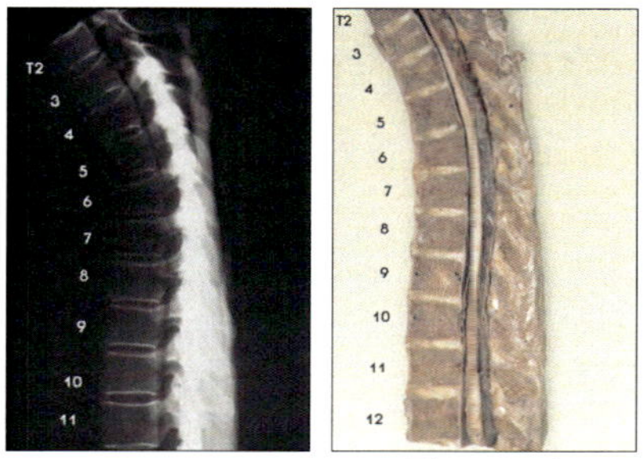

Plates 4-8 A & B
THORACIC UPPER POSTERIOR AND LOWER ANTEROLISTHESIS

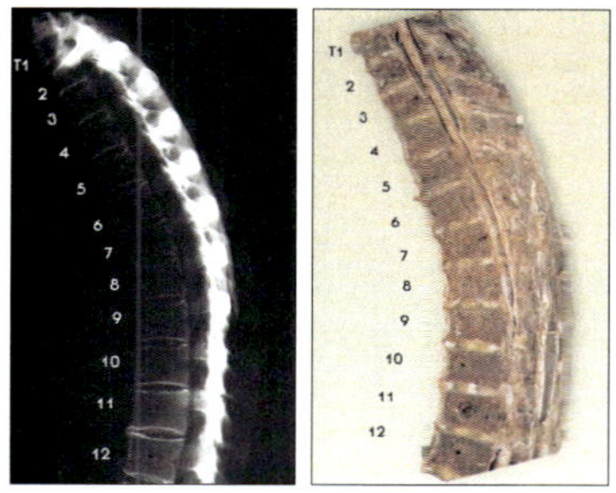

Plates 4-9 A & B
THORACIC SPINE - ANTEROLISTHESIS UPPER AND LOWER VERTEBRAE

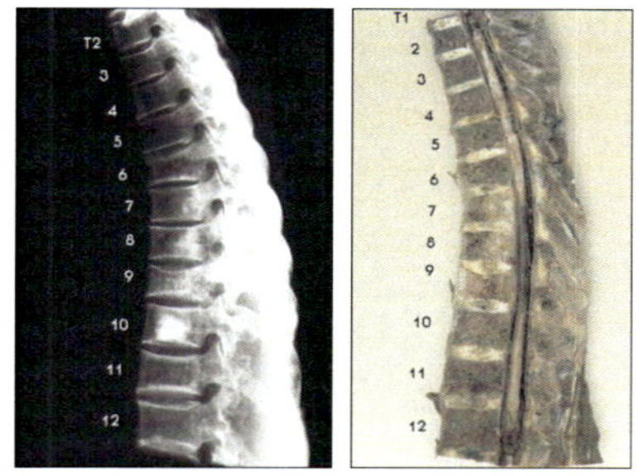

Plates 4-10 A & B
THORACIC SPINE: UPPER AND LOWER ANTEROLISTHESIS

SECTION V:

Hyperkyphosis of the thoracic curve (3 pairs)

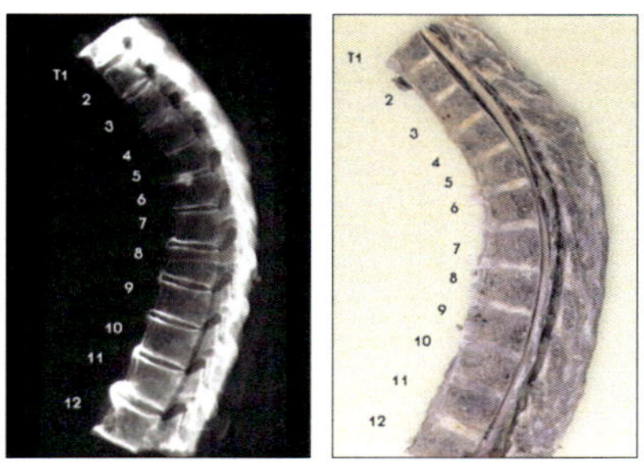

Plates 4-11 A & B
HYPERKYPHOSIS
THORACIC SPINE: PROGRESSIVE SPURRING WITH OSTEOPOROSIS AND HYPERKYPHOSIS

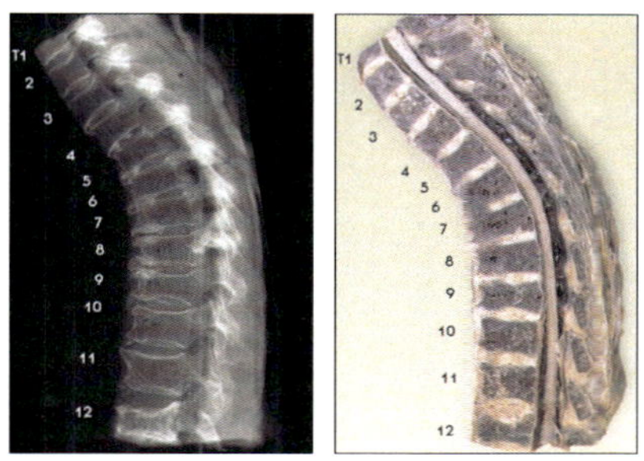

Plates 4-12 A & B
PROGRESSIVE SPURRING WITH HYPERKYPHOSIS CAUSED BY OSTEOPOROSIS

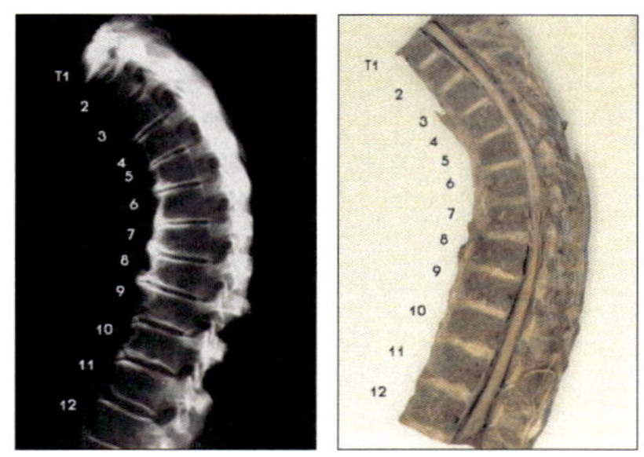

Plates 4-13 A & B
PROGRESSIVE SPURRING AND HYPERKYPHOSIS

Additional X-rays and MRIs

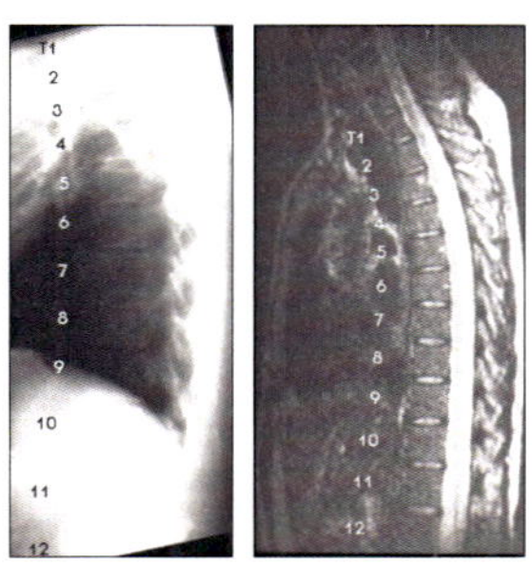

Plates 4-14 A & B
THORACIC SPINE: X-RAY AND MRI OF PATIENT WITH CORD TETHERING DUE TO ALTERED CURVES

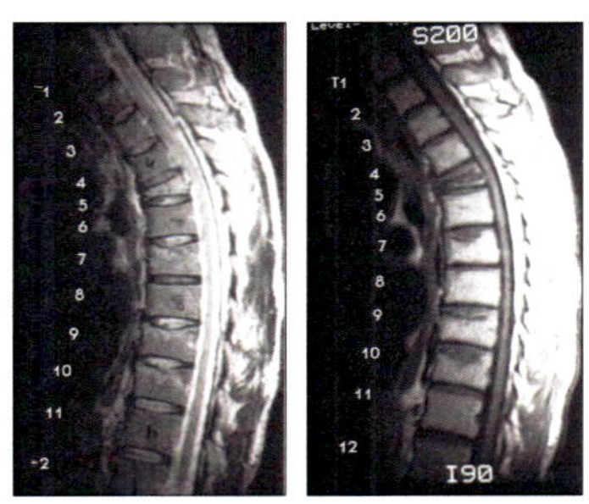

Plates 4-15 A & B
HYPERKYPHOSIS DUE TO COMPRESSION FRACTURE

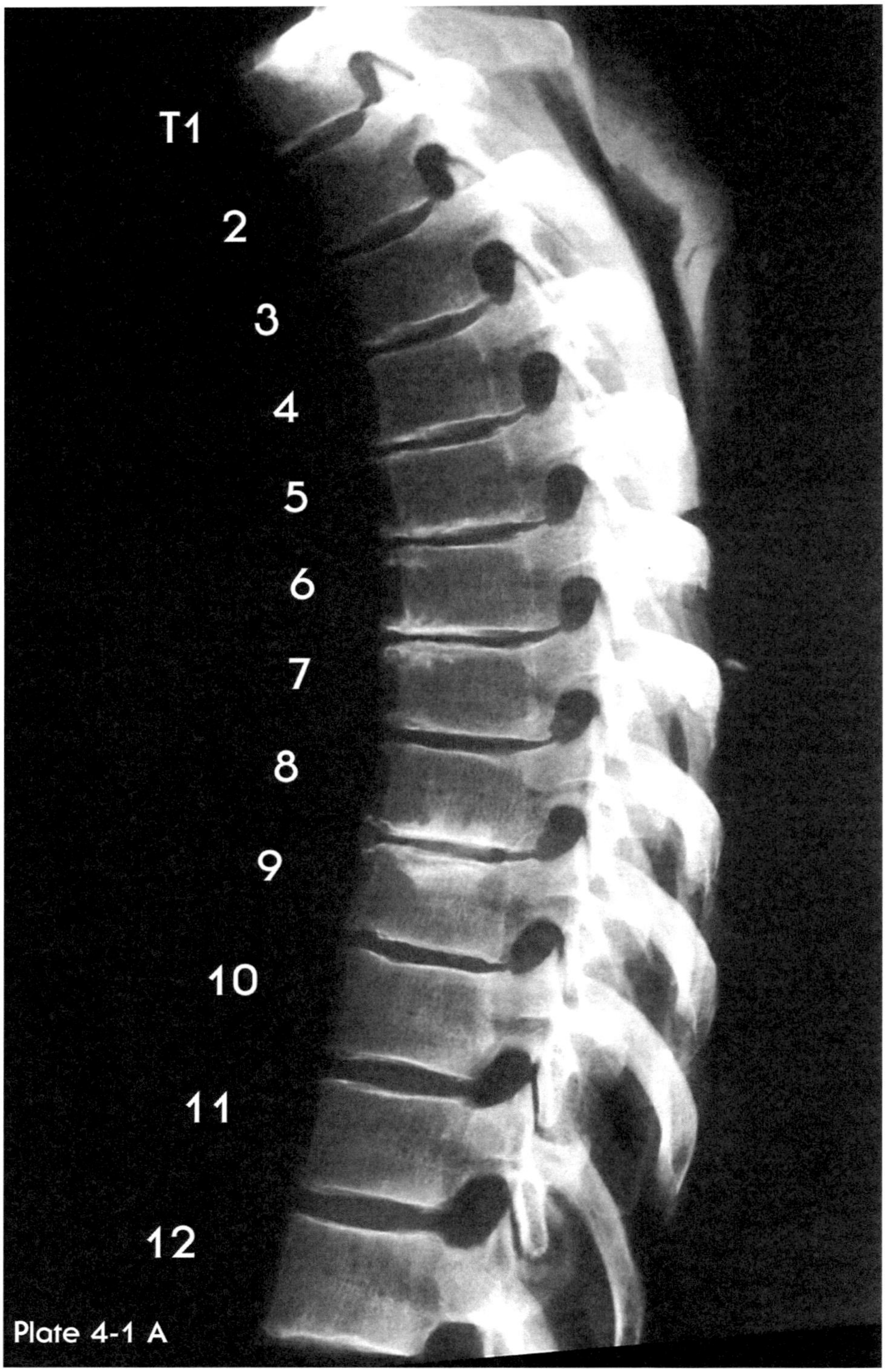

Plates 4-1 A & B
SUBLUXATIONS WITH A NORMAL KYPHOTIC CURVE
This shows the thoracic spine with minor compression fractures and multiple disc herniation.

All the discs in this specimen show anterior brown degeneration indicating poor imbibition (fluid exchange) and chronically low hydration of that part of the disc. Signs of trauma are seen in the endplate disturbances of the inferior body of T3 down to the superior endplate of the body of T10. This is a result of the subluxations of T1 to T10

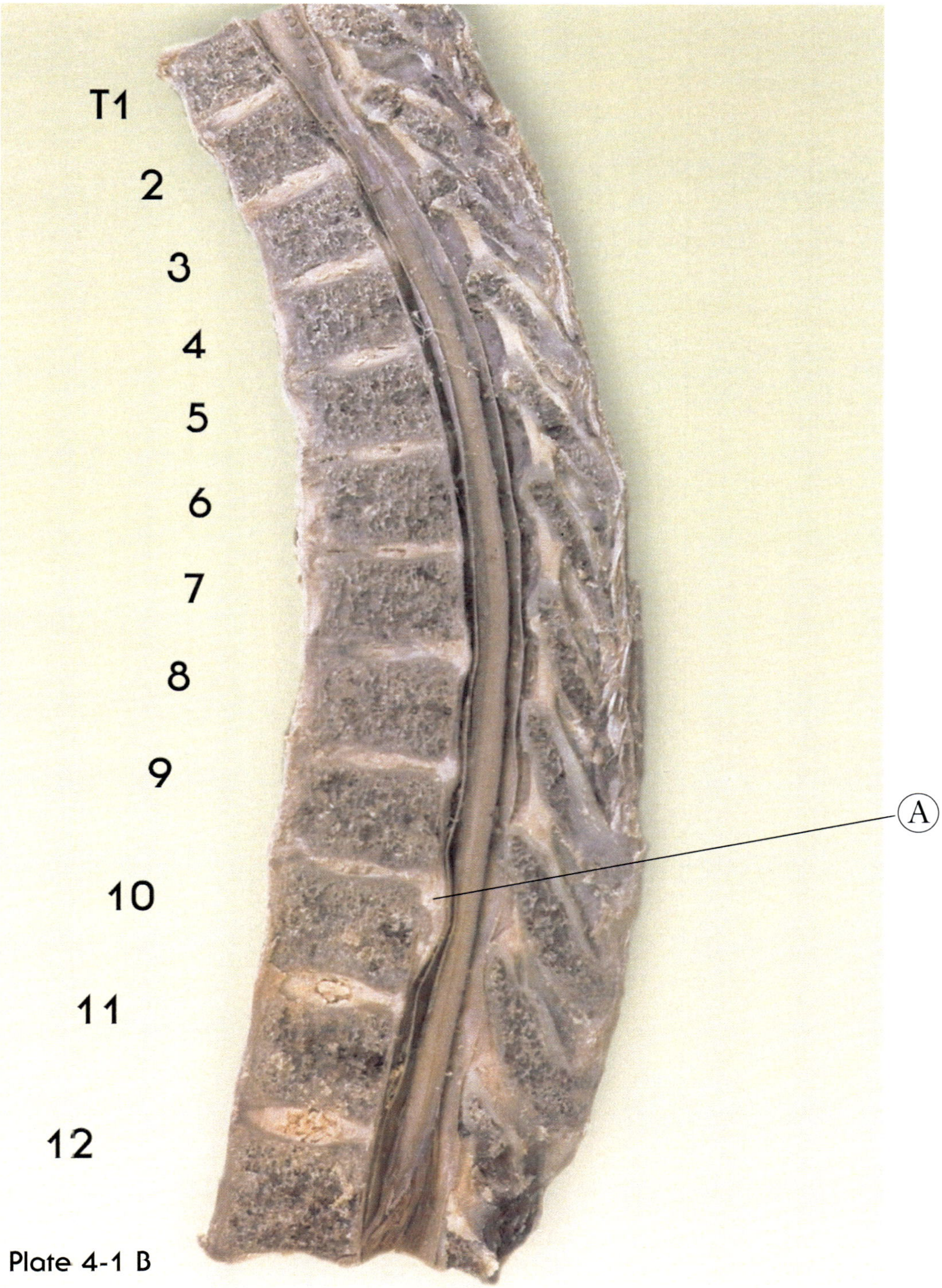

Plate 4-1 B

and the resulting osteophyte development of the affected segments.
T2 is retro to T1 with disc bulging slightly; T3 is retro to T2 with disc herniation and cord contact; T4 is anterior to T3 with signs of compression and misalignment of T5 to T9. T8 anterior to T7 with disc herniating and mild cord contact;T9-T10 disc herniating with cord contact; note normal alignment and appearance of T11 and T12.
(A) Disc herniation

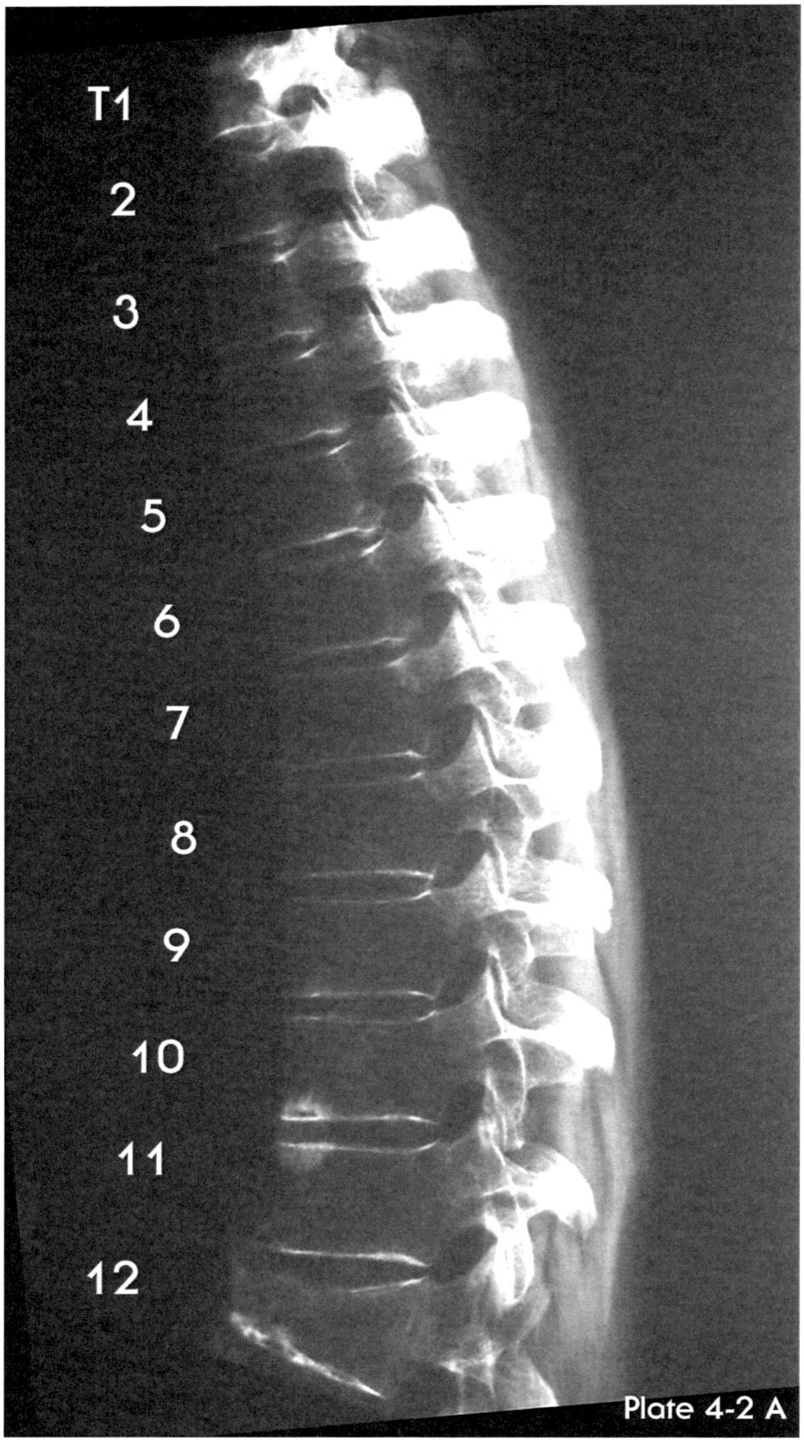

Plates 4-2 A & B
REVERSED UPPER THORACIC CURVE
Anterolisthesis Upper Thoracics

The compression fracture of T12 has created a wedge shaped vertebral body. The reversal of the normal kyphotic curve between T2 and T5 could be an adaptive response to this trauma or a posterior to anterior force occurring in this area. This has resulted in a 'dishing' or indentation of

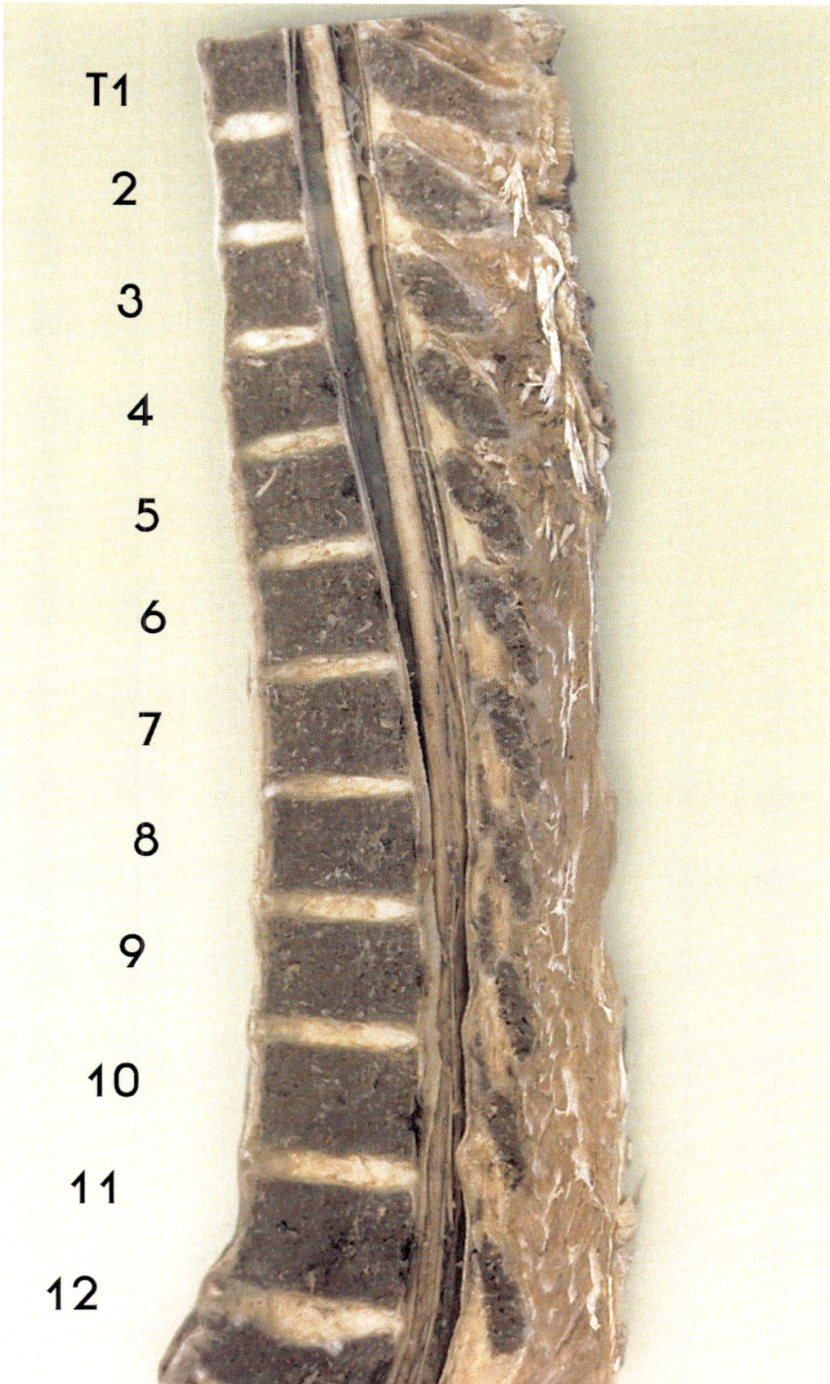

Plate 4-2 B

this portion of the thoracic spine. T4 is a complete anterolisthesis and the apex of this curve reversal ; From the T4-T5 disc and below, there is anterior brown degeneration that indicates poor hydration in this portion of the discs. T6-T11 looks aligned except for T10-T11 with slight anterior spurring. The T6-T11 area is slightly off the sagittal plane.

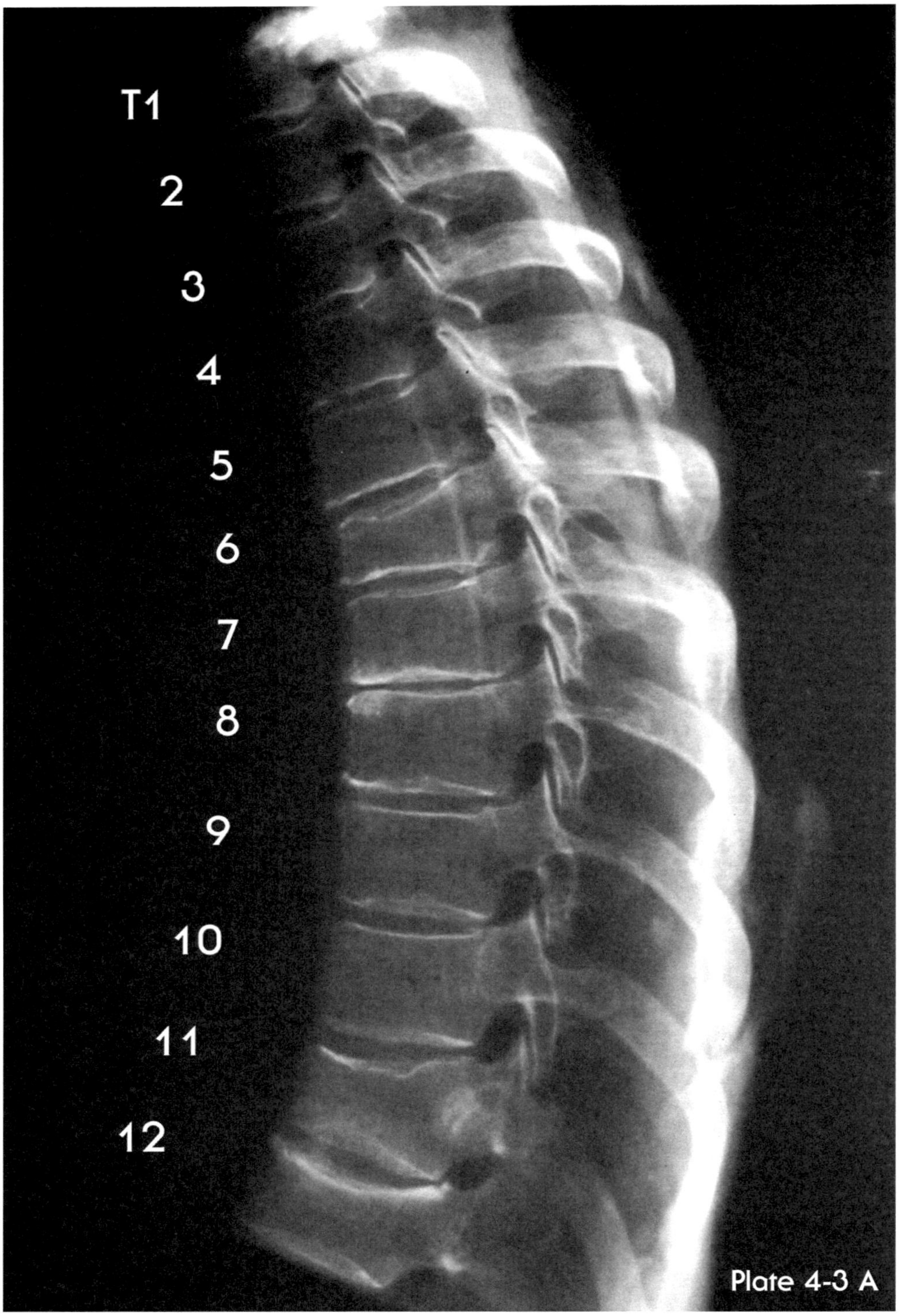

Plates 4-3 A & B

Thoracic Anterolisthesis: Upper Thoracic

This specimen has definite signs of trauma with compression fractures from T6 through T8 and T11-T12. There is a disc herniation at T11-T12 with cord contact. The upper thoracic curve reversal could be from an adaptive response to the lower thoracic trauma and resulting deformity, or to a direct posterior to anterior event.

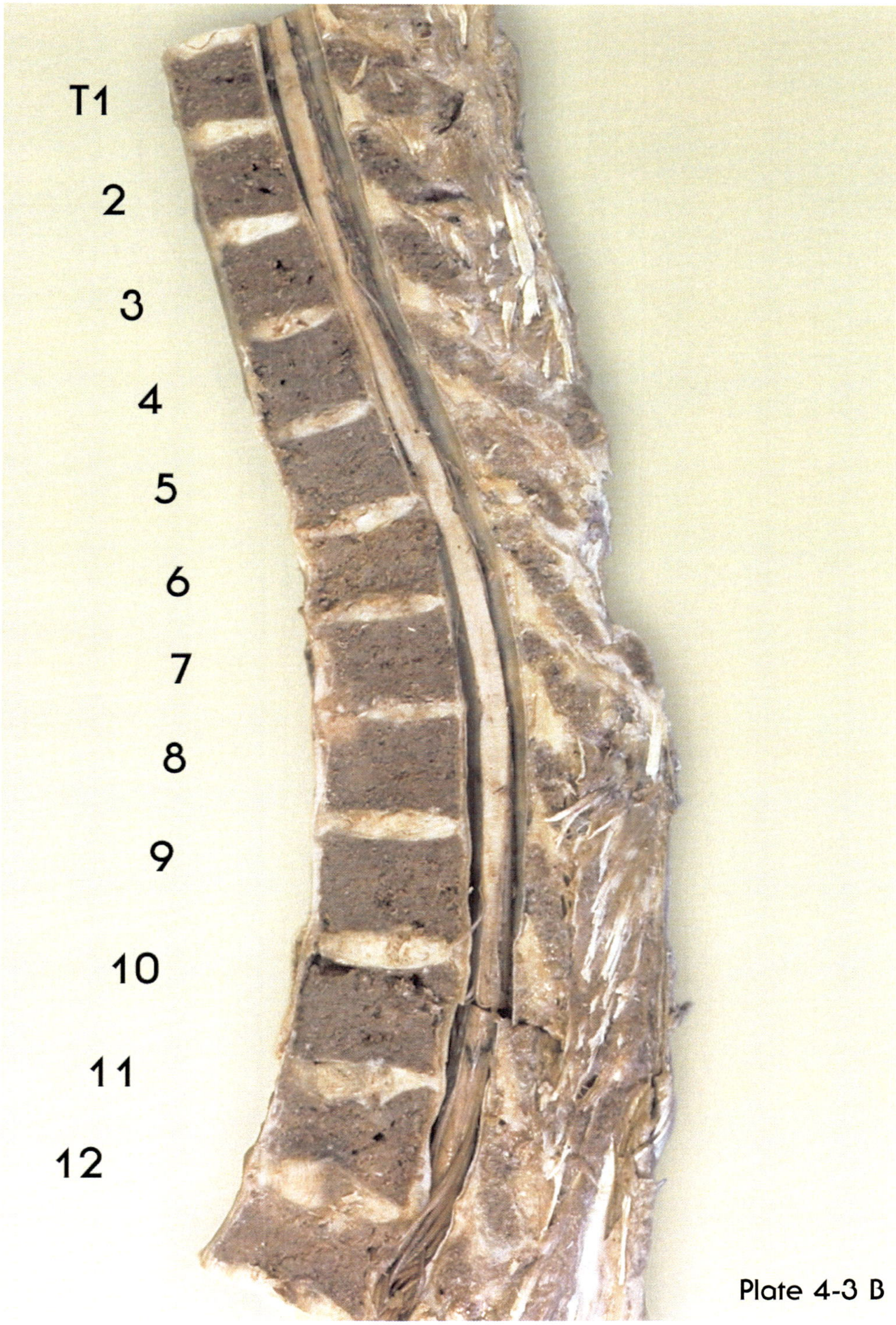

The anterior reverse apex is at T4-T5 with a anterolisthesis of T5. Despite the compression fractures a kyphotic curve returns to the lower thoracic spine.

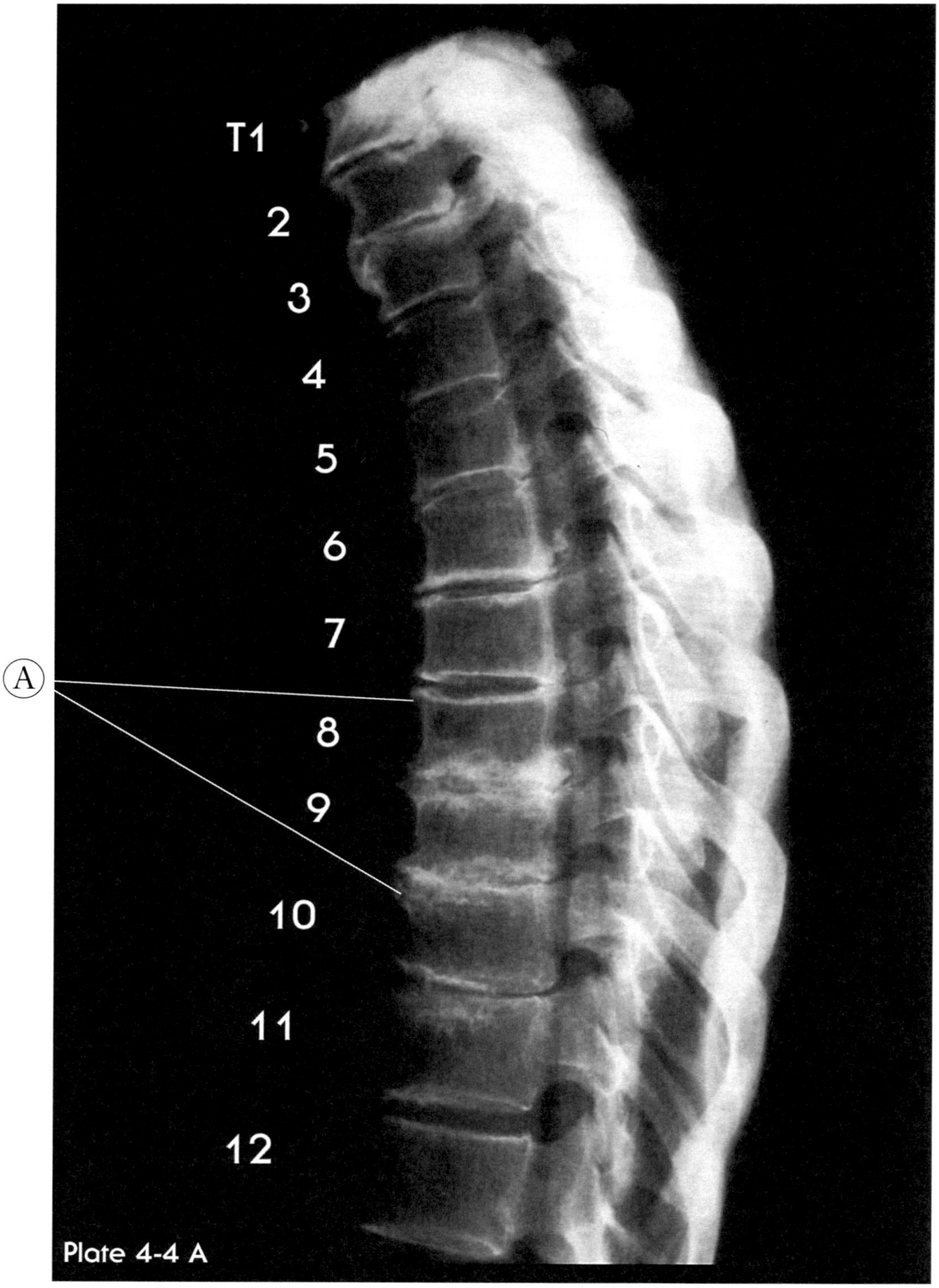

Plates 4-4 A & B

Thoracic Spine: Anterolisthesis: Upper Thoracic

This specimen has signs of old trauma with multiple segments compressed and sclerotic. There is loss of normal disc height and spurring anteriorly and posteriorly. The curve reversal has an anterior apex of T3-T4, with stair stepping subluxations of T4 to T12. Disc degeneration has advanced to near fusion of T8-T9 and T9-T10 with posterior bulging

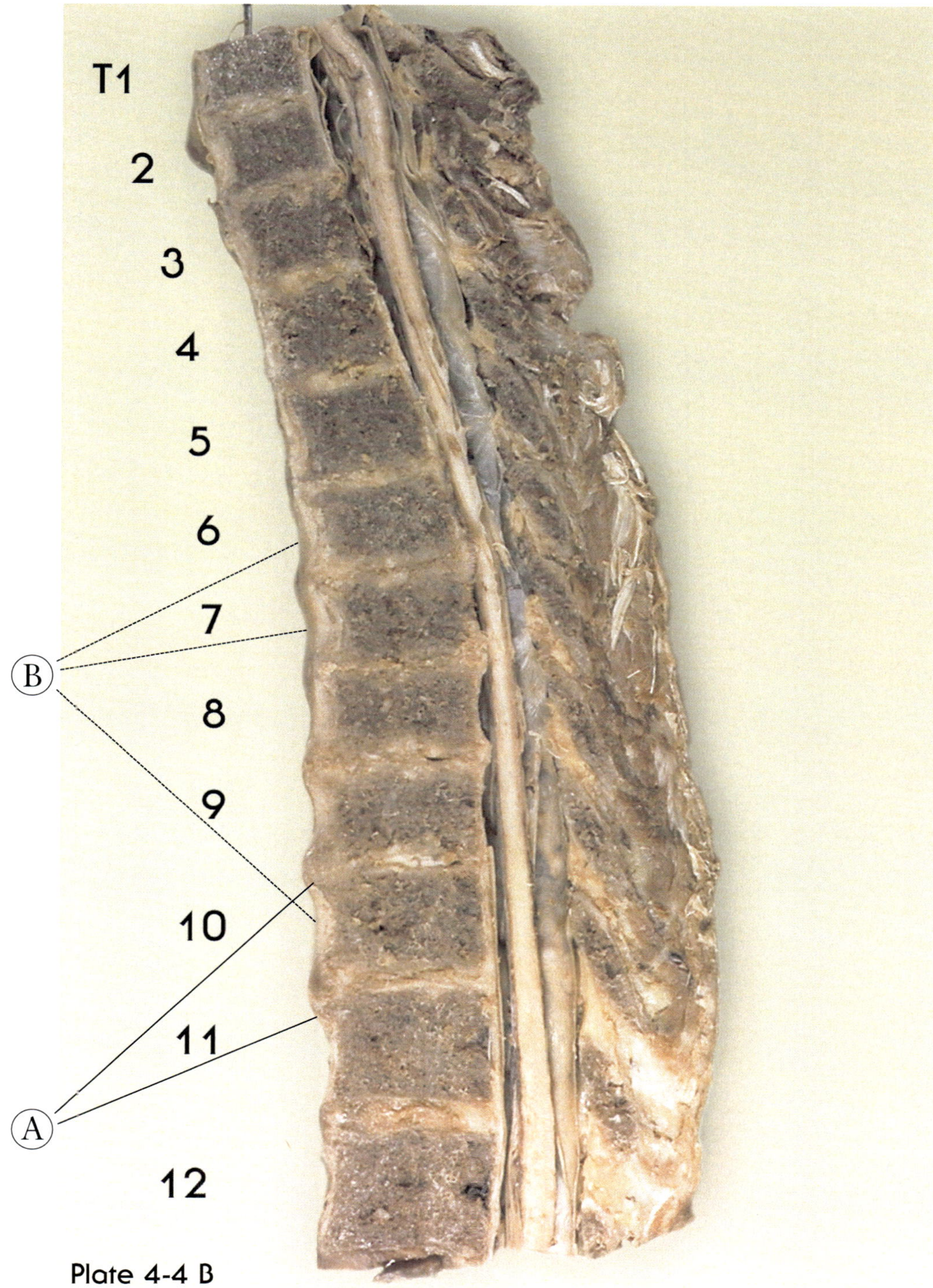

Plate 4-4 B

near cord contact in the neutral position. (This means that flexion of any part of the vertebral column could make those posterior disc protrusions clinically significant.) The anterior endplate spurring and disc bulging is associated with anterior longitudinal ligament thickening from T5 to T11.

(A) Anterior spurs and endplate changes.
(B) Hypertrophy of Anterior Longitudinal Ligament

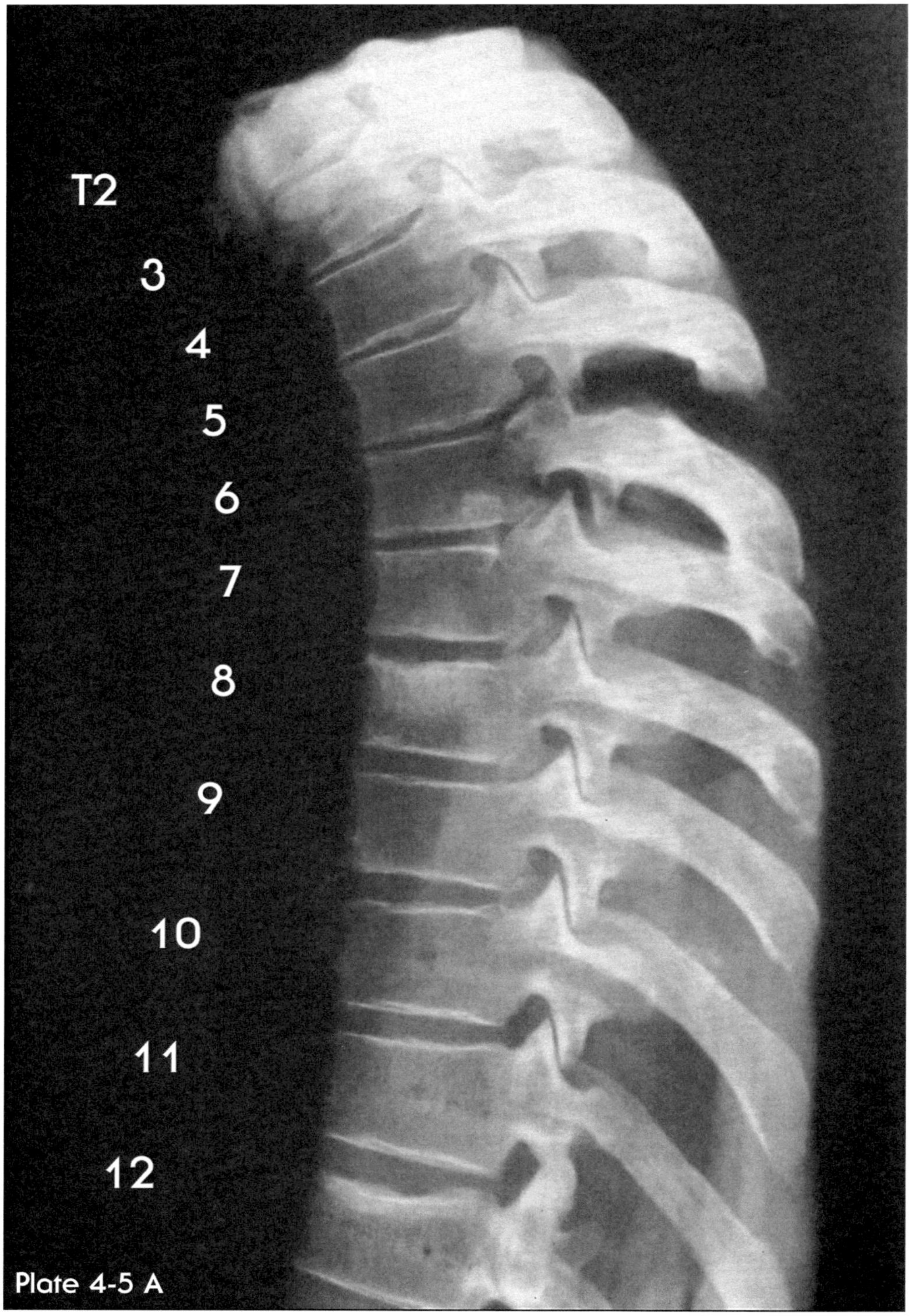

Plates 4-5 A & B
REVERSED LOWER THORACIC CURVE (T7-T11)
Thoracic Spine : Anterolisthesis lower thoracics

T2-T6 appear normal except for endplate damage with slight spurring anteriorly with all segments, indicating an anterior weight bearing posture. There is a mild reversal of the

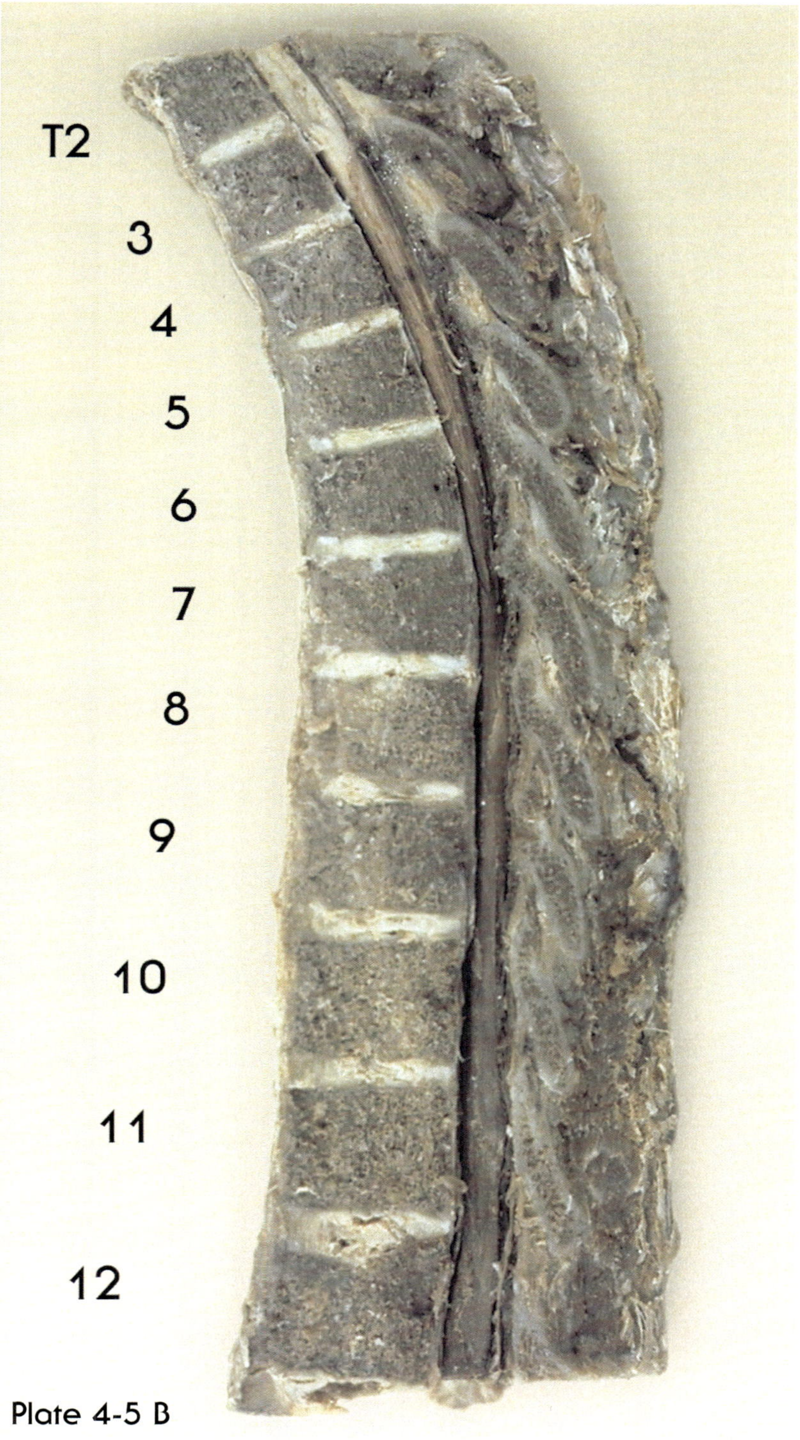

Plate 4-5 B

thoracic curve with an anterior apex at T10. Compression damage from T7 to T12 and all endplates have signs of repair. All discs have anterior brown degeneration with a Schmorl's node in the superior T8 endplate; T12 vertebral body has suffered a compression fracture. Near normal alignment was maintained and disc pathology is only moderate to absent.

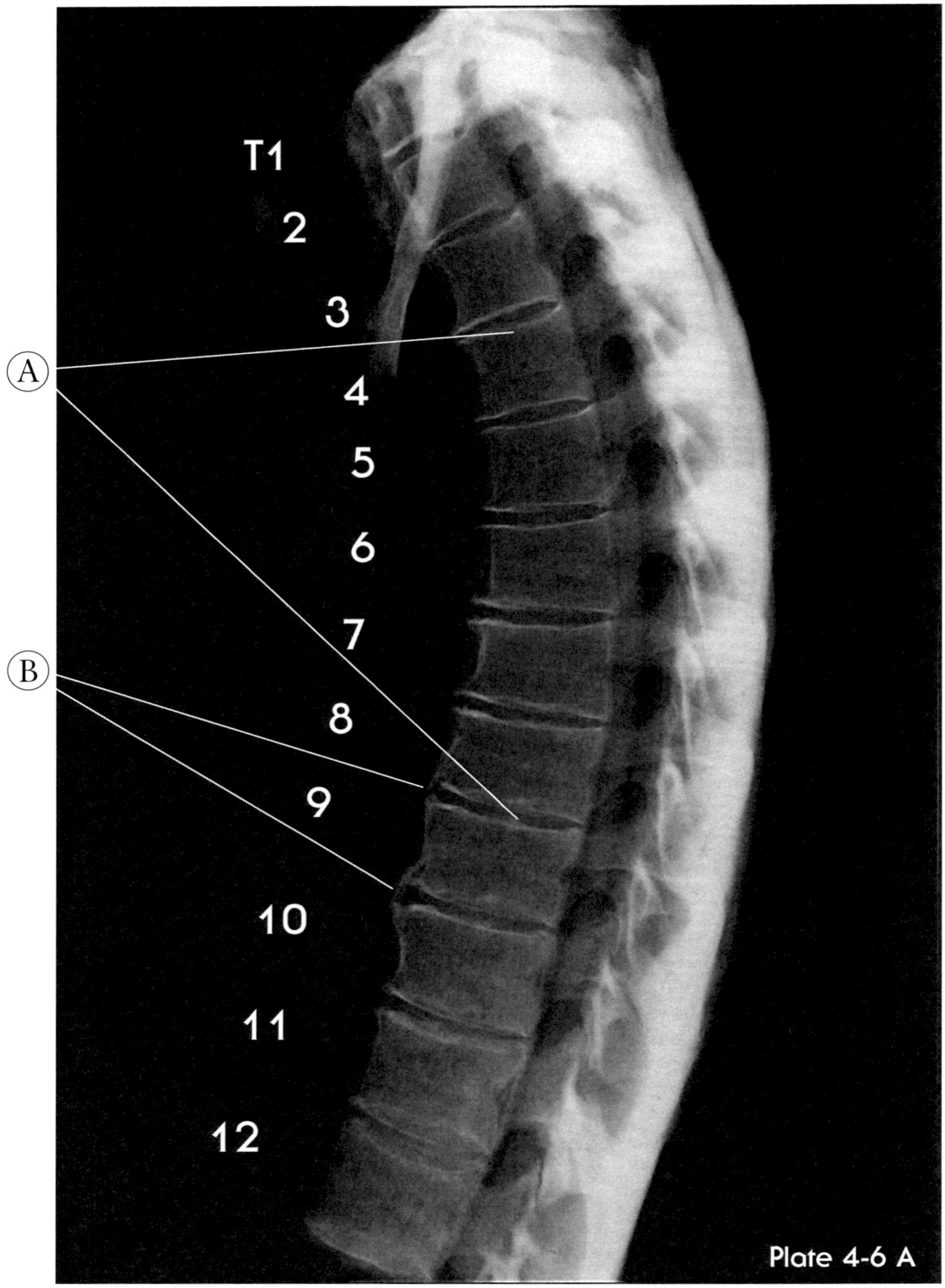

Plates 4-6 A & B

REVERSED LOWER THORACIC CURVE

Thoracic Spine: Anterolisthesis of lower thoracics

This specimen has a moderate reversal of the kyphotic curve from T8 to T11 with an anterior apex at T9. T1-T2 disc looks OK with slight brown degeneration of disc; T3 retro to T2 with anterior spurring of T2-T3 with slight disc tearing and bulging. From T3 to T12 there is anterior spurring, loss of disc height anteriorly with brown degeneration; T6 retro to T7 with compression of T6 or Schmorl's node on the inferior endplate of T6; T7-T8 tearing with

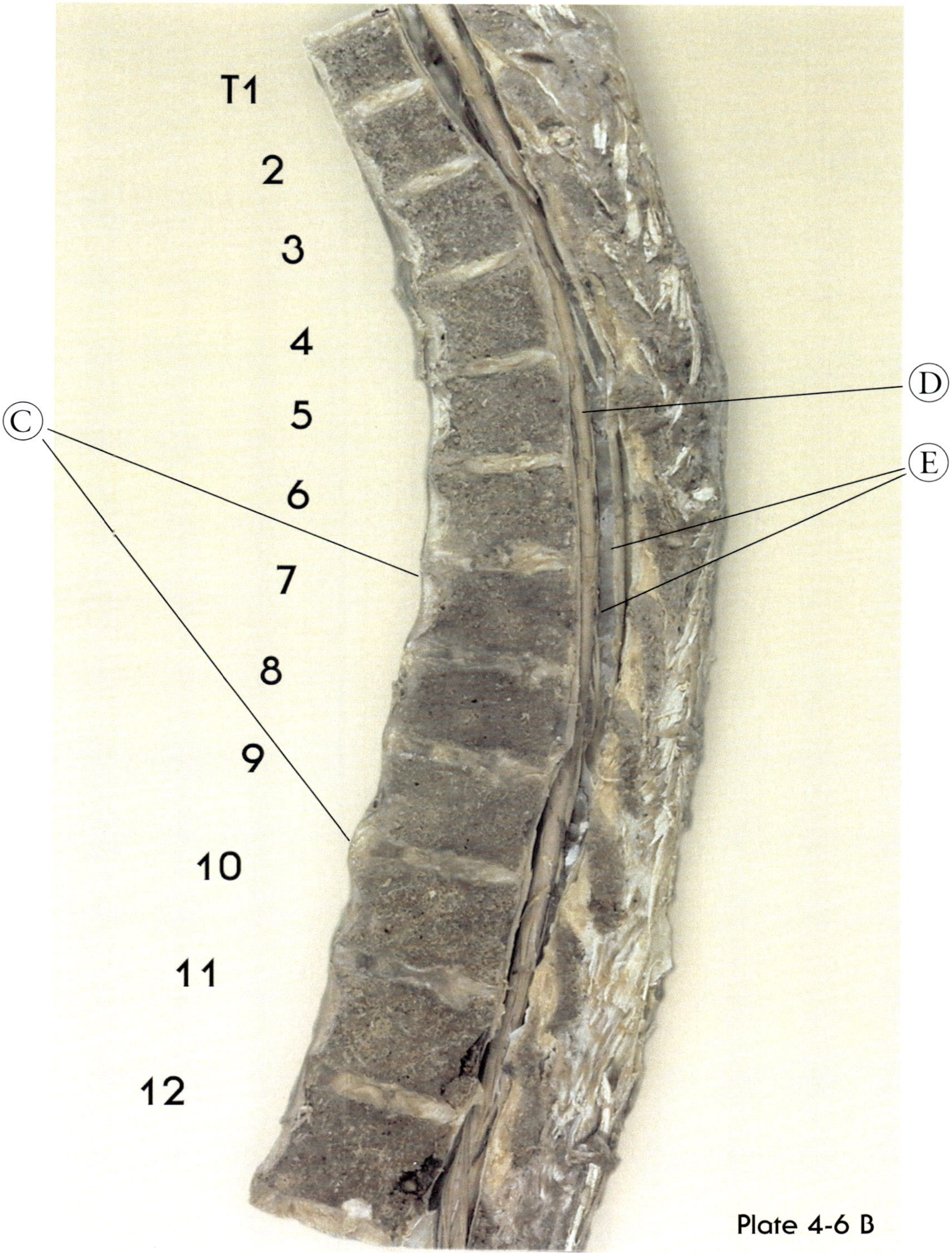

Plate 4-6 B

degeneration; T7-T11 are aligned with marginal and non-marginal osteophytes. All endplates appear to have repaired from significant axial loading.

(A) All endplates appear disrupted in various degrees.
(B) Para-spinal osteophytes, T8-T9, T9-T10; ossification of Anterior Longitudinal Ligament
(C) Appearance of hypertrophy of Anterior Longitudinal Ligament T7-T9.
(D) Spinal cord. Note anterior position in canal.
(E) There are intrathecal or subarachnoid adhesions on the dorsal aspect of the cord with nerve and vascular entrapment.

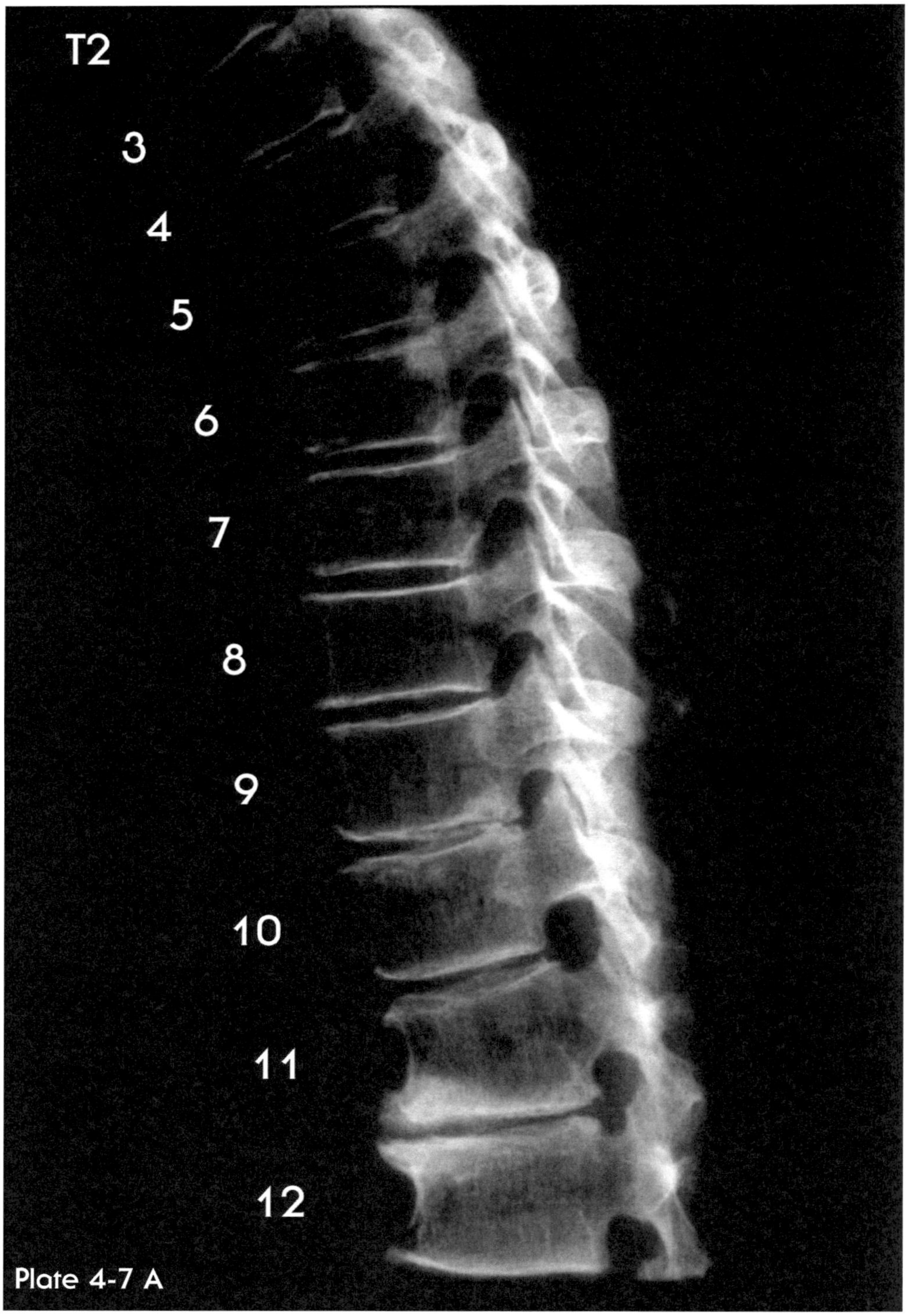

Plate 4-7 A

Plates 4-7 A & B

REVERSED LOWER THORACIC CURVE

This specimen has a reversed kyphotic curve from T7 to T11 with an anterior apex at T9. T2-T6 look normal except for the anterior disc degeneration. There are subluxations of T7 to T12 with varying degrees of degeneration, anterior spurring, endplate sclerosis and

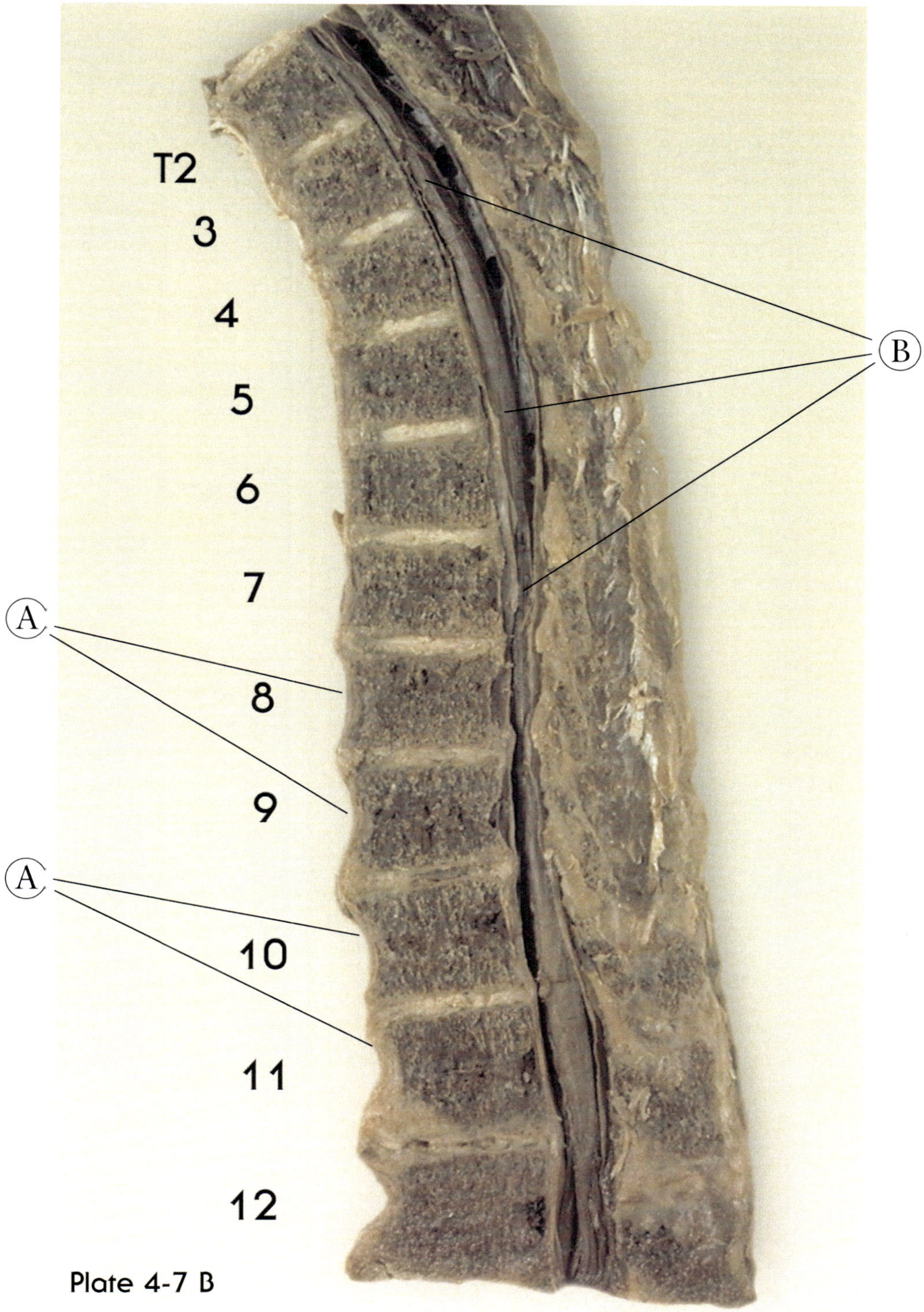

Plate 4-7 B

anteriorly bulging discs. T11 is a complete retrolisthesis with T12 having signs of compression repair, anterior spurring, and slight posterior spurring. There is severe DJD with cavitation of the disc.

(A) Hypertrophy of the Anterior Longitudinal Ligament from T8 to T11

(B) The spinal cord is anteriorly displaced from T2-T7.

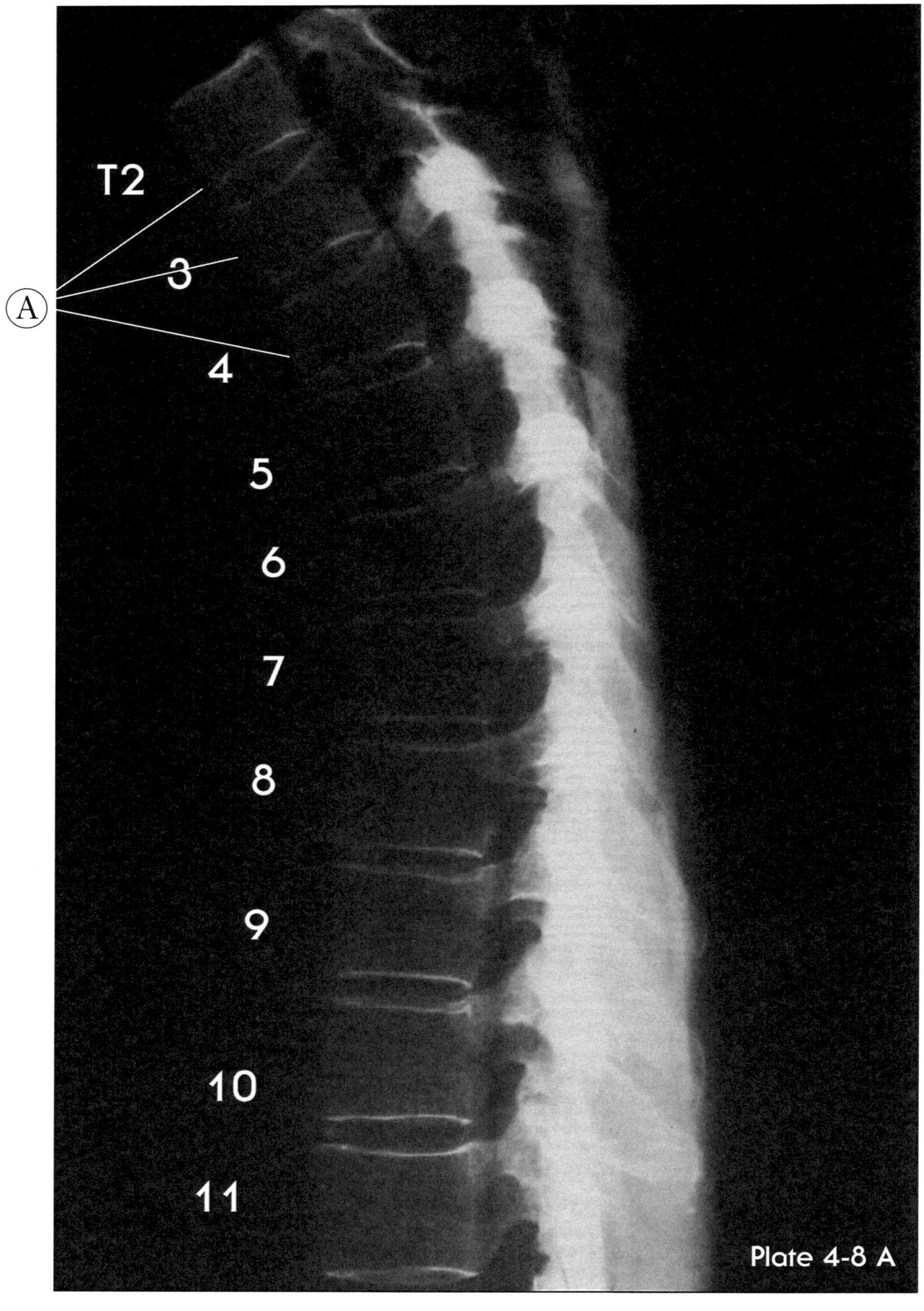

Plates 4-8 A & B

THORACIC UPPER POSTERIOR AND LOWER ANTEROLISTHESIS

T3 is retro to T2 with compression of T3 anteriorly, loss of the vertebral body height anteriorly and degeneration of the anterior disc T2-T3. Note cord in anterior canal to T7; T4 antero to T5; compression fracture of T5 of anteriorly results in loss of vertebral bodies' height with disc degeneration in anterior; T6 is retro to T5 with anterior disc bulge and degeneration; T7

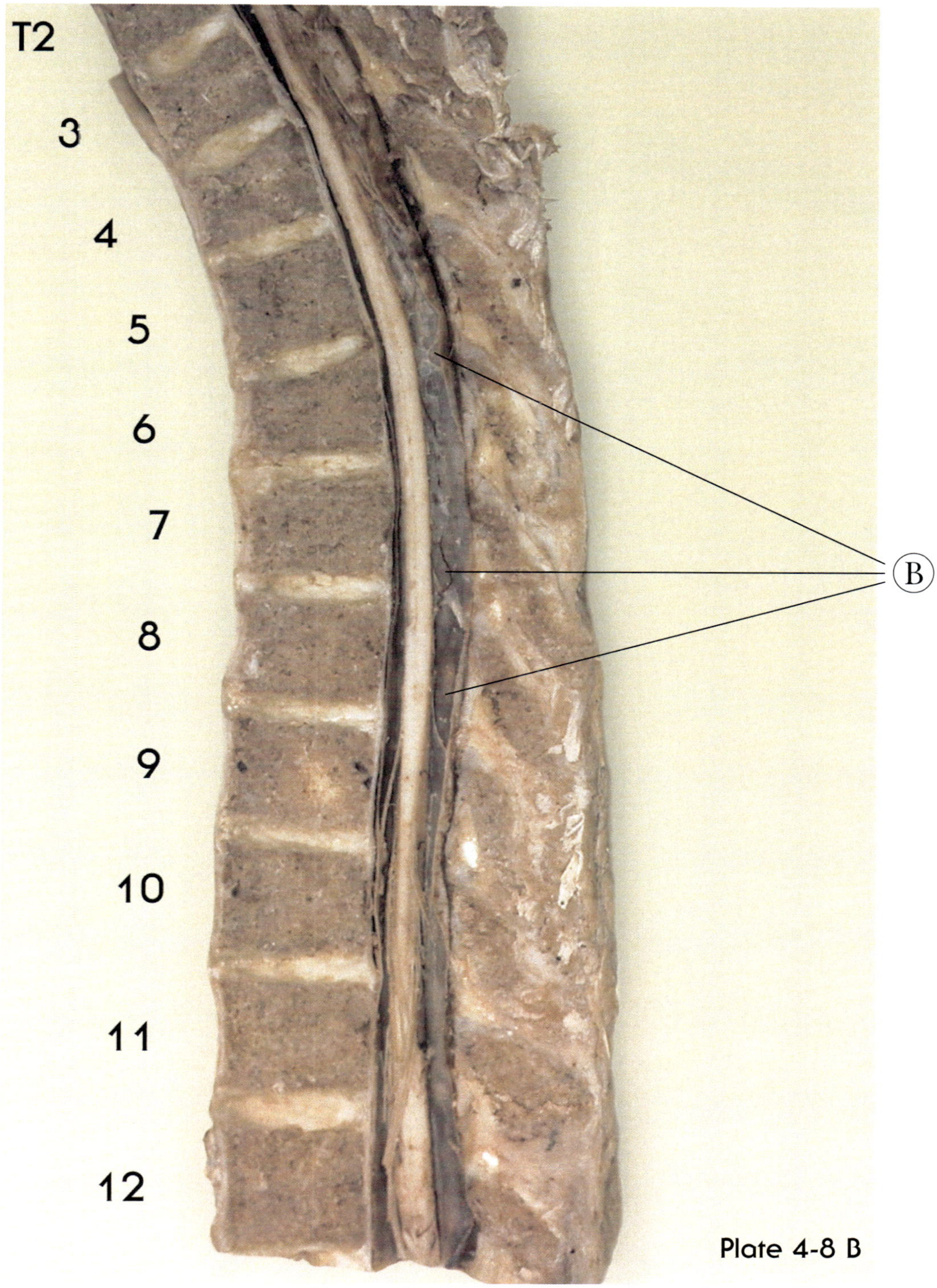

Plate 4-8 B

is anterior to T8 with anterior disc degeneration; T9 retro to T8 with anterior disc degeneration with very slight posterior disc bulge; T10 is retro to T9 with anterior disc degeneration and very slight posterior disc bulge T11 is retro to T10; T11-T12 is normal except for slight dehydration and degeneration.

(A) T2-T4 appear to have slight nuclear compressions.

(B) The intrathecal adhesions entrapping nerve roots and blood vessels.

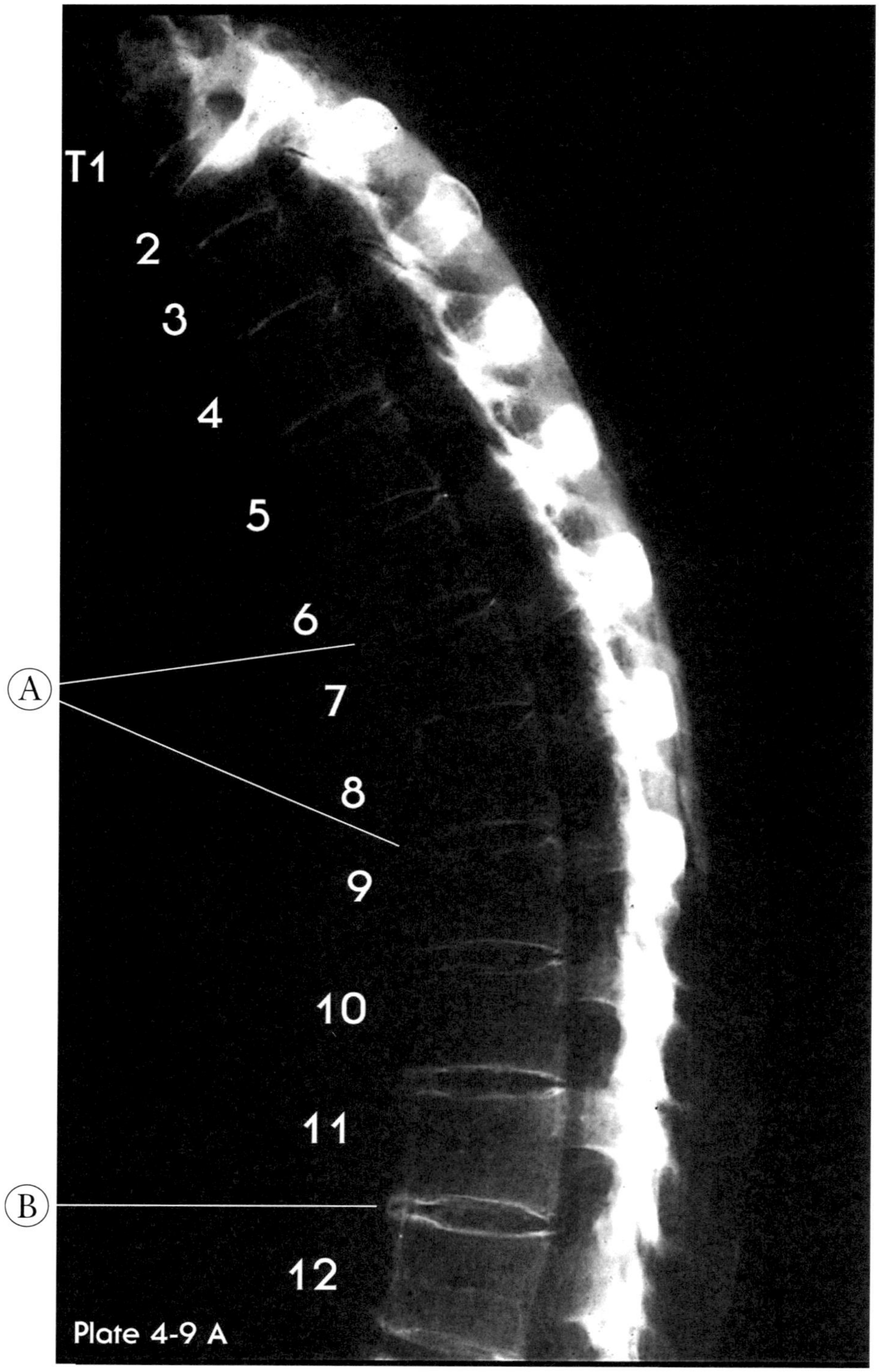

Plates 4-9 A & B
THORACIC SPINE - ANTEROLISTHESIS
UPPER AND LOWER VERTEBRAE

T1-T2 look normal with slight brown degeneration; T3 is retro to T2 showing disc tearing with anterior and posterior bulging ; T4 is retro to T3, with slight anterior spurring (marginal osteophyte); T5 is retro to T4. There is slight brown degeneration on all discs.

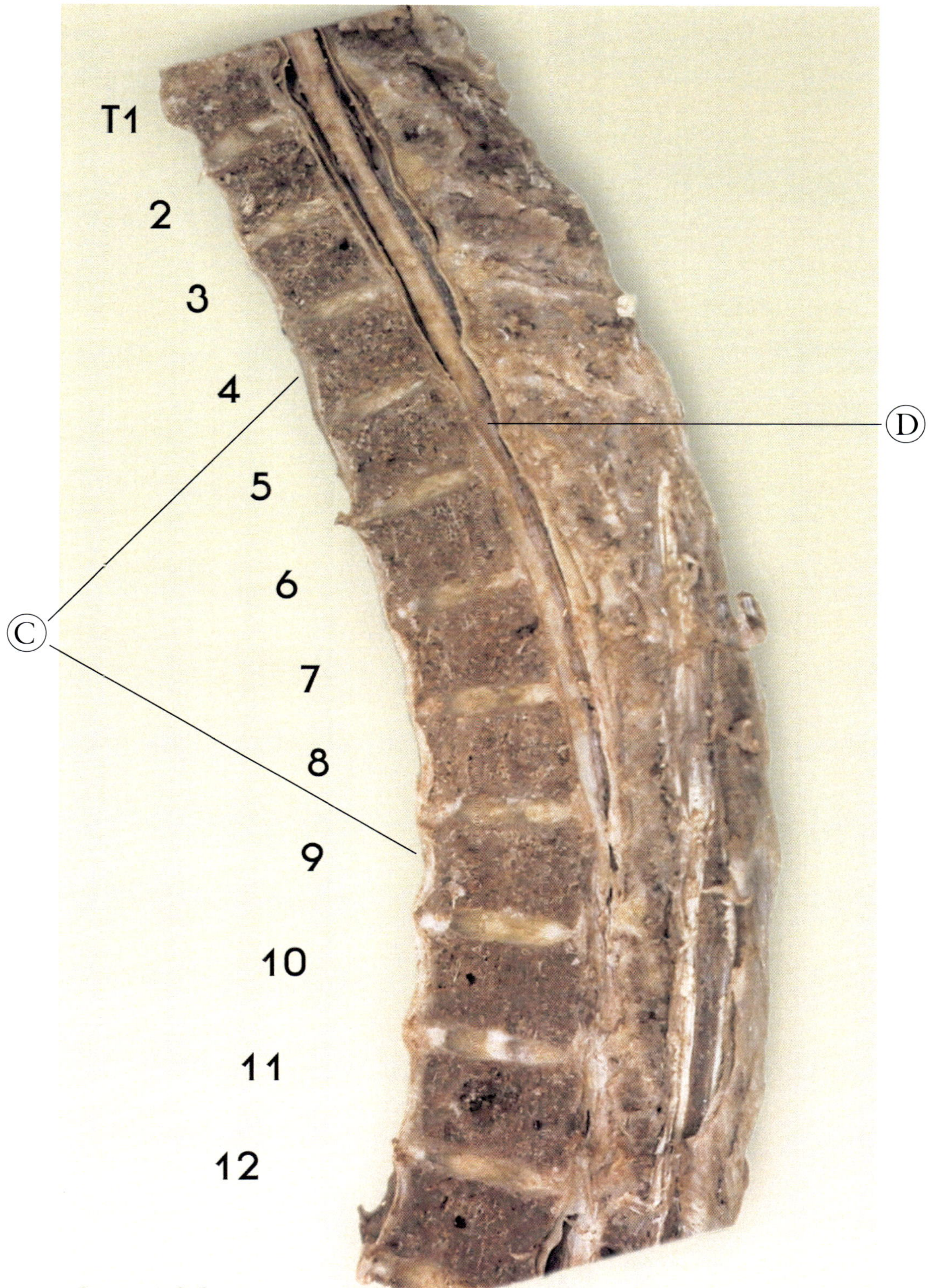

Plate 4-9 B

There is loss of the mid-sagittal plane at T3 and below exposing part of the outside and inside edge of the thecal sac.

(A) Beginning of calcification of discs T6-T7 to T1ˉ-T12.
(B) Para-spinal osteophytes of T10-T12.
(C) Hypertrophy of anterior longitudinal ligament from T4 to T9.
(D) Spinal cord on anterior wall of canal.

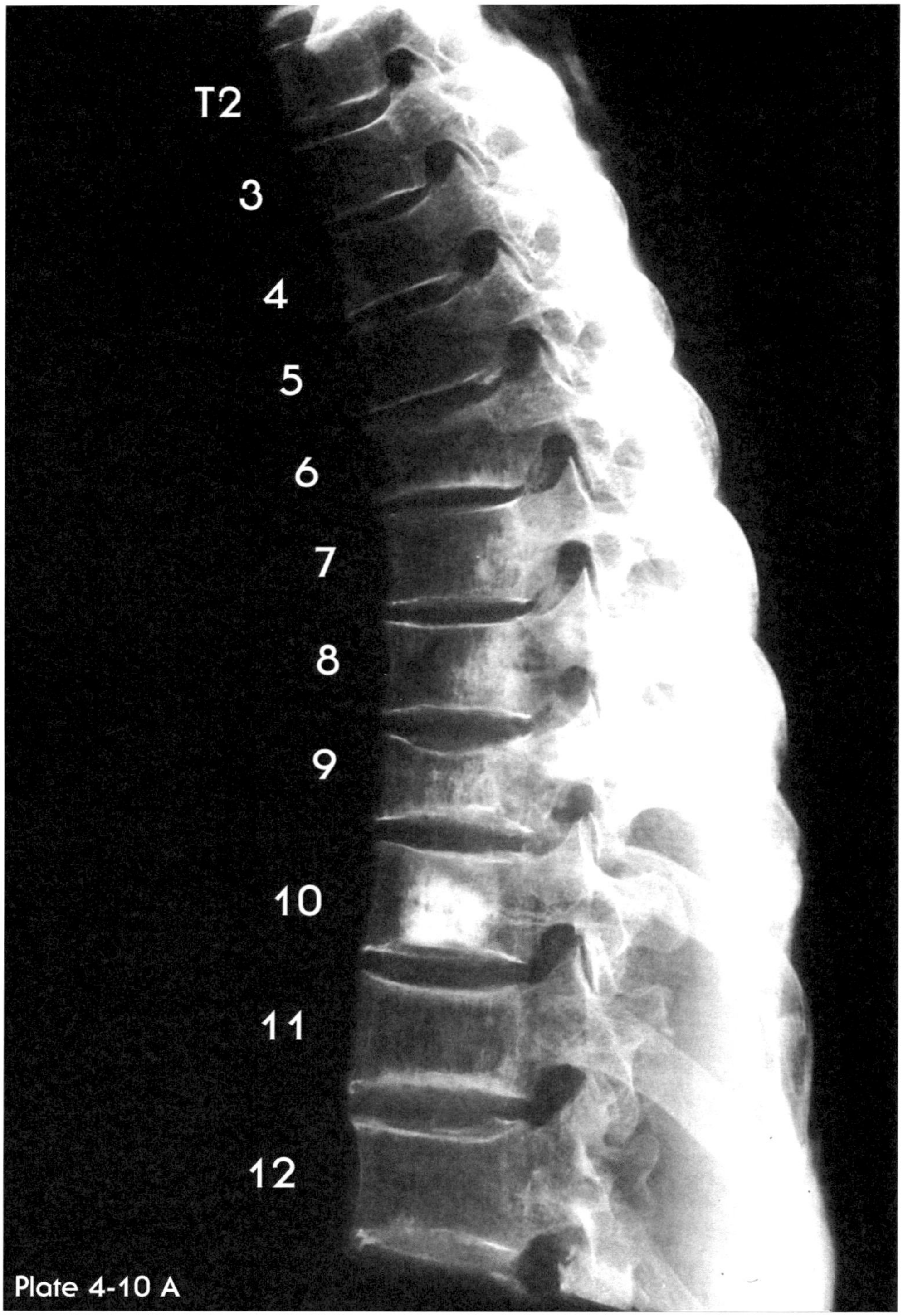

Plates 4-10 A & B

THORACIC SPINE: UPPER AND LOWER ANTEROLISTHESIS

There are compression fractures with loss of height of T6 and T9.
Vertebrae aligned throughout. All discs have slight to moderate DJD.

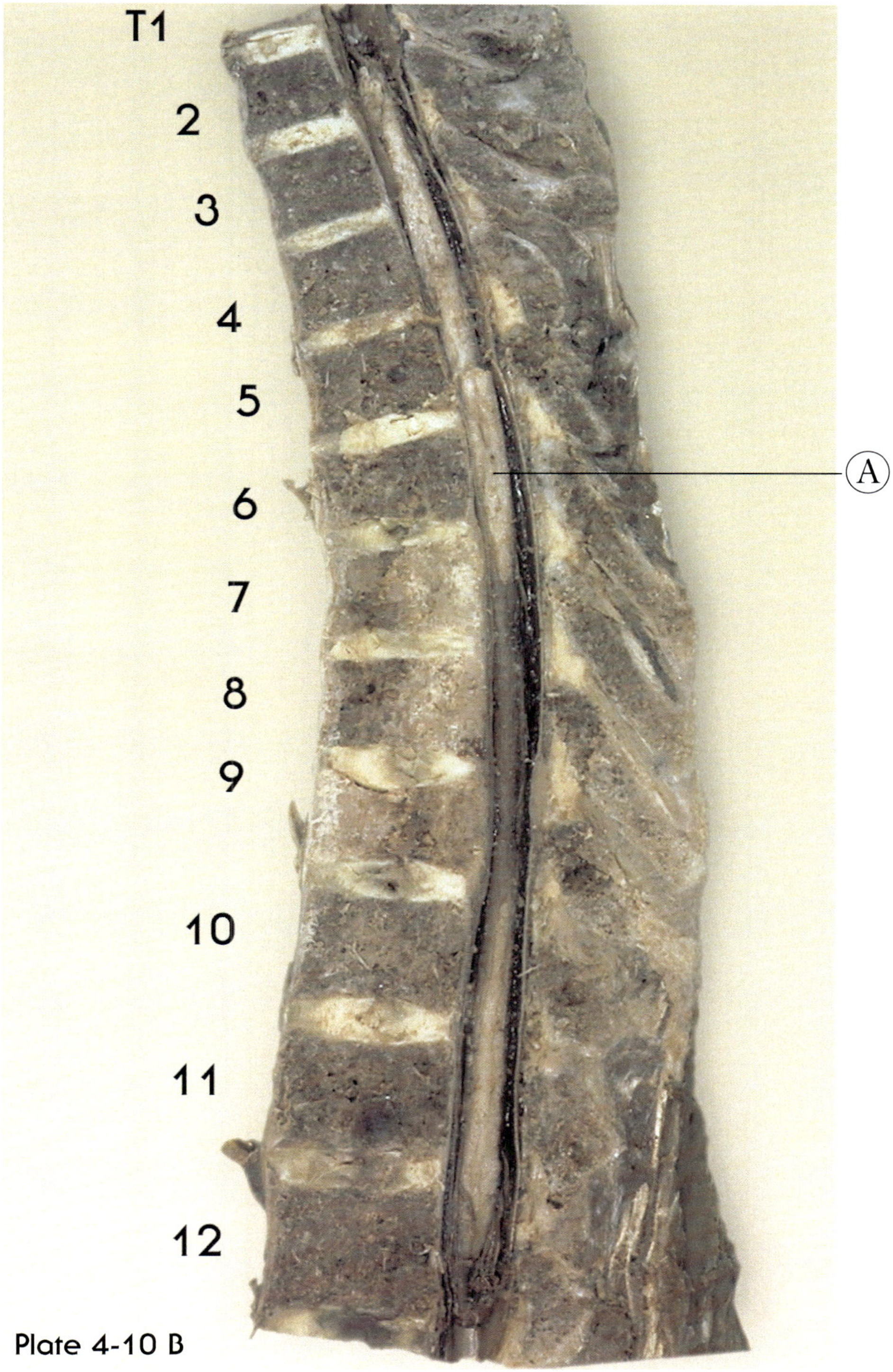

Plate 4-10 B

Compression fracture of T9, not a Schmorl's node; T9-T10 cavitation;T10-T11 tearing; T11 is a slight but complete anterolisthesis; T12 is retro to T11 with disc tearing, slight cavitation, and DJD.

(A) Spinal cord

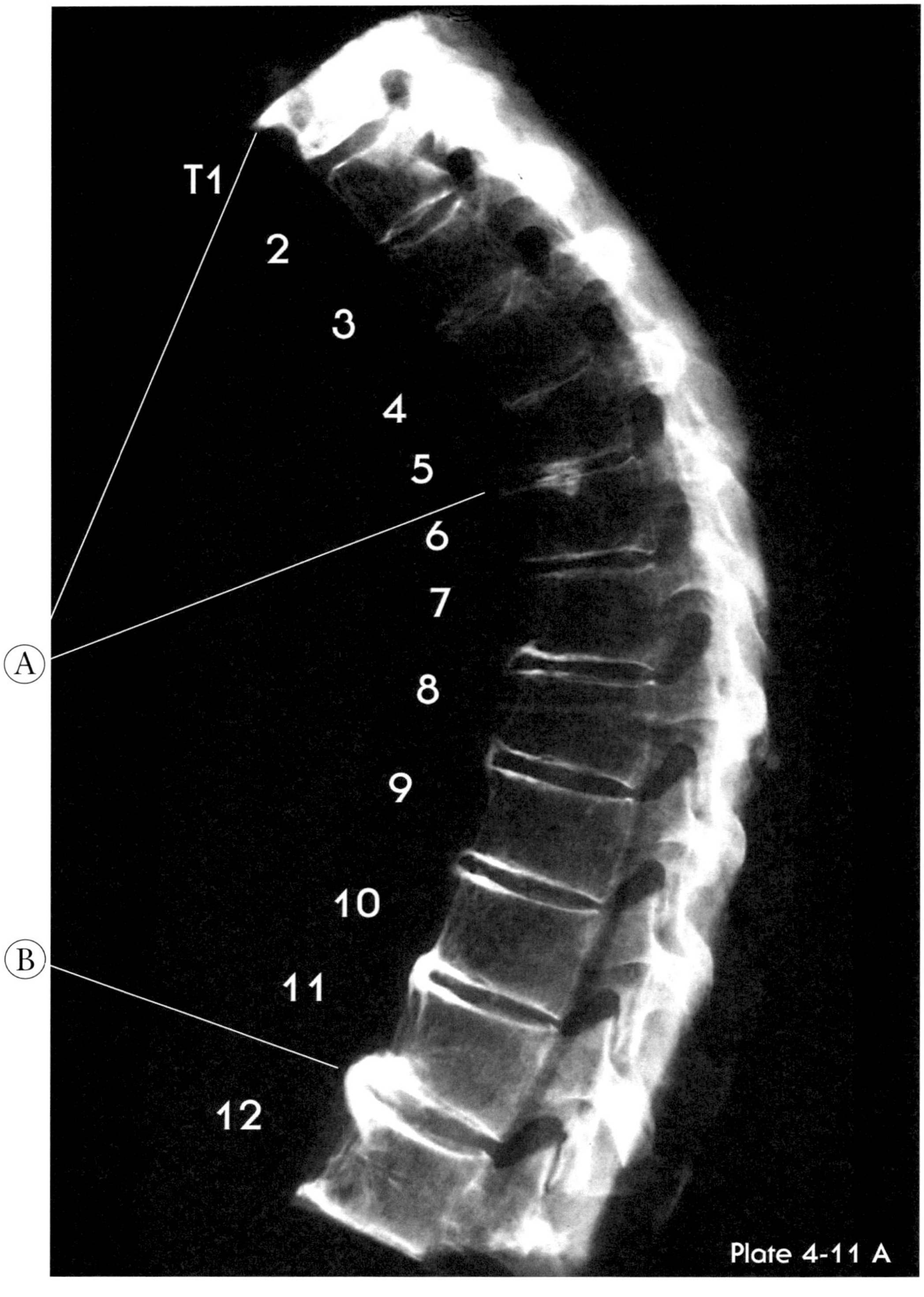

Plates 4-11 A & B
HYPERKYPHOSIS
Thoracic Spine: Progressive Spurring with Osteoporosis and Hyperkyphosis

This specimen has an increase in the kyphotic curvature with signs of trauma and calcification of part of the anterior longitudinal ligament. Almost all of the endplates are disrupted, with anterior disc narrowing from T2 to T7, and brown degeneration throughout. T3-T11 look aligned.

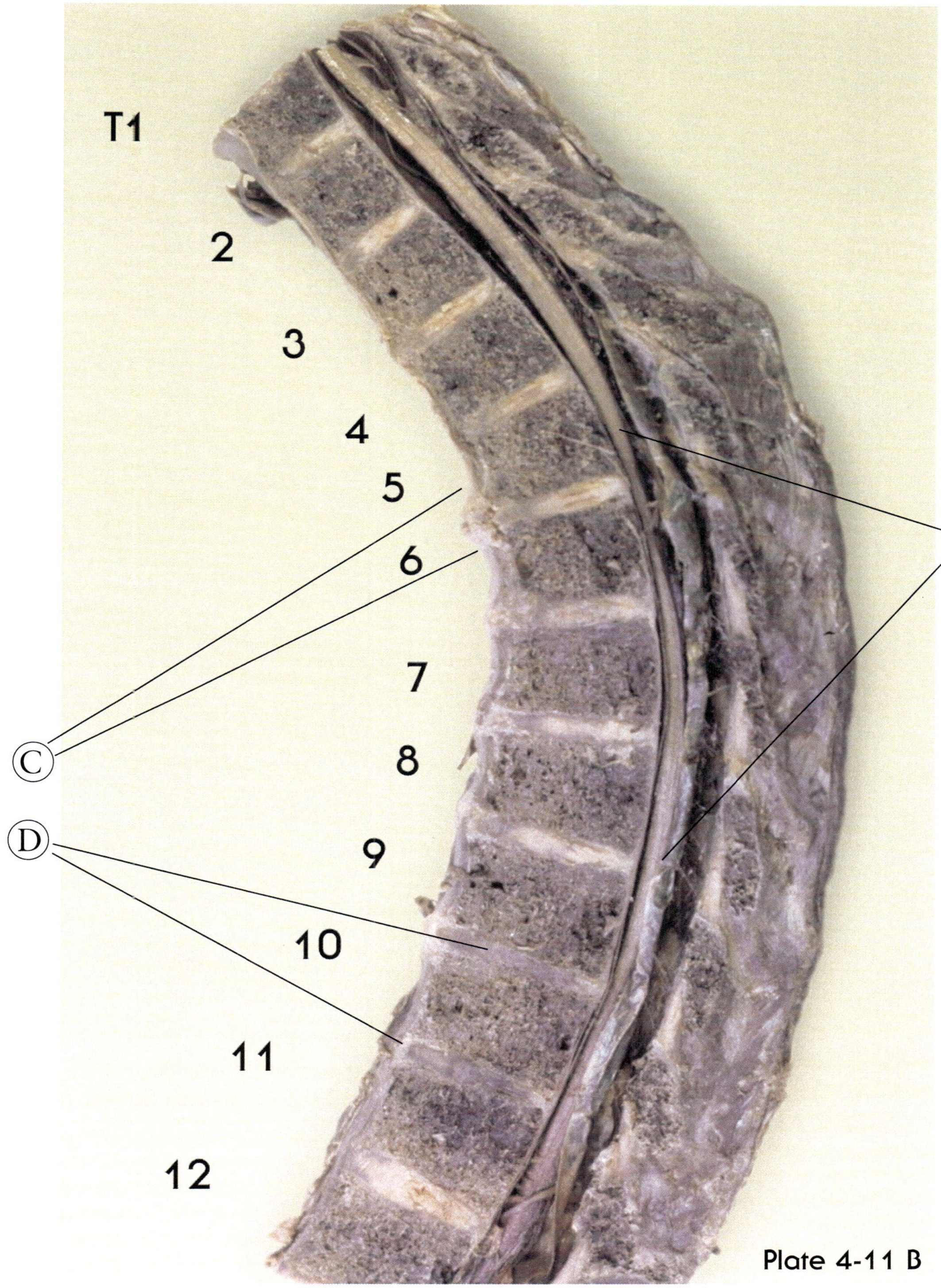

(A) Major marginal osteophytes at T1 and T5-T6.
(B) T11-T12 has significant calcification of anterior disc and A.L.L..
(C) The hypertrophy of the A.L.L. from T4-T8, only part is calcified. T3-T4 and inferior segments have hypertrophy of the A.L.L. as a result of compression and stress.
(D) T9-T10 and T10-T11 have significant disc dehydration and calcification.
(E) Note anterior placement of cord T5-T9. This condition of the A.L.L. hypertrophy from T3-T12 could qualify as "DISH" (Diffuse Idiopathic Skeletal Hyperostosis) because more than three consecutive segments involved. (An early stage?)

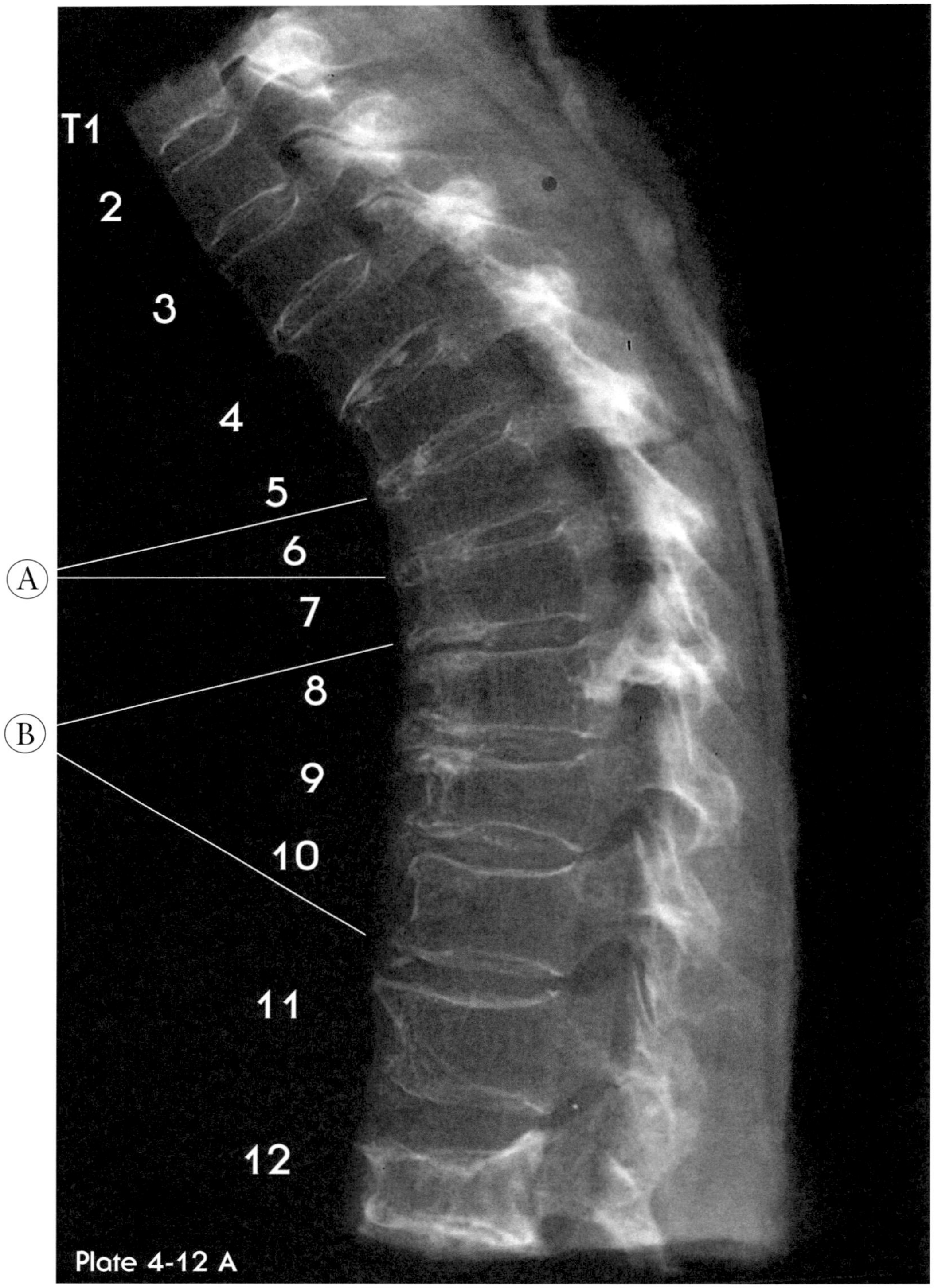

Plate 4-12 A

Plates 4-12 A & B
PROGRESSIVE SPURRING WITH HYPERKYPHOSIS
CAUSED BY OSTEOPOROSIS

This specimen has an increase in the kyphotic curvature as a result of subluxations, compression fractures, and loss of anterior disc height between T4 and T9. There is a very slight compression fracture of T4. T5 is retro to T4 with very slight compression fracture of

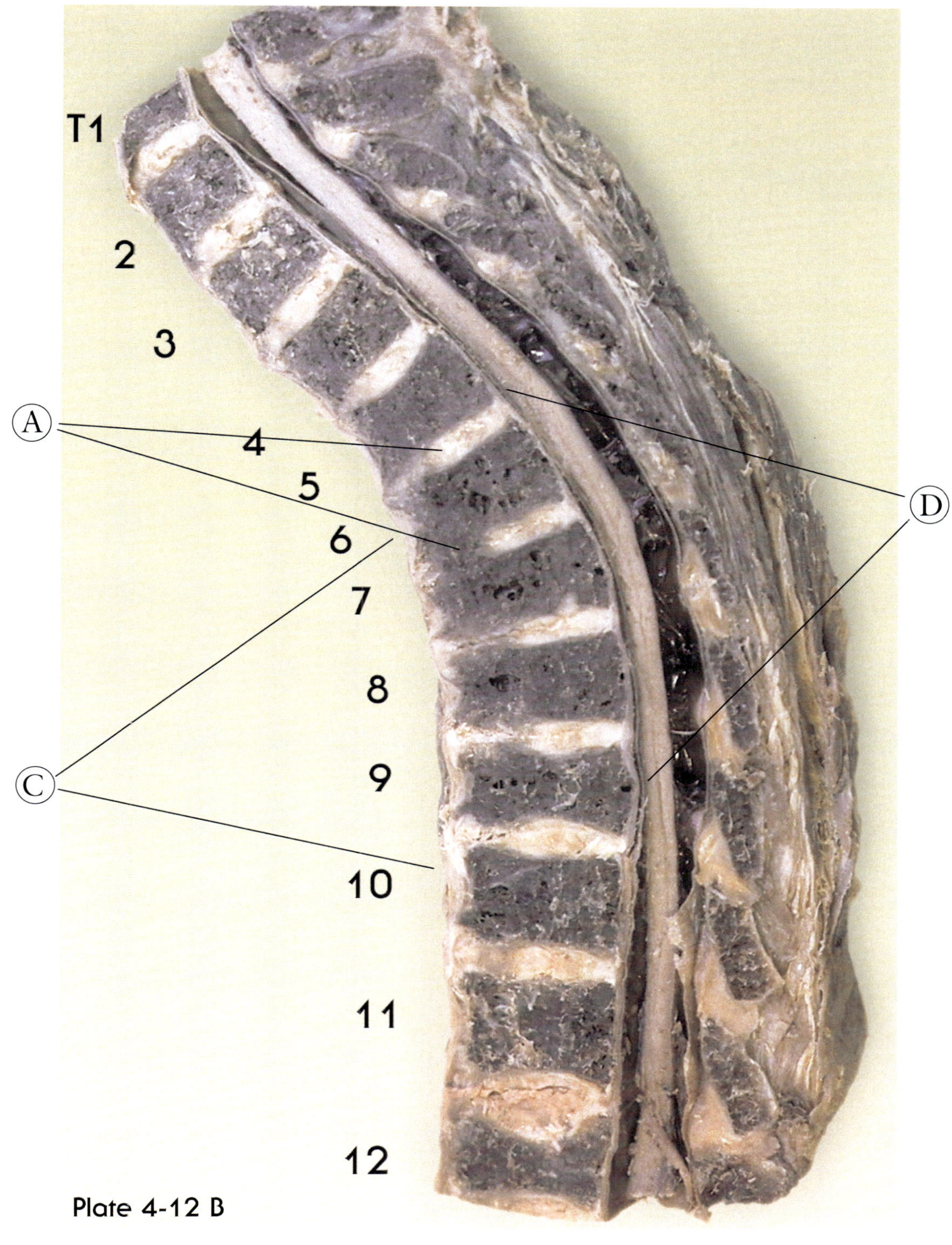

Plate 4-12 B

T5 with calcification of the disc. T6-T12 have normal alignment but changes due to compression fractures of T6-T12.

(A) Some discs have dark brown areas that correspond to calcified appearance on X-ray.
(B) There is anterior vertebral body spurring from T3 to T12.
(C) Hypertrophy of A.L.L. from T5-T12.
(D) There is spinal cord-canal contact from T5 to T9.

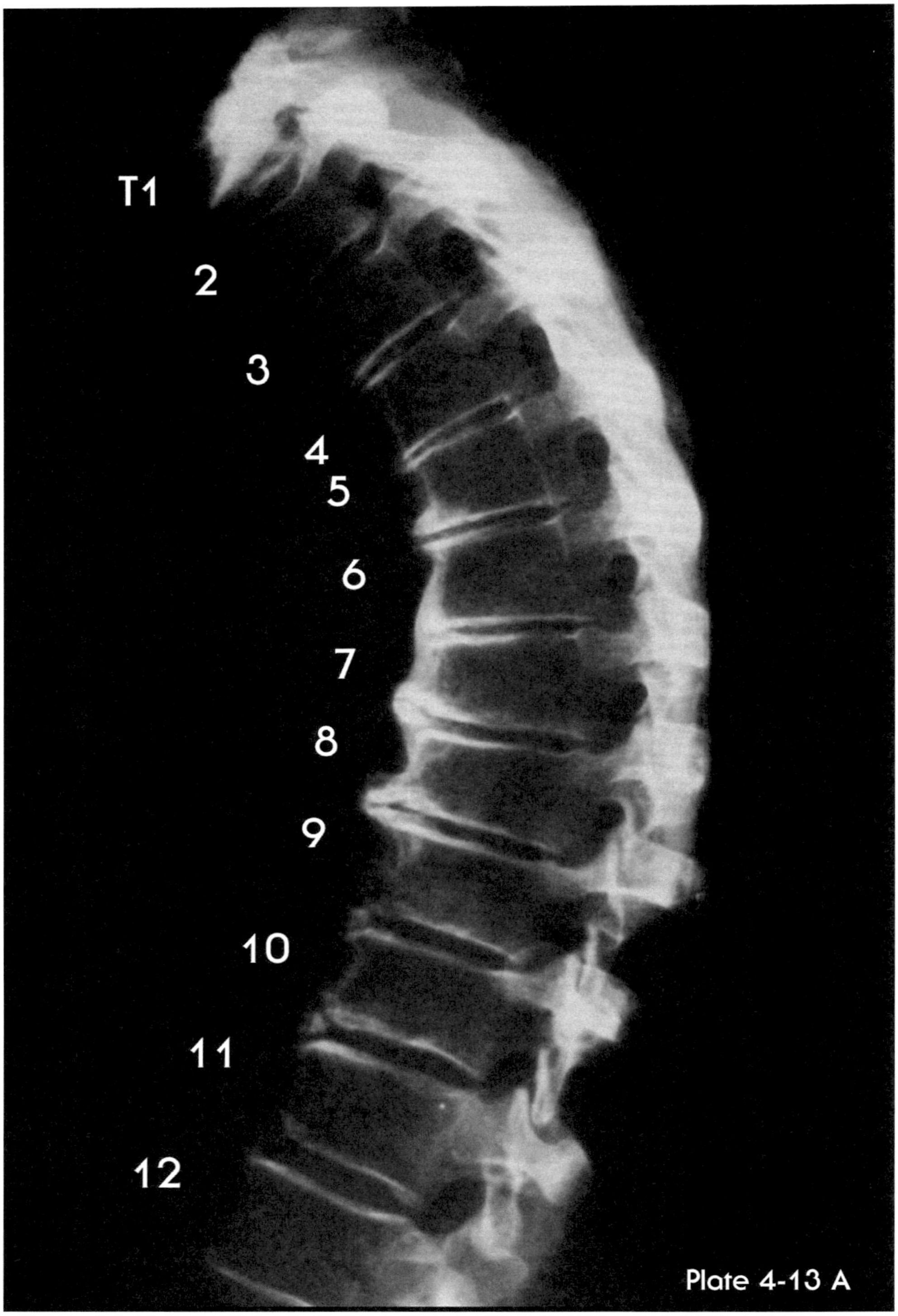

Plates 4-13 A & B

PROGRESSIVE SPURRING AND HYPERKYPHOSIS.

There appear to be no anterior/posterior subluxations. The hyperkyphosis is due to compression fractures of T5 to T11 with some loss of disc height. T6 to T9 has an anterior fusion with para-spinal osteophytes of four segments [DISH].

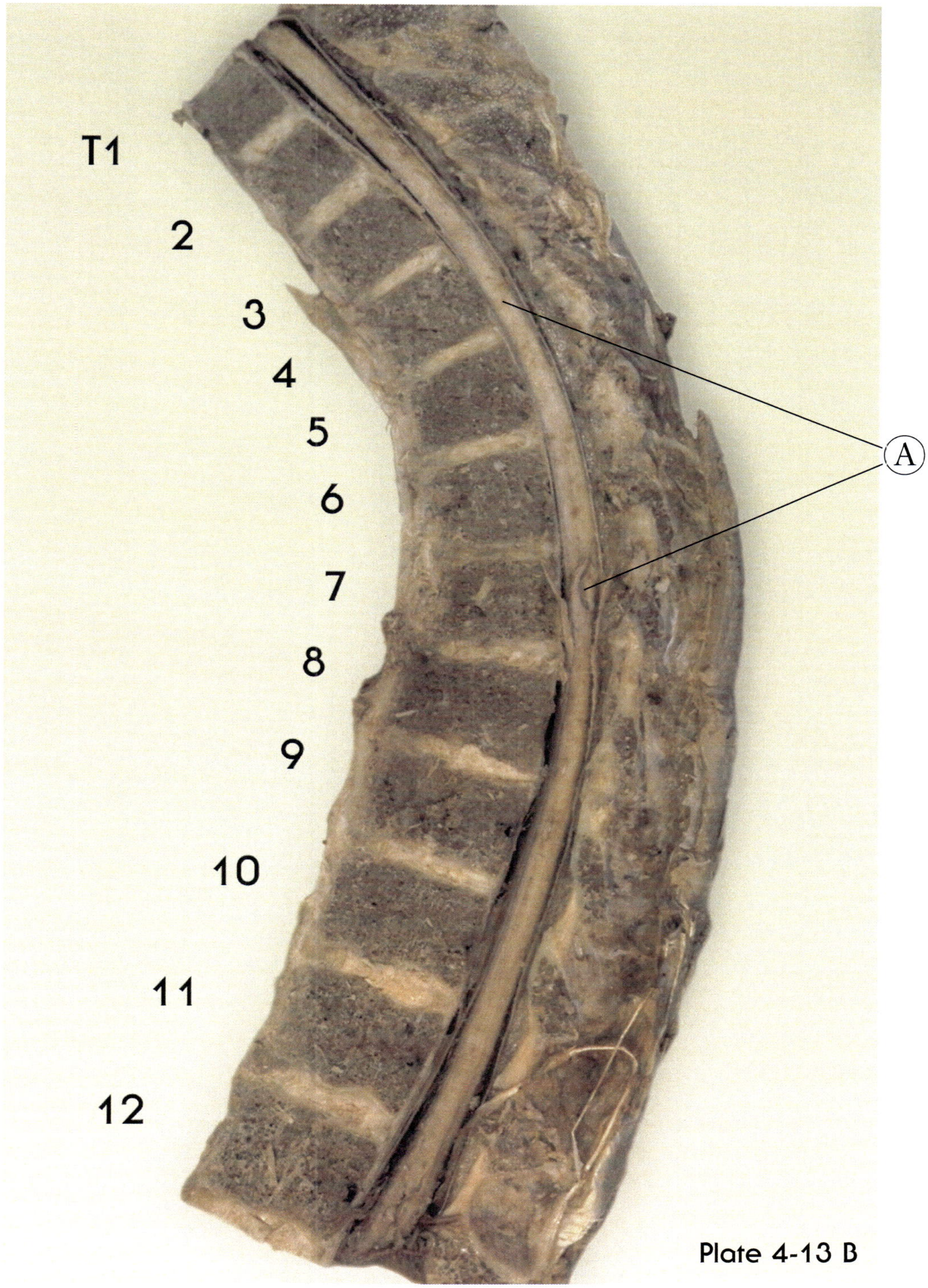

(A) Cord-canal contact. Note: This individual had a near normal cervical curve and lumbar curve.

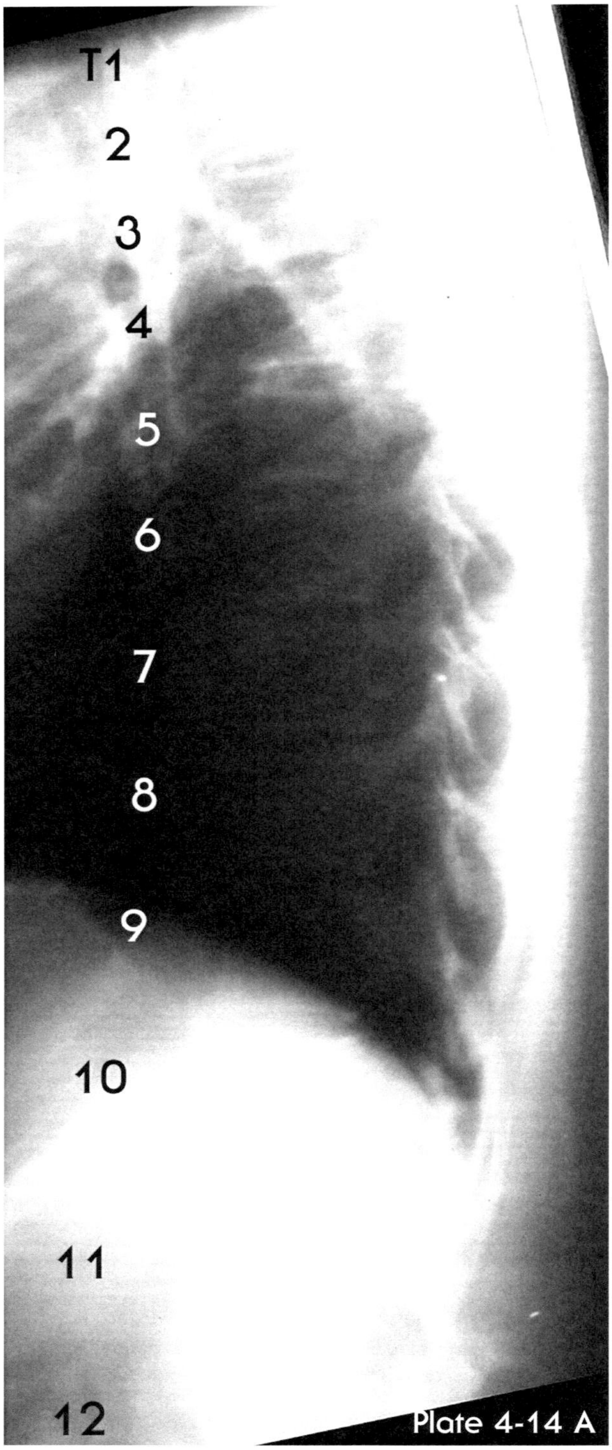

Plates 4-14 A & B

THORACIC SPINE: X-RAY AND MRI OF PATIENT WITH CORD TETHERING DUE TO ALTERED CURVES

Note the hypokyphosis and cord-canal contact from T3 to T9.

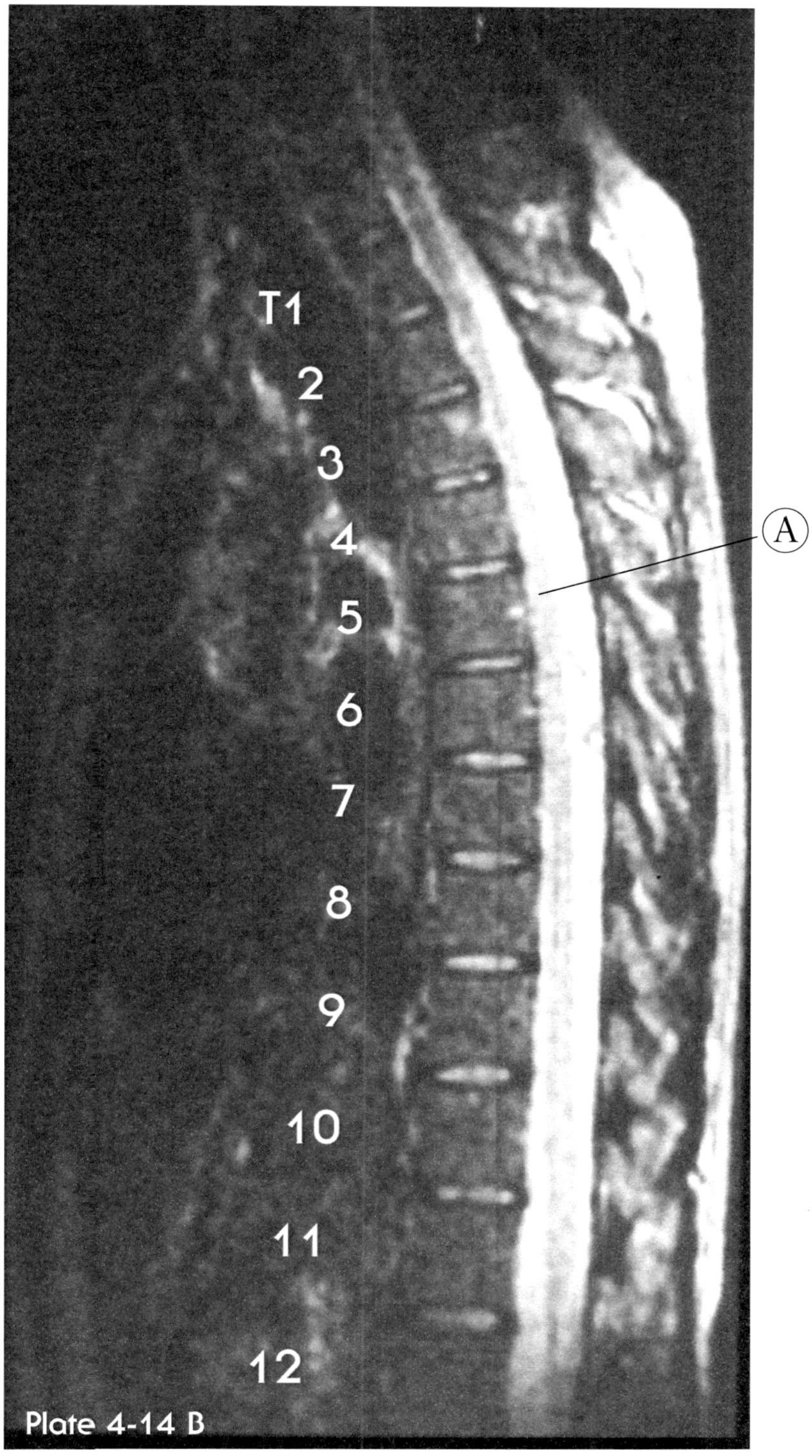

This patient has many internal organ symptoms that are worsened by sitting at her desk. When she is away from work her digestion, ulcer, bowel and bladder complaints "mysteriously" go away.

(A) Spinal cord

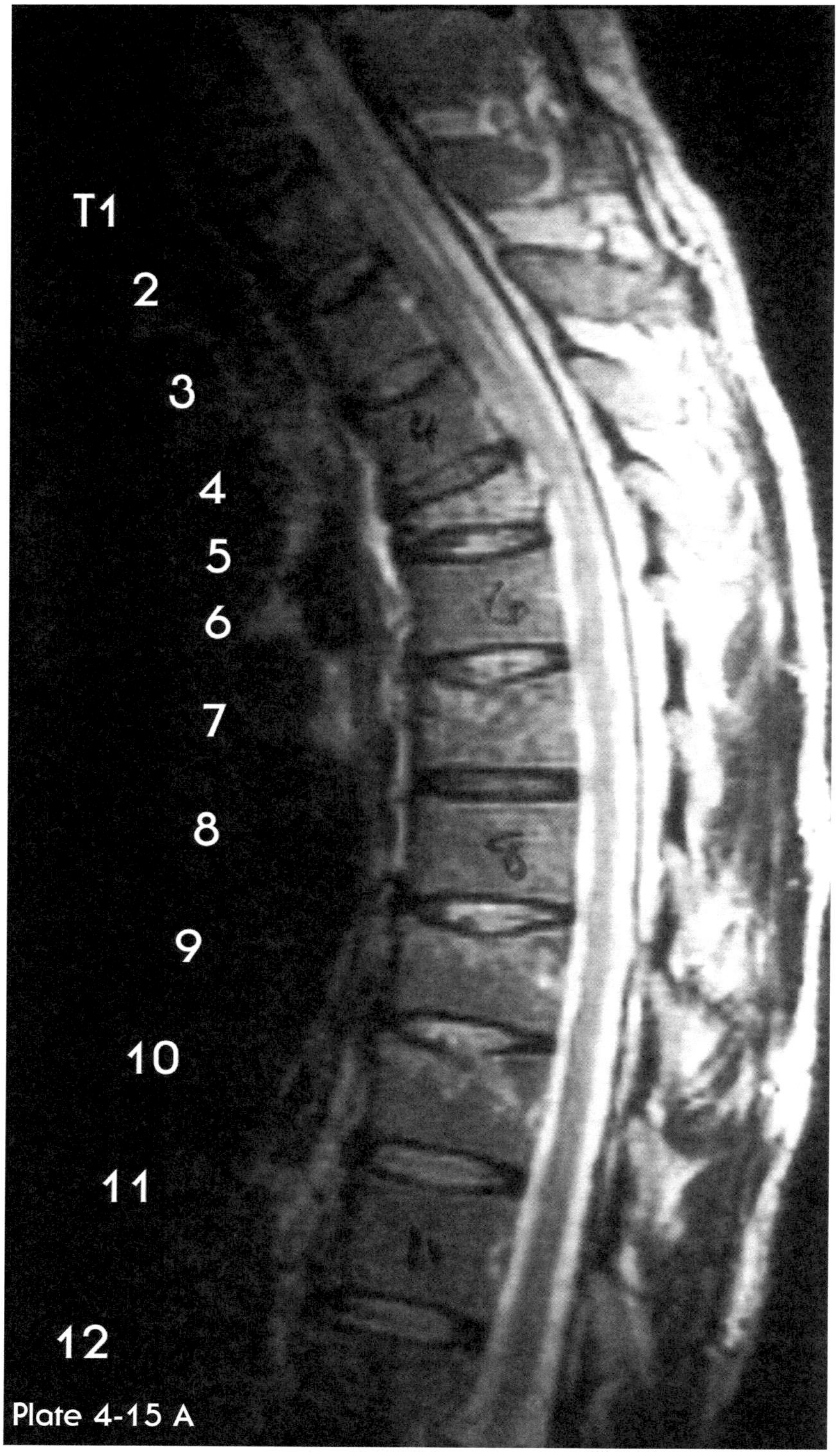

Plate 4-15 A

Plates 4-15 A & B

HYPERKYPHOSIS DUE TO COMPRESSION FRACTURE

Here are two MRIs of the same individual with different contrasts or "signals". There are compression fractures of T5, T7, T9, and T10, with only T5 suffering a major change of shape. There is a moderate retropulsion of T5 into the canal, with spinal cord contact in the supine positition.

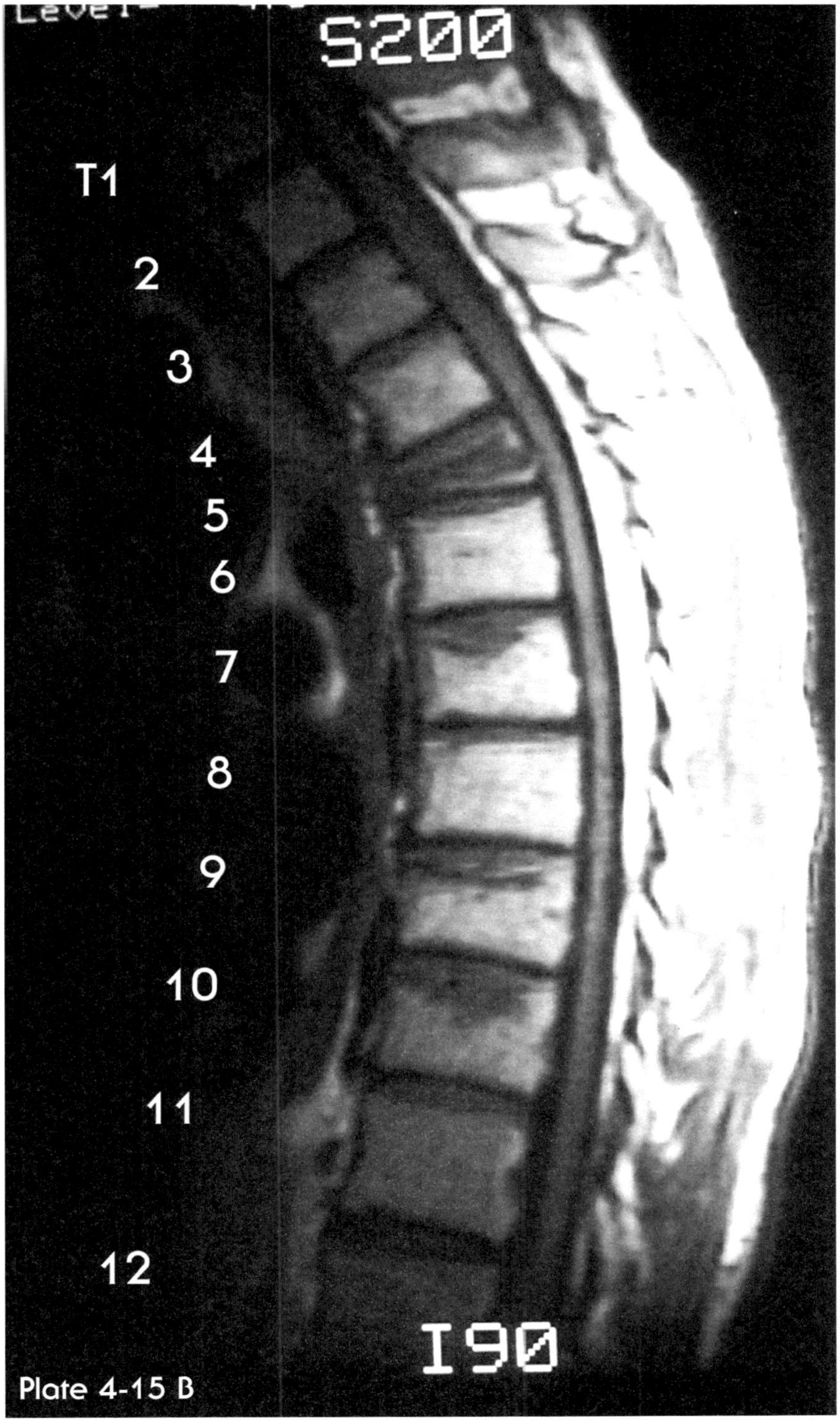

Plate 4-15 B

Certain flexed positions caused moderate to severe radiating rib and chest pain in the T5-T6 area. Cervical hypolordosis adversely affects the spinal cord after an injury to the thoracic spine. There is tractioning of the cord from T3-T9 caused by cervical hypolordosis and hyperkyphosis of the thoracic spine. This image is taken in the recumbent position which gives the patient relief. The symptoms appear while sitting and worsen with neck flexion.

CHAPTER FIVE

Subluxations Of The Lumbar Spine

Discussion

The lumbar spine bears more of the body's weight than any other part of the vertebral column, as its massive body and robust facets indicate. Normally, a lordotic curve is present or should be present in the lumbar spine. Both the angles of the facets and the angle between the pedicles and vertebral bodies necessitate this curvature. A three point weight bearing system exists with the two pairs of facets and vertebral bodies each bearing roughly a third of the gravitational load. Separations of the spinous processes and facets (flexion) increase the length of the posterior wall of the spinal canal and put all the weight bearing on the discs. Anatomical studies of trabecular patterns of the bone clearly indicate that the facets are weight-bearing joints.[1,2,3,4,5] In **Figure 5-1** a CT Scan of L4 shows hypertrophy of the left articular facets and loss of joint space, common features of subluxation.

Alteration of the curve of the lumbar spine can cause these articular facets to separate or hyper load. Shifting of most of the gravitational load to the discs and vertebral bodies occurs with an unequal loading of the articular facets. Note the osteophytes and altered joint space is on the left in **Figure 5-1**. Chronic subluxation of the lumbar spine stops normal motion of the discs and interrupts their hydraulic function (**see Figure 5-2**). This specimen has three levels of disc degeneration. Notice the alignment of L1 and L2 and the condition of the disc. There is misalignment of L3 posteriorly to L2, with wedging, tearing, and bulging of the disc. This condition is caused by subluxation and the resulting loss of normal motion and hyper loading. The L3-L4 disc is even more distressed, which is caused by the retrolisthesis of L4. There is significant dehydration, tearing, cavitation, and loss of disc height.

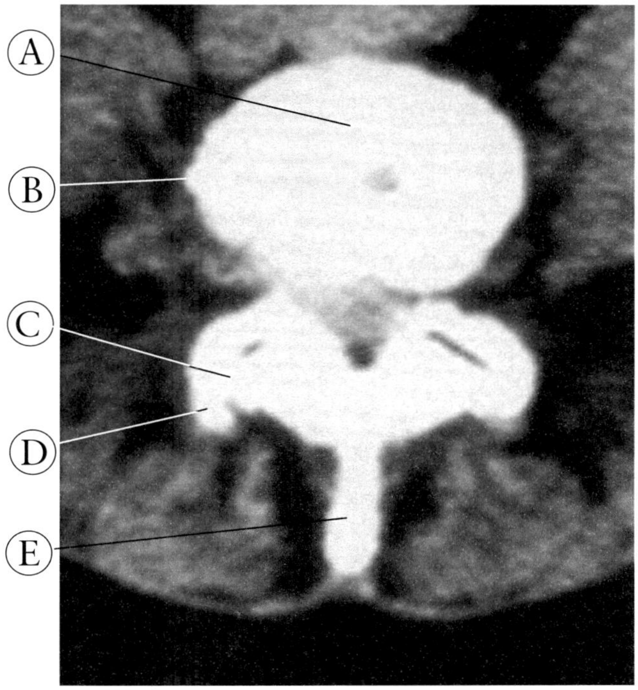

Figure 5-1
CT SCAN OF L4 IN AN INDIVIDUAL WITH CHRONIC LUMBAR SUBLUXATIONS AND OSTEOARTHRITIS.
The altered weight bearing has affected the facets and body of the vertebra. Note that the hypertrophy of the vertebra in the body and articular facet is on the left.

(A) Body of vertebra
(B) Osteophytes or "spurs"
(C) Diminished joint space
(D) Altered facet
(E) Spinous process

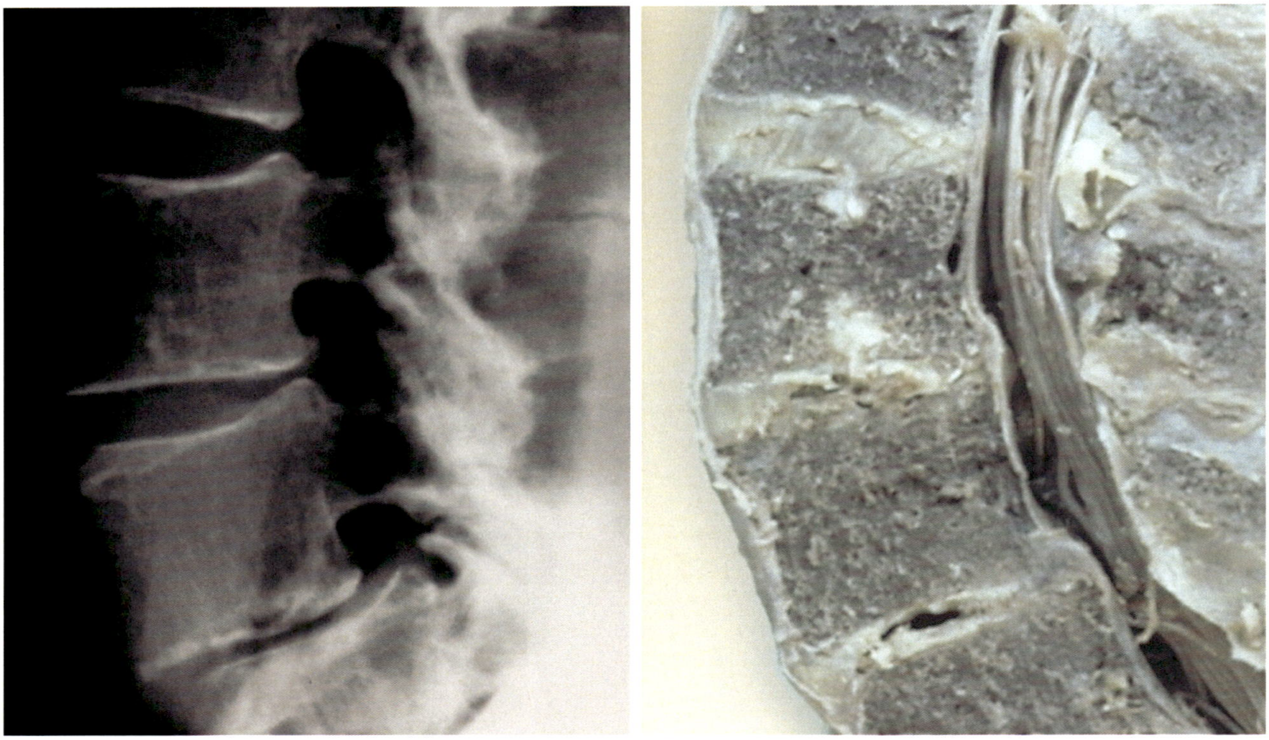

Figure 5-2
A VIEW OF VARYING DEGREES OF DISC HEALTH.
Note the different conditions of the discs in the same individual. The subluxations and disc degeneration are intimately related. When normal alignment is maintained the disc can be in good health regardless of age. All the discs in this specimen are the same age but only the subluxated motor units degenerate.

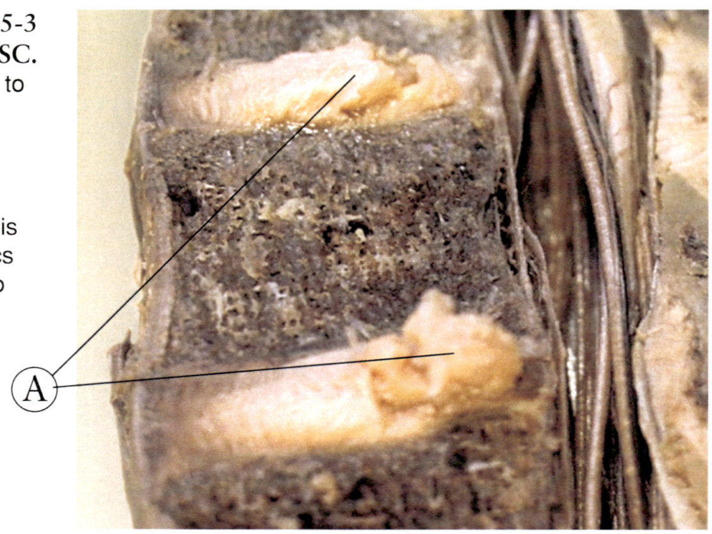

Figure 5-3
THE HYDROPHILIC DISC.
The L2-L3 and L3-L4 discs have been exposed to tap water after the lumbar spine was cut in a sagittal plane. The nucleus pulposus in this cadaver have absorbed the water and have bulged. This is an expected phenomenon. The annular walls and endplates normally contain this water absorbing glycoprotein matrix. These discs convey motion between and transmit the load to the vertebrae.

(A) Nucleus pulposus

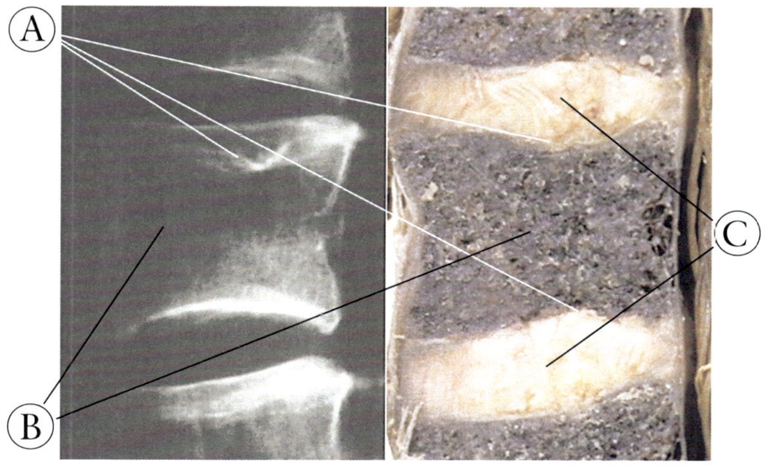

Figure 5-4
THE SHOCK ABSORBING VERTEBRAL BODY.

The superior and inferior endplates have been damaged and repaired with the deforming force being absorbed by the L2 vertebral body. Under the load the endplates deflect more than the annular walls. Notice the discs have remained relatively healthy and that the alignment was not disturbed by the trauma.

(A) Damaged endplates
(B) Vertebral body
(C) Discs

The lumbar intervertebral disc is the largest avascular structure in the body. To remain healthy, it is dependent upon the constant, slow influx of fluid.[6,7,8,9] In **Figure 5-3** the hydrophilic nature of the nucleus pulposus is demonstrated in near normal discs. After exposure to water the newly cut edge of the nucleus pulposus bulged out with the absorbed water. The normal disc has between 76 to 89% volume of water.[10]Many studies have been conducted on the subject, but the latest research indicates that loading and unloading during normal spinal motion is the primary mechanism for disc nutrition and fluid exchange.[11,12,13] This exchange primarily takes place through the top and bottom endplates and not, as previously thought, through the annular walls.[14,15,16]

Discs are not Shock-Absorbers.

Additional studies indicate that the disc, contrary to popular belief, is not primarily a shock absorber.[17] To demonstrate this point, **Figure 5-4** shows an anatomical specimen and its lateral X-ray. The vertebral bodies, the endplates, and the medullary bone in particular, deflect more during loading than the annular rings.[18] In other words, the bulging of the annular rings is less than the bowing and bending of the endplates into the medullary bone of the vertebral bodies during loading. The nucleus pulposus is not spherical in shape, contrary to the impression created by illustrators (**see Figure 5-5**). In the lumbar spine it has a kidney bean shape in cross section, and in coronal section, is uniform in height, and resembles a column. The whole nucleus pulposus is wider than it is high.

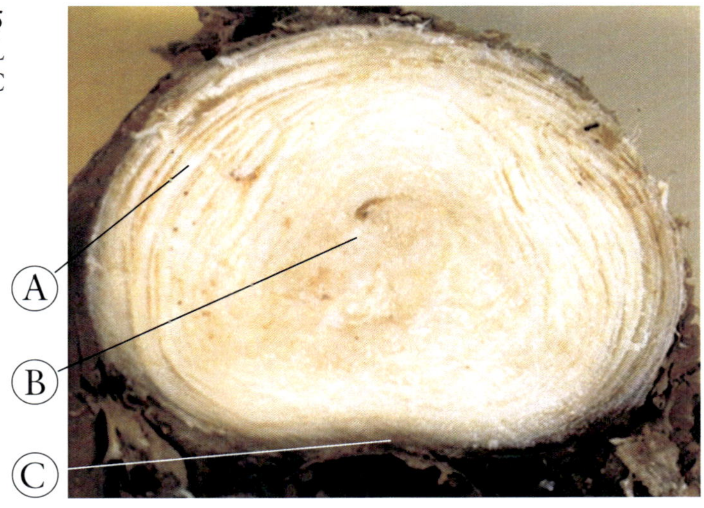

Figure 5-5
CROSS SECTION OF A NORMAL LUMBAR DISC

The lumbar discs and vertebrae have a kidney bean shape, with a slight impression at the posterior side. The nucleus pulposus is in the posterior portion of the disc.

(A) Annulus fibrosus (annular rings)
(B) Nucleus pulposus
(C) Posterior impression

The lumbar spine in **Figure 5-6** shows that although the L2 vertebra has sustained a compression fracture, the adjacent discs have remained intact, with the alignment near normal. The L2 vertebral body and endplates have taken the brunt of the force, deforming to the point of crushing. The disc is, for mechanical purposes, a closed hydraulic system, as only a small amount of fluid (about 11%) is lost during normal compression. The remaining disc fluid is not deformable, since the annular rings are normally inelastic. The endplates do deform, compressing the trabeculae of the medullary bone.[19,20] This is the mechanism for the vertebrae to absorb force. The science of hydraulics shows that force introduced at one

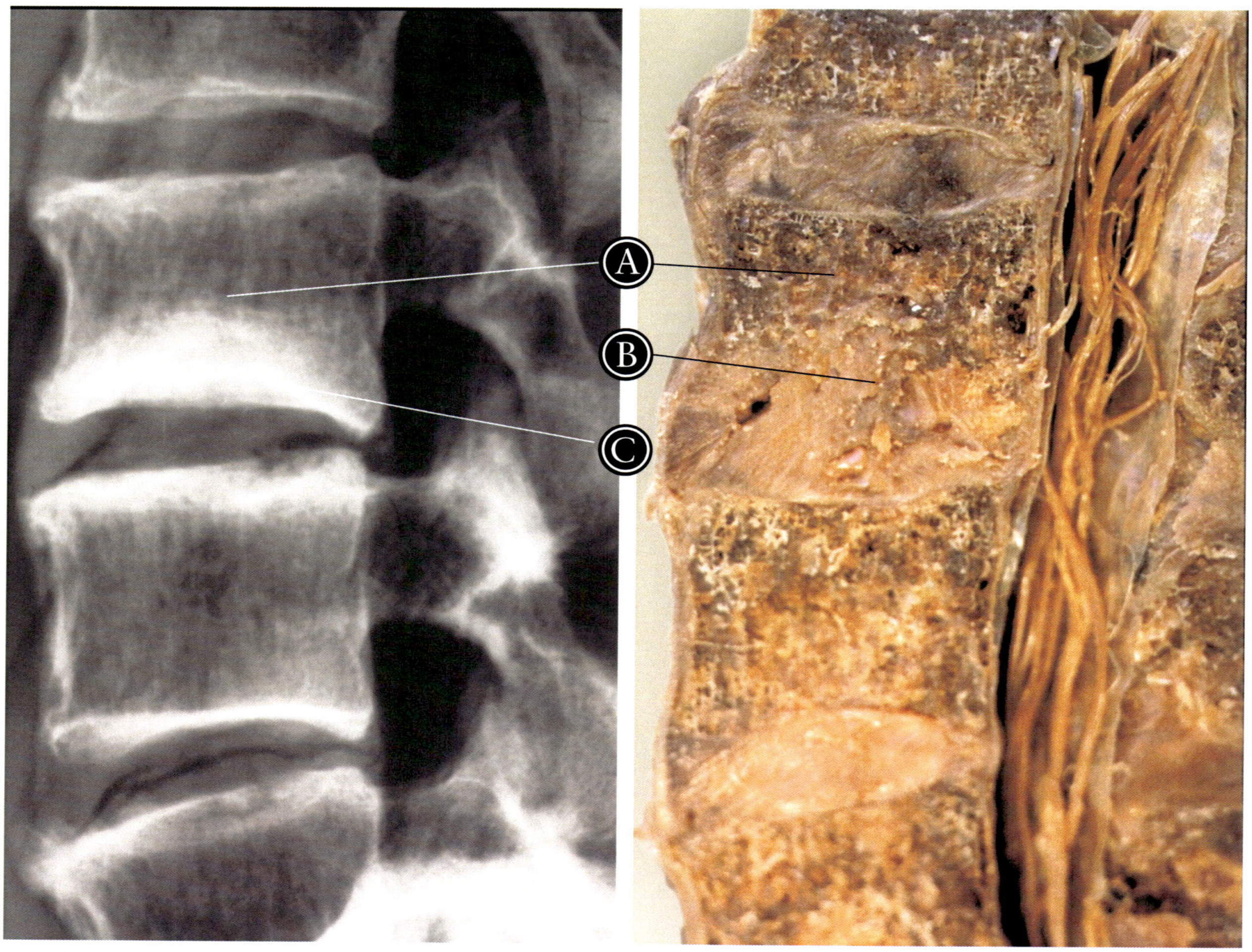

Figure 5-6
A LARGE NUCLEUS PULPOSUS PROTRUSION INTO L2.

The L2-L3 disc has protruded up into L2. Note on the X-ray a bone repair has taken place that happened some time ago. This is another example of the vertebral body absorbing the deforming force of trauma with the nucleus pulposus expanding into the vertebral body of L2.

(A) L2 vertebral body
(B) Nucleus pulposus
(C) Repaired compression injury to L2

end of a fluid filled system is automatically transferred to the other end of that system; that is, the force is transmitted, not absorbed. Thus, when the lumbar spine is compressed, the force is transmitted to the vertebral bodies so that they absorb the load (or shock). As **Figure 5-7** demonstrates, when the force is too great, the vertebral bodies can actually collapse. The vertebral bodies of L2 through L5 have all suffered compression fractures but the A to P alignment was not significantly altered and the discs have remained relatively healthy. The discs, being hydrophilic, create an osmotic pressure that will cause the disc to expand to fill the available space (see **Figures 5-6** and **5-7**).

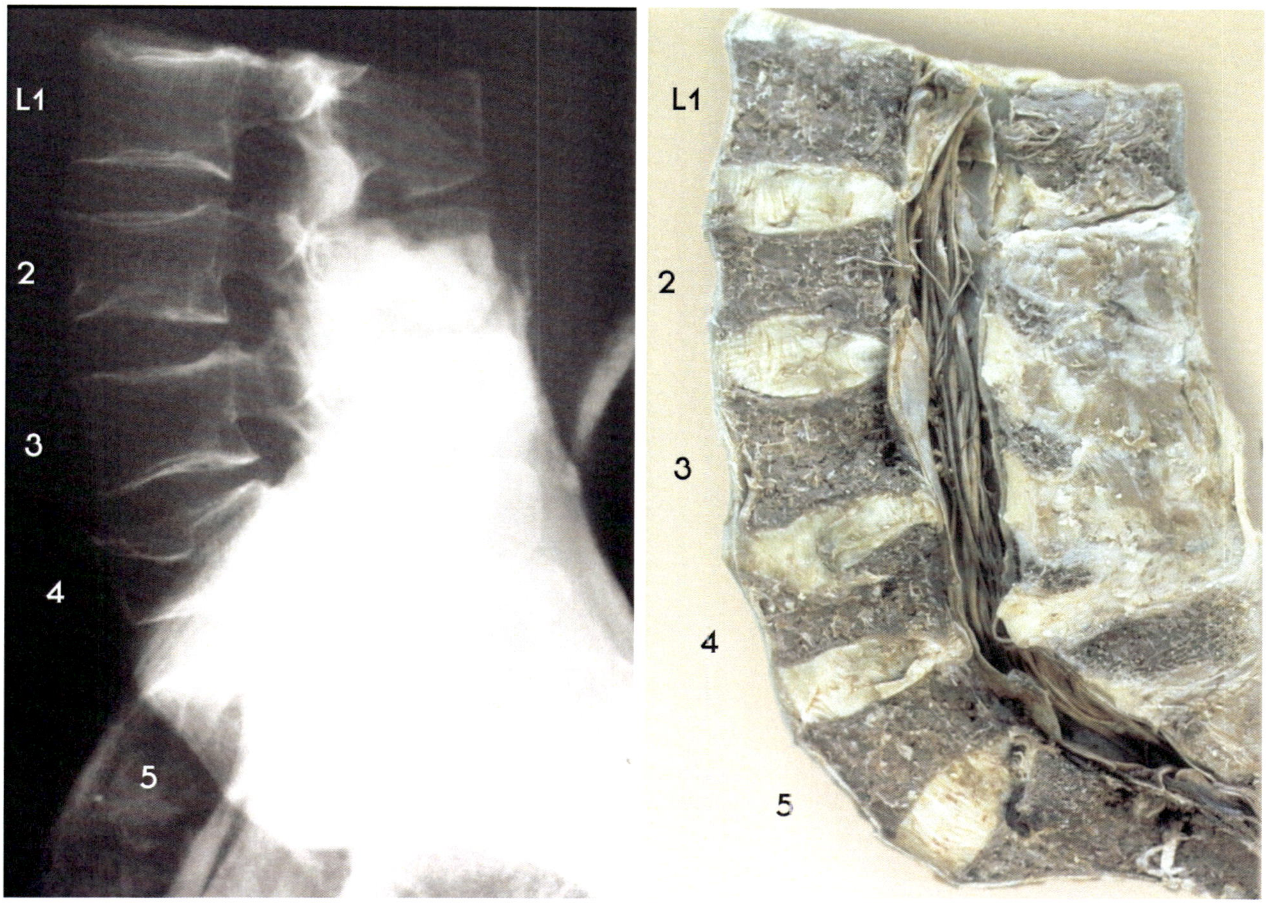

Figure 5-7

COMPRESSION FRACTURES OF THE LUMBAR SPINE WITH NEAR NORMAL ALIGNMENT

This specimen has compression fractures of L2,L 3, L4, and L5. The lordotic curve and the A to P alignment have been maintained despite the trauma. Notice that the disc height has actually increased in certain areas.

Types of Lumbar Subluxations

The subluxations of the lumbar spine are classified according to the changes in architecture. The lordotic curve of the lumbar spine is an essential architectural feature. Subluxations generally cause less neural involvement if the lordotic curve is maintained. **Figure 5-8** is a comparison of lumbar spines. In **Figure 5-8a,** L5 is anterior to L4 with disc tearing and other signs of degeneration. L5 has moved posteriorly to the sacrum and the disc has totally desiccated, indicating an old, long standing condition. Note the lack of osteophytic spurs and canal stenosis. The lordotic curve preserved normal weight bearing of most of the joints and major bony changes did not occur.

In **Figure 5-8b** the lordosis is lost with the subluxation of L3 and L4 and widening of the vertebral bodies has taken place. This occurs at the site of the subluxation only. Note the change in spinal canal width at the subluxation and overall canal length.

Figure 5-8c shows a lumbar spine with the characteristic "stair-stepping" of vertebral bodies that have buckled under deforming stress. There clearly is a loss of normal alignment between L3-L4 and L4-L5 resulting in a reversal of the lordotic curve. The vertebral segments have undergone chronic degeneration as a result of the altered weight bearing. Displacement of opposing endplates causes a shearing of the annulus and nucleus. The uncoupling of facets, stress on facetal capsules, or hyper-loading, and stress on the disc annulus, cause a proprioceptive reflex resulting in guarding by the paraspinal muscles and the intrinsic muscles of the vertebral column. This locks the vertebrae into the buckled position, and thus interrupts the pumping motion that is necessary for normal flow of fluid in and out of the discs. The discs, of course, begin a slow process of dehydration and degeneration.[21,22]

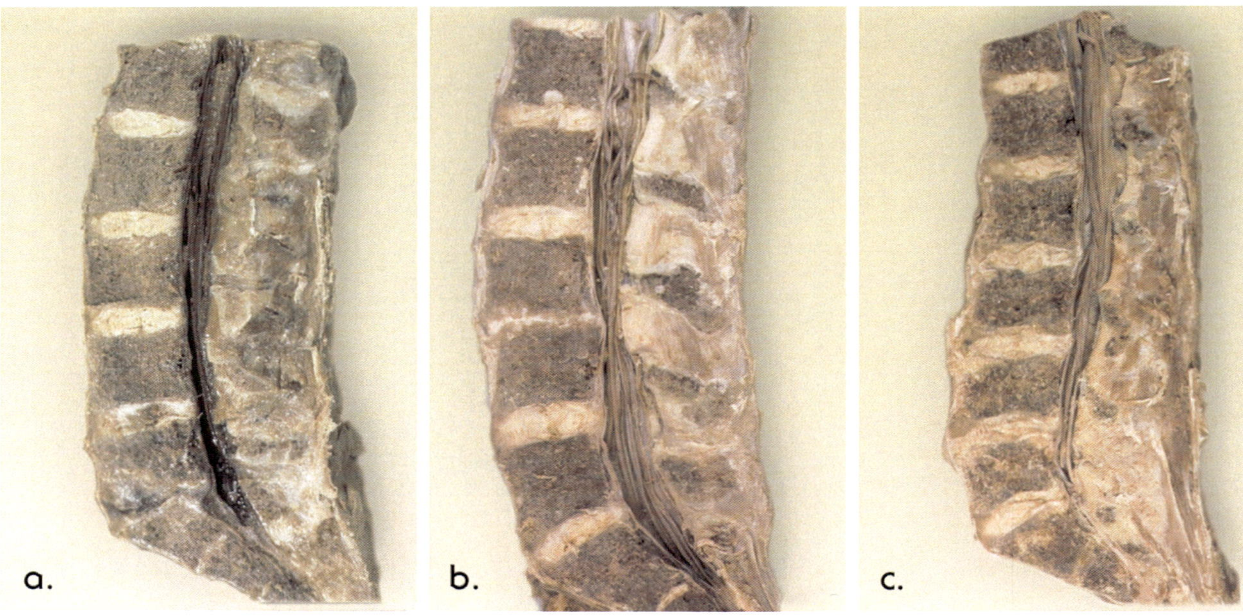

Figure 5-8

A COMPARISON OF SUBLUXATIONS WITH A LORDOTIC CURVE, WITHOUT A CURVE AND A REVERSED CURVE.

In this small set of lumbar spines the curve and the shape of the canal are closely related. In comparing (a) to (b), the difference in the spinal canal length can be noted, the longer being in (b). The spine in (c) has an even longer spinal canal than (a) or (b). Also the patterns of degeneration are different. Subluxations occurring with the curve intact have milder degenerative changes. In (b) the canal stenosis is apparent and in (c) the vertebral body widening and spurring are obvious. (See **Figure 1-7** on page 6.)

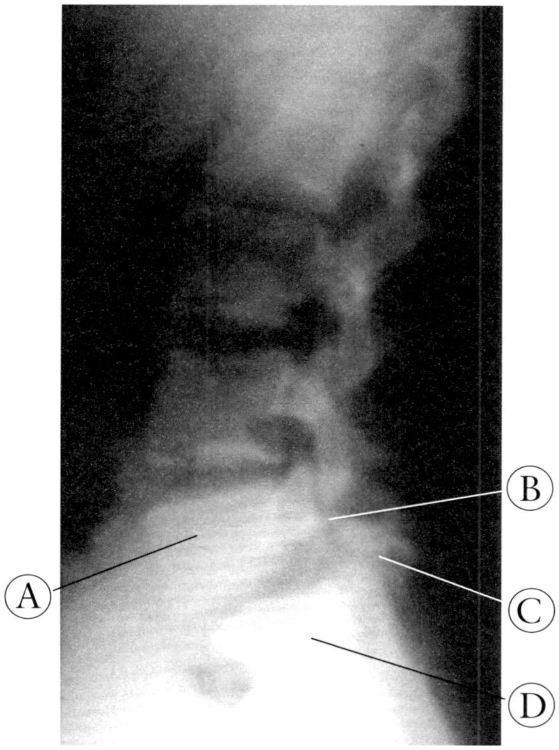

Figure 5-9

LATERAL LUMBAR X-RAY OF A 20 YEAR OLD WITH L5 SPONDYLOLISTHESIS.

The fifth lumbar vertebra is broken and separated because of a pars defect. The entire spine including the L5 vertebral body and superior articular joint have subluxated anteriorly.

(A) Body of L5 vertebra
(B) Break in articular arch of L5
(C) Inferior articulations of L5
(D) Sacrum

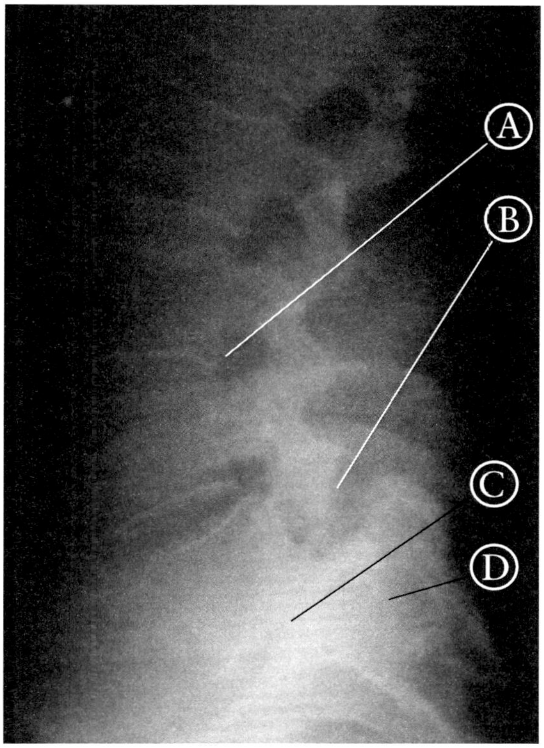

Figure 5-10

LATERAL LUMBAR X-RAY OF 75 YEAR OLD WITH SPONDYLOLISTHESIS.

The fifth lumbar vertebra is broken and separated. The fifth lumbar vertebral body is fused to the sacrum. Patient denies chronic pain. Note maintenance of Lumbar curve.

(A) L3-L4 subluxation
(B) Break in L5 vertebra
(C) Fused L5-S1 joint
(D) Sacrum

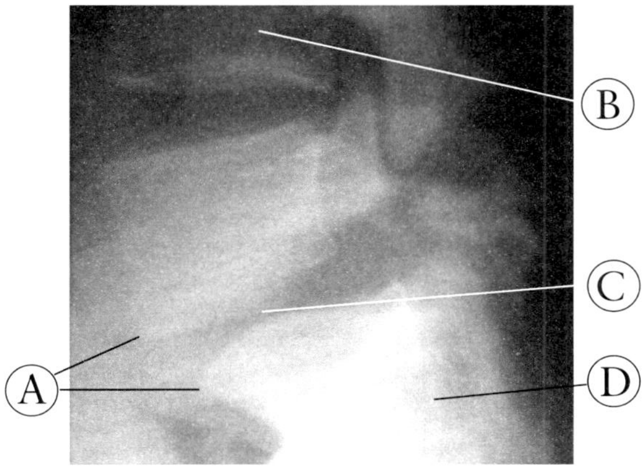

Figure 5-11

CLOSE-UP OF L5 SPONDYLOLISTHESIS IN 20 YEAR OLD.

This injury occurred at age 6. The fifth lumbar disc is sheared by the shifted endplates and signs of anterior spurring are present. The loss of disc height adds to the picture of a chronic injury in a young person.

(A) Anterior spurs
(B) L4 subluxated posteriorly to L5
(C) Narrowed L5-S1 disc
(D) Sacrum

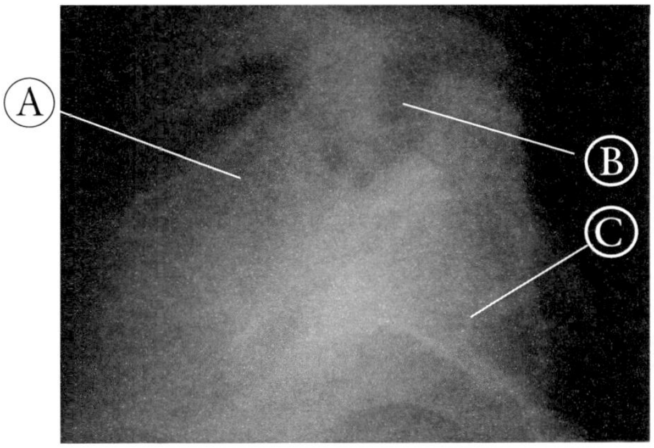

Figure 5-12

CLOSE-UP OF SPONDYLOLISTHESIS IN A 75 YEAR OLD.

Note the L5 vertebra has fused in the anterior position relative to the sacrum. The gap between the anterior part of L5 and the posterior part is still visible.

(A) L5
(B) Gap in L5
(C) Sacrum

This study shows the etiology of osteoarthritis of the spine is subluxation. Loss of the normal curves increases the forces that change the vertebrae. Subluxation increases the weight-bearing on the vertebral body, which then increases the vertebral body loading. Wolf's Law suggests this will cause an increase in the cross-sectional area of the vertebral bodies (**see Figure 5-8c**). This enlargement of the vertebral bodies and endplates manifests as spurs, osteophytes, encroachment into the spinal canal (stenosis), and encroachment of the intervertebral foramen, often leading to damage and stress in the nervous system. This study of the human spine indicates that the degenerative changes of subluxations cause less stenotic change to the intervertebral foramen and spinal canal if the normal lordotic curve is maintained.[23]

Lumbar and sacral subluxations can be fixed with contracture of the lumbo-sacral aponeurosis or thoraco-lumbar fascia (**see Figures 5-9 – 5-13**). Soft tissue adaptation to a subluxation complex can restrict motion of nearby joints. For example, the superior displacement of the apex of the sacrum can become permanent with a shortening of the 5 to 7 mm. thick anchoring of the lumbosacral fascia and tendinous attachments of the erector spinae musculature to the lower sacrum. This would alter and restrict the normal motion of the facets of at least the lower lumbar spine. A condition created by subluxations results in what is commonly referred to as degenerative arthritis, degenerative disc disease, or spondylosis. In osteoarthritis of the spine, the primary agent is the subluxation which causes altered weight bearing. This study and others demonstrate that the subluxation occurs traumatically, either instantly or repetitively, and that increased degeneration takes place over time at those levels.[24]

This long term process will eventually involve the sympathetic structures that travel along the side of the lower spine. Note in **Figures 5-14** and **5-15** that the bulging discs and osteophytes are stretching the lumbar splanchnic nerve, a rami of the sympathetic chain. This nerve has been associated with vascular function of the leg.

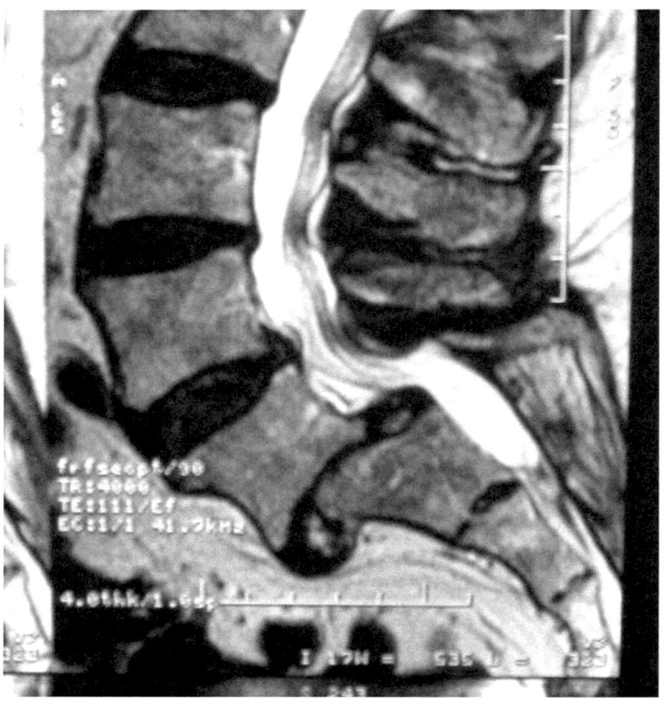

Figure 5-13
MRI study of the same individual in Figures 5-10 and 5-12.

Note the appearance of some soft tissue at the L5-S1 disc.

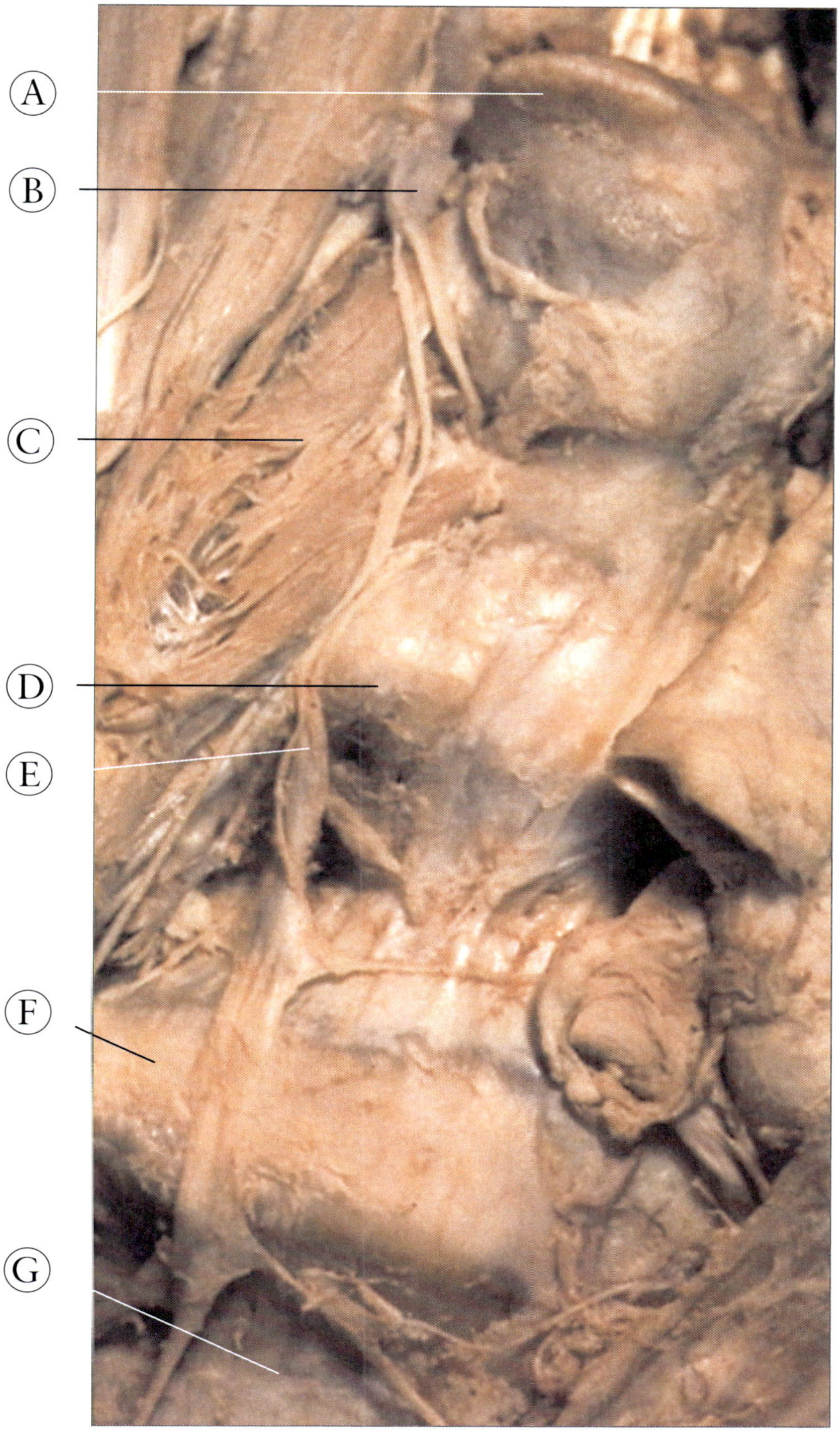

Figure 5-14
Anterior view of lumbar degeneration

This is the anterior view of L3 to Sacrum of a degenerated lumbar spine and the Lumbar Splanchnic Nerve being stretched.

A. L3-L4 osteophyte
B. Lumbar sympathetic ganglion
C. Psoas
D. L4-L5 disc bulge
E. Lumbar sympathetic nerve
F. L5-S1 disc bulge
G. Sacrum

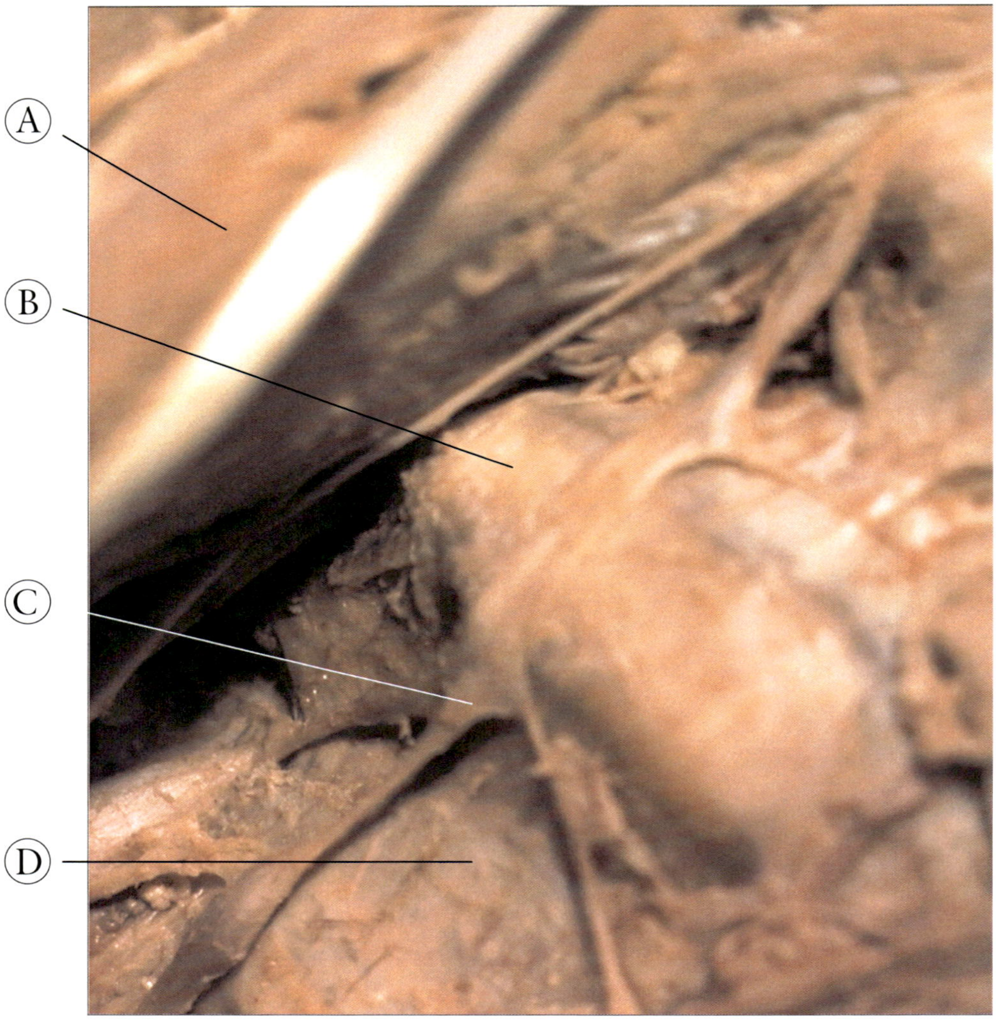

Figure 5-15
Close up of anterior view of the lumbar spine and sympathetic nerve.

A. Psoas
B. L5-S1 anterior disc bulge
C. Sympathetic splanchnic nerve
D. Sacrum

CHAPTER FIVE — EXPANDED TABLE OF CONTENTS

Atlas of Subluxations of the Lumbar Spine

SECTION I

Subluxations of the lumbar spine with a lordotic curve (14 pairs)

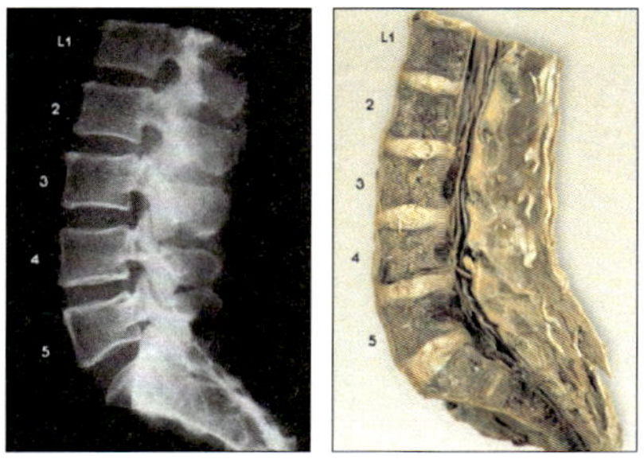

Plates 5-1 A & B
LUMBAR SPINE - near normal, slight subluxations

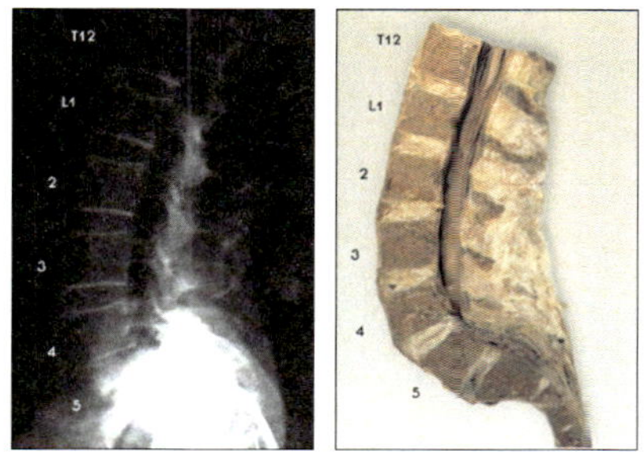

Plates 5-2 A & B
LUMBAR SPINE - variations in "normal" lumbar curve

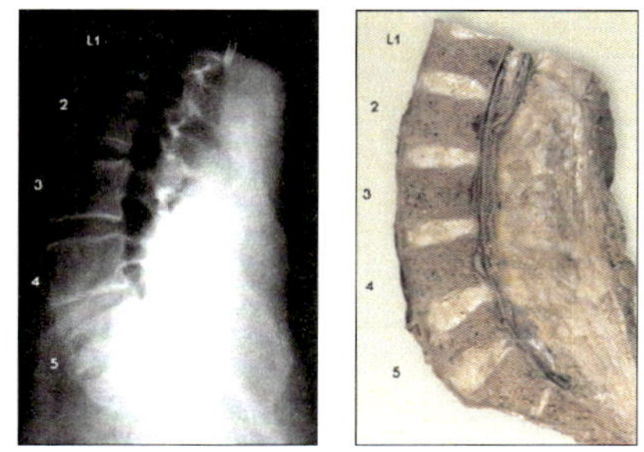

Plates 5-3 A & B
LUMBAR SPINE - L5 has a compression fracture with sclerosis and healthy discs.

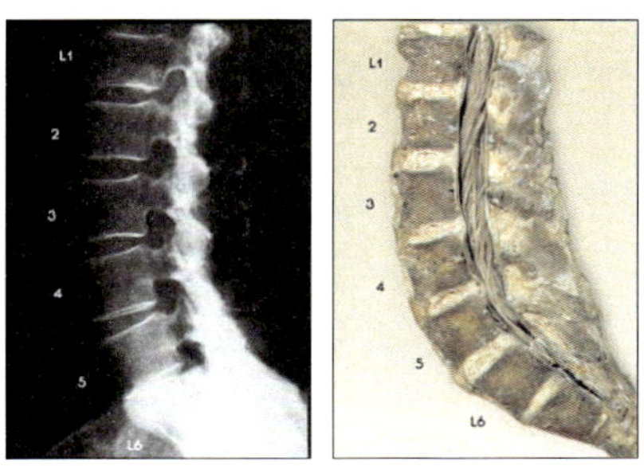

Plates 5-4 A & B
LUMBAR SPINE - Variations in the "normal" lumbar curve

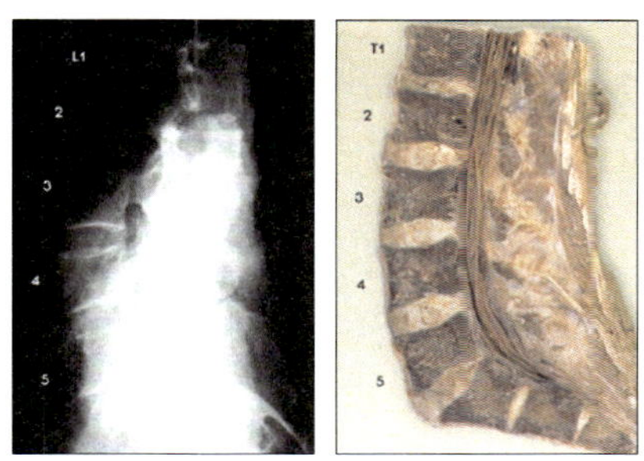

Plates 5-5 A & B
LUMBAR SPINE - A near normal lordotic curve with L5-sacral wedging

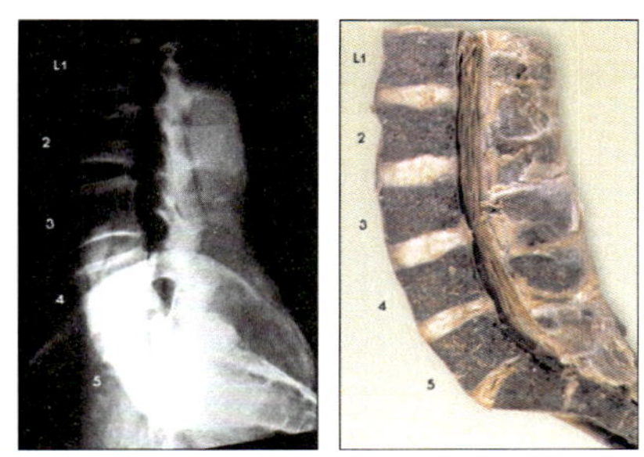

Plates 5-6 A & B
LUMBAR SPINE - This shows variations in a"normal" lumbar curve

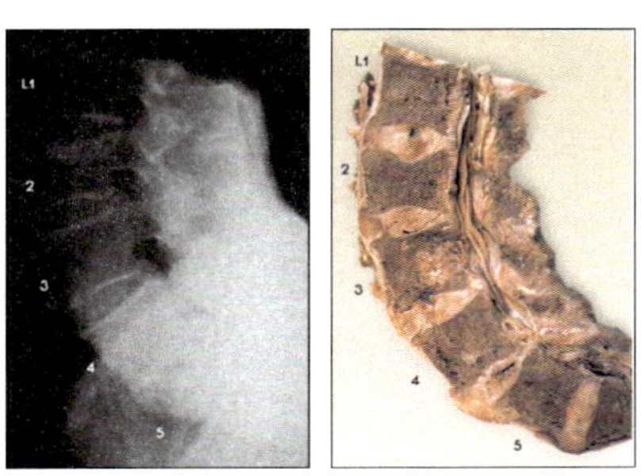

Plates 5-7 A & B
LUMBAR SPINE - This specimen has subluxated segments with the curve maintained

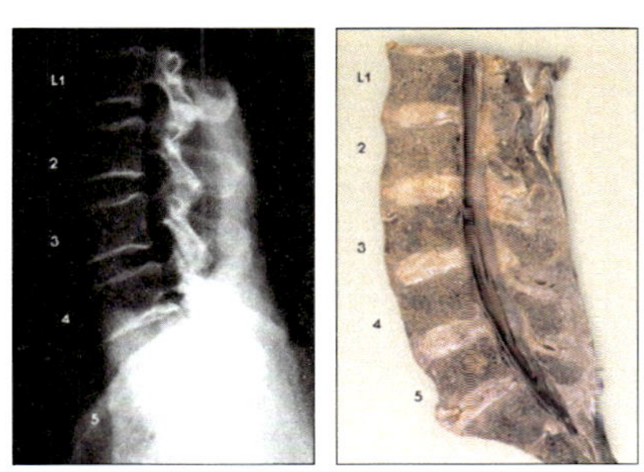

Plates 5-8 A & B
LUMBAR SPINE - variations in "normal" lumbar curve -I

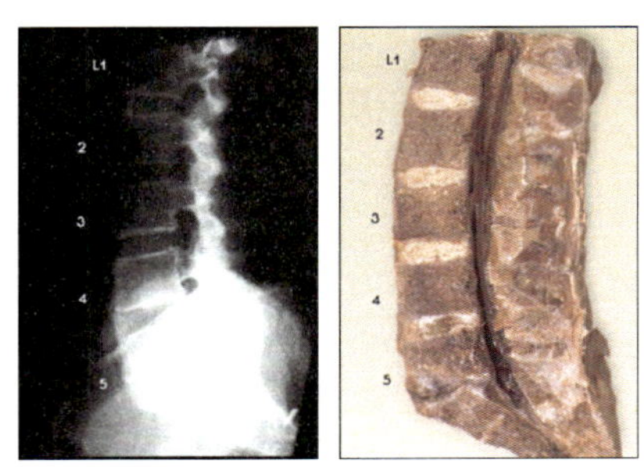

Plates 5-9 A & B
LUMBAR SPINE - Normal discs above a major subluxation with damaged discs

CHAPTER FIVE — EXPANDED TABLE OF CONTENTS

Atlas of Subluxations of the Lumbar Spine

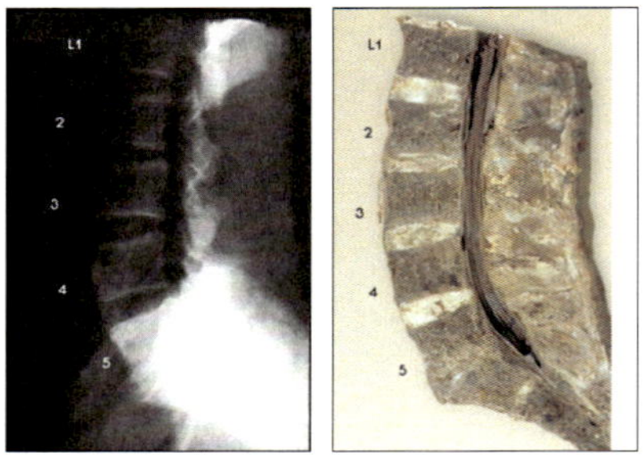

Plates 5-10 A & B
LUMBAR SPINE - This demonstrates L5-sacrum wedging with anterior displacement of the sacrum

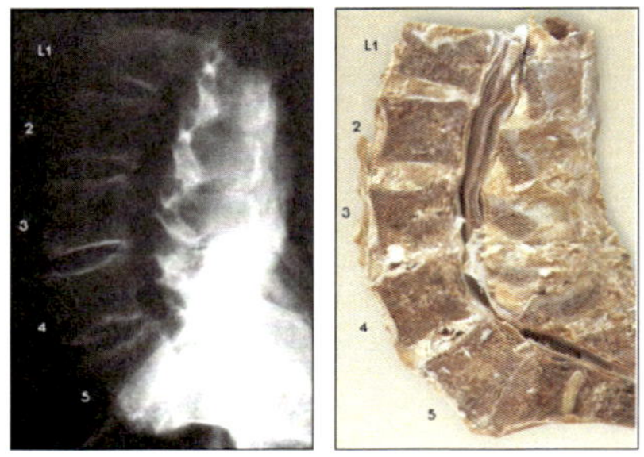

Plates 5-11 A & B
LUMBAR SPINE - This shows complete anterolisthesis of L4 and partially of L5 and S1 with end stage fusion

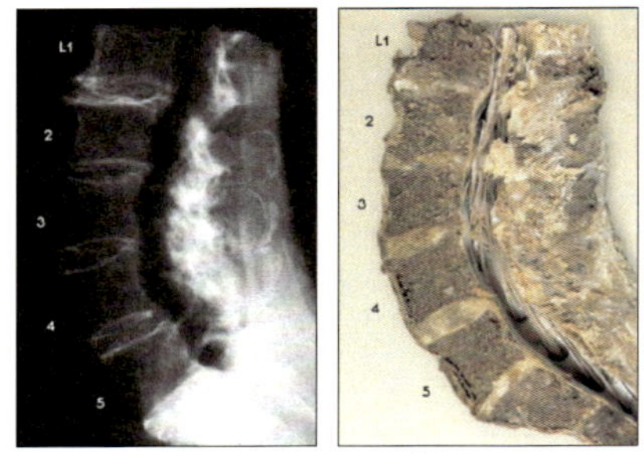

Plates 5-12 A & B
LUMBAR SPINE - This illustrates normal discs below damaged discs with lordosis maintained

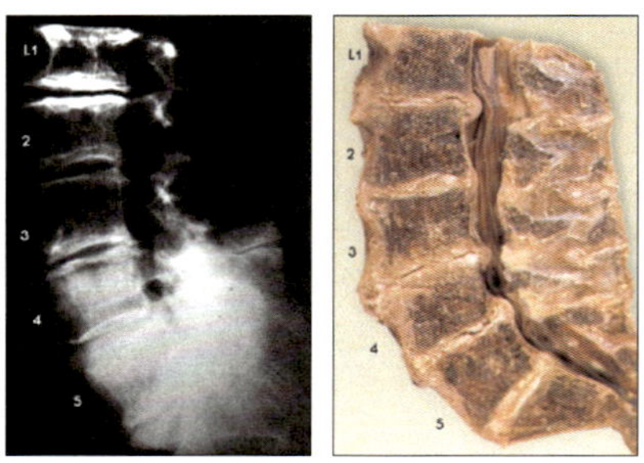

Plates 5-13 A & B
LUMBAR SPINE - The end-stages of degeneration, post trauma

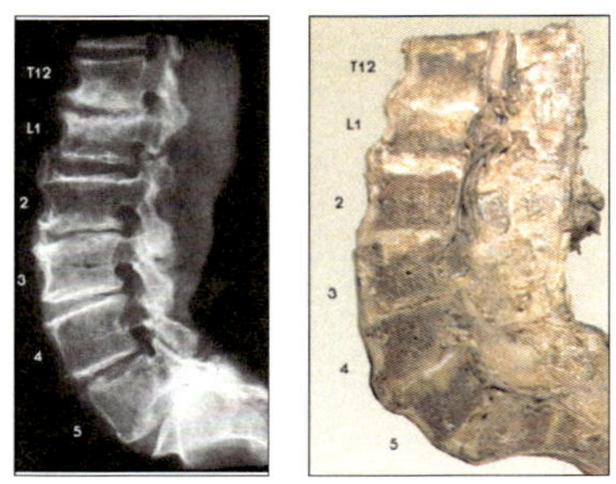

Plates 5-14 A & B
LUMBAR SPINE - This has subluxated segments with the curve maintained, sequential retrolisthesis to the segment below, or stairstepping

SECTION II:

Subluxations of the lumbar spine with a loss of lordotic curve (6 pairs)

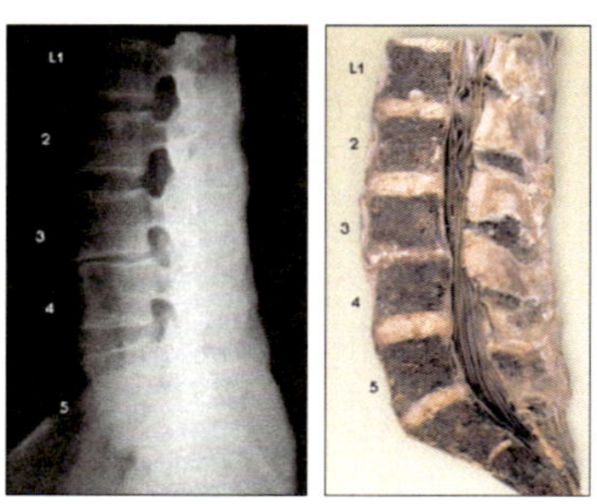

Plates 5-15 A & B
LUMBAR SPINE - This shows hypolordosis with one significant subluxation

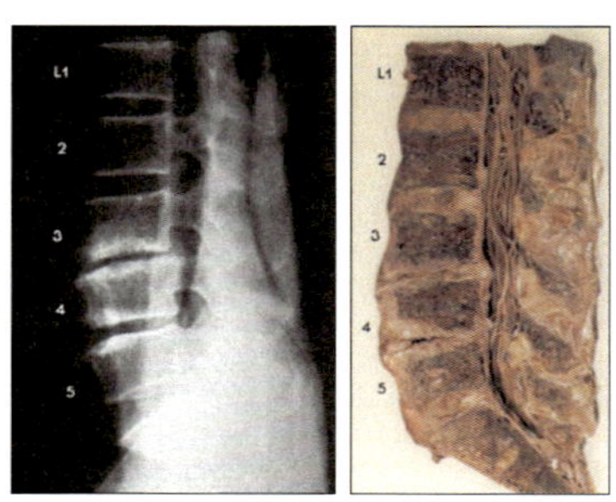

Plates 5-16 A & B
LUMBAR SPINE - This illustrates subluxations with a loss of lordotic curve and various stages of disc degeneration

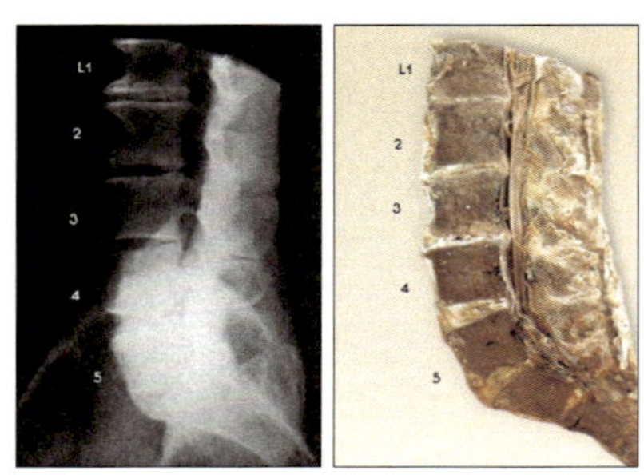

Plates 5-17 A & B
LUMBAR SPINE - The subluxation complex of this specimen involves the entire lumbar spine

CHAPTER FIVE — EXPANDED TABLE OF CONTENTS

Atlas of Subluxations of the Lumbar Spine

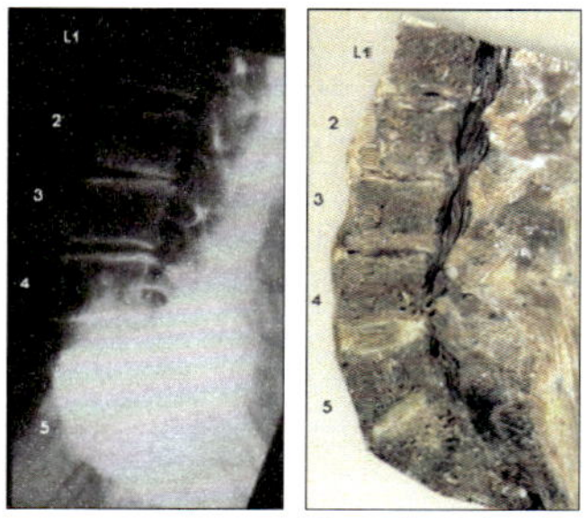

Plates 5-18 A & B
LUMBAR SPINE - This shows multiple subluxations with loss of curve

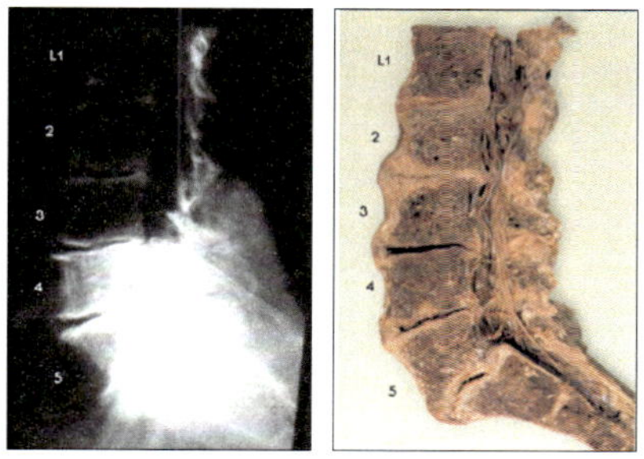

Plates 5-19 A & B
LUMBAR SPINE - This illustrates subluxations in end-stages of degeneration with a loss of lordotic curve

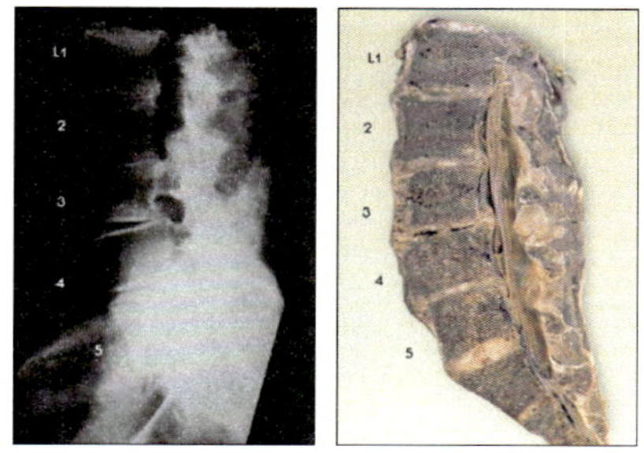

Plates 5-20 A & B
LUMBAR SPINE - This specimen has multiple subluxations and the end-stages of degeneration

SECTION III:

Subluxations of the lumbar spine with a reversed lordotic curve (4 pairs)

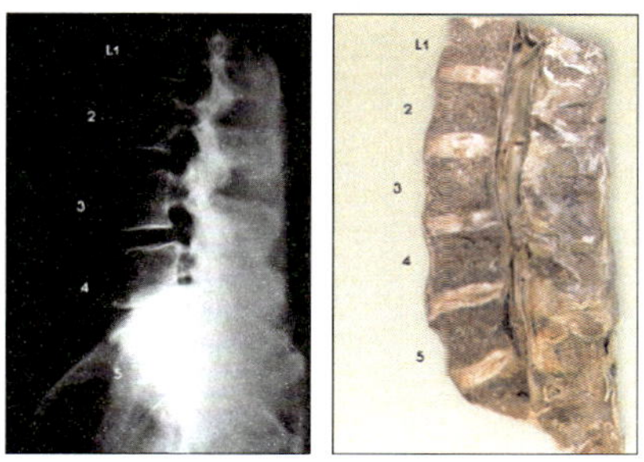

Plates 5-21 A & B
LUMBAR SPINE - This individual has a reversed lumbar lordotic curve with complete retrolisthesis of L4

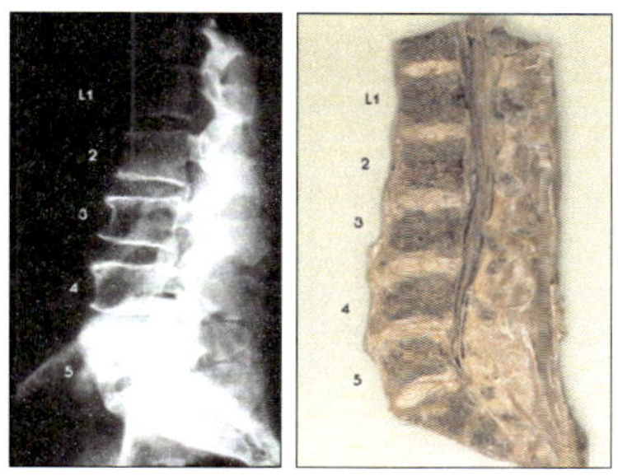

Plates 5-22 A & B
LUMBAR SPINE - Sequential retrolisthesis forming a 'stairstepping' of L1-L5 into a reversed lordotic curve

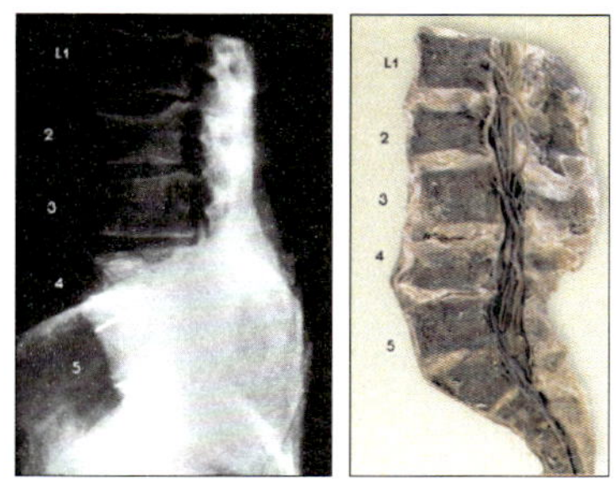

Plates 5-23 A & B
LUMBAR SPINE - L3 is a complete retrolisthesis creating a reversed lordotic curve

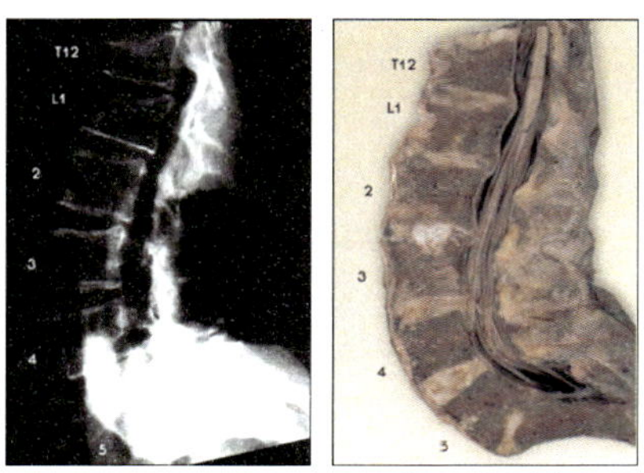

Plates 5-24 A & B
LUMBAR SPINE - This shows a reversed lordotic curve in the upper lumbar spine

Additional X-ray/MRI Comparison

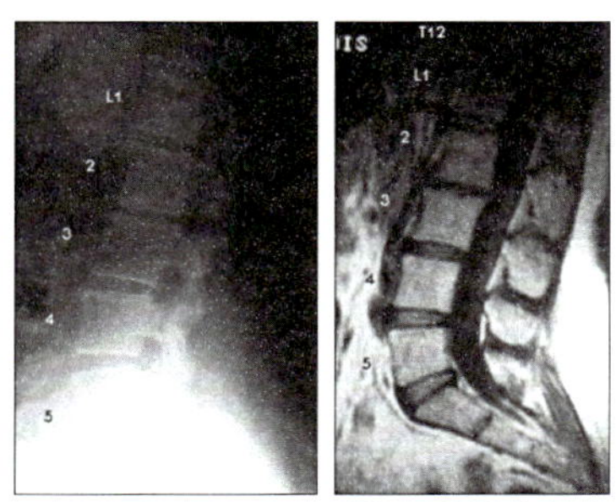

Plates 5-25 A & B
LUMBAR SPINE WITH A LOSS OF LORDOTIC CURVE
An X-ray and MRI comparison

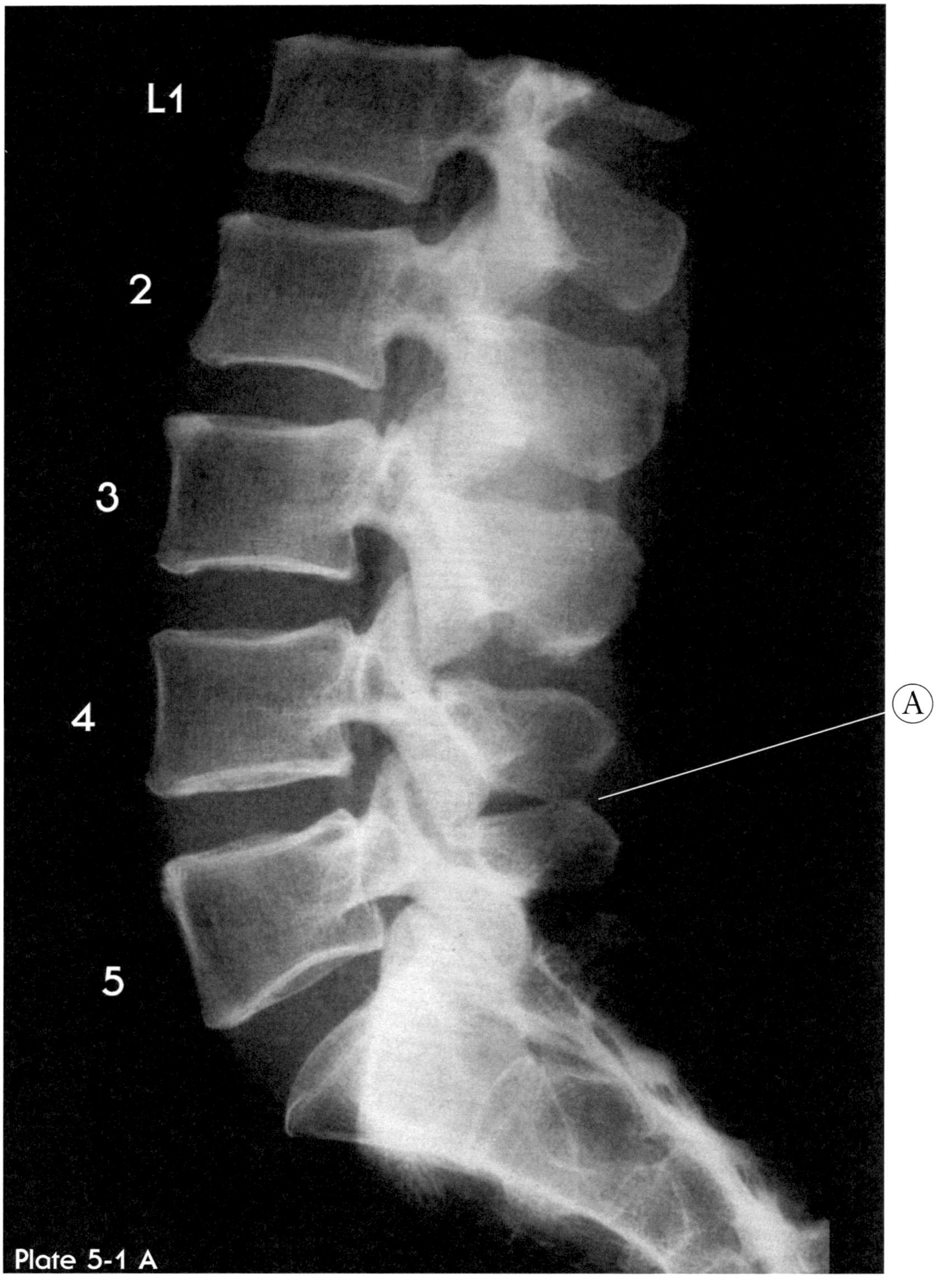

Plates 5-1 A & B

LUMBAR SPINE - near normal, slight subluxations

Some of the lordotic curve in this specimen has been maintained.

L1 and L2 look aligned. The rest of the spine is a reversed stair stepping with each vertebra being posterior to the next inferior vertebra. L2 is slightly retro to L3 with slight disc bulging.

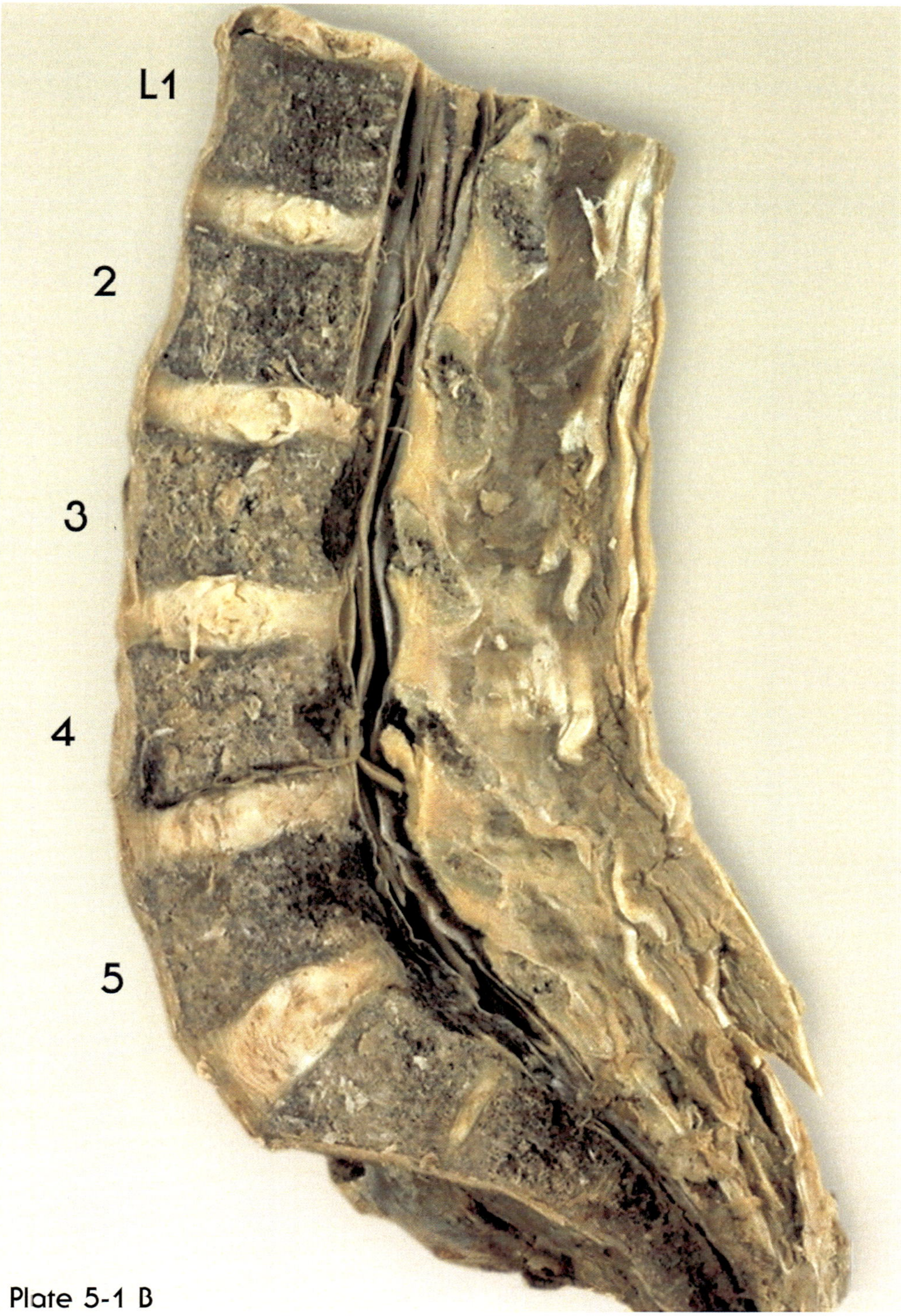

Plate 5-1 B

L3 slightly retro to L4 with disc bulge; L4 retro to L5 with disc wedging; L5 is slightly retro to the sacrum with disc wedging and bulging.

(A) L4-L5 spinous processes contact each other.

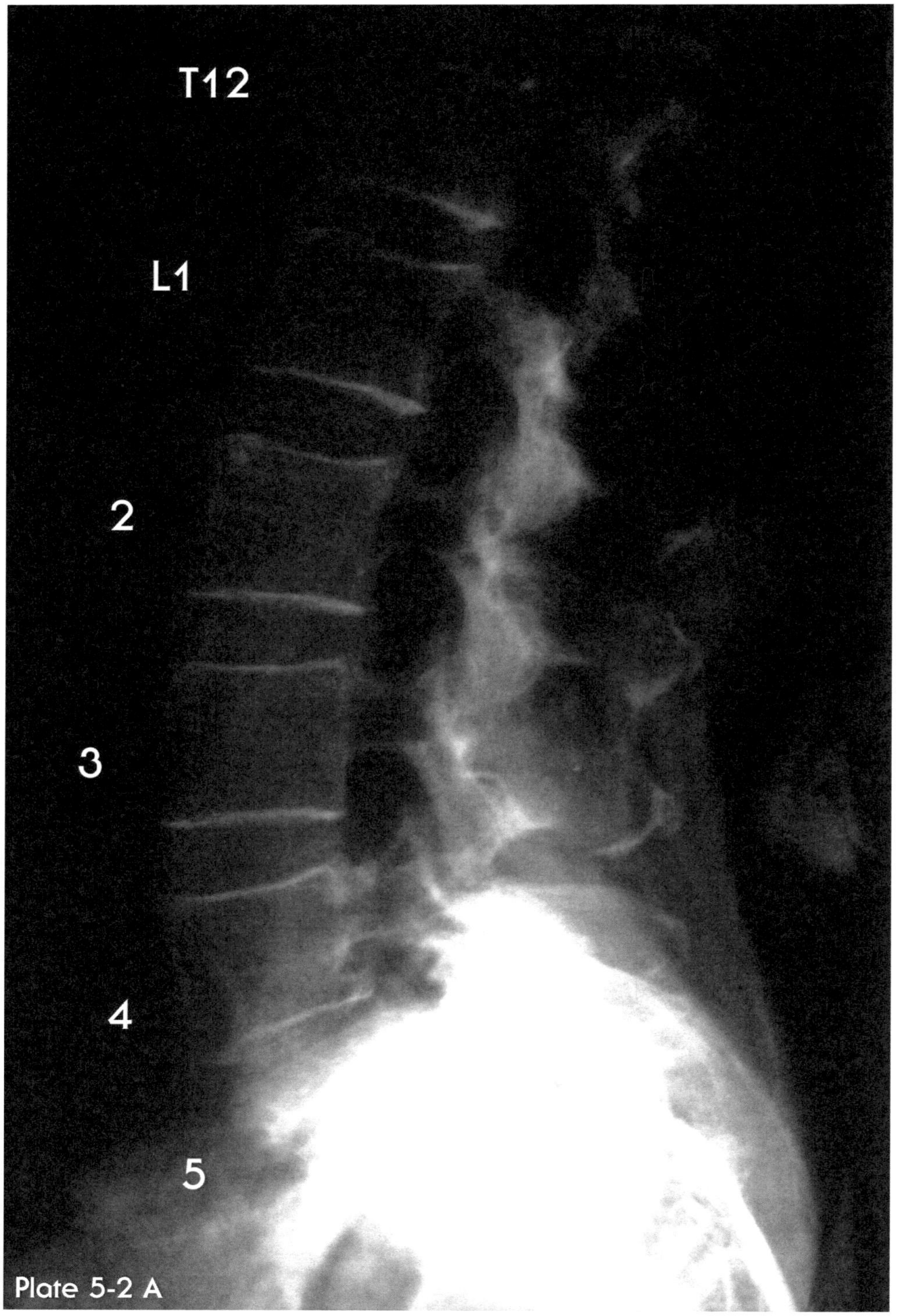

Plates 5-2 A & B
LUMBAR SPINE - variations in normal lumbar curve

This is a good example of slight degeneration processes in the discs with minor antero and retro displacement.

T12 is slightly retro to L1 with a small posterior bulge, slight tearing, and the beginnings of brown degeneration anteriorly. L1 is slightly retro to L2 with slight tearing and anterior

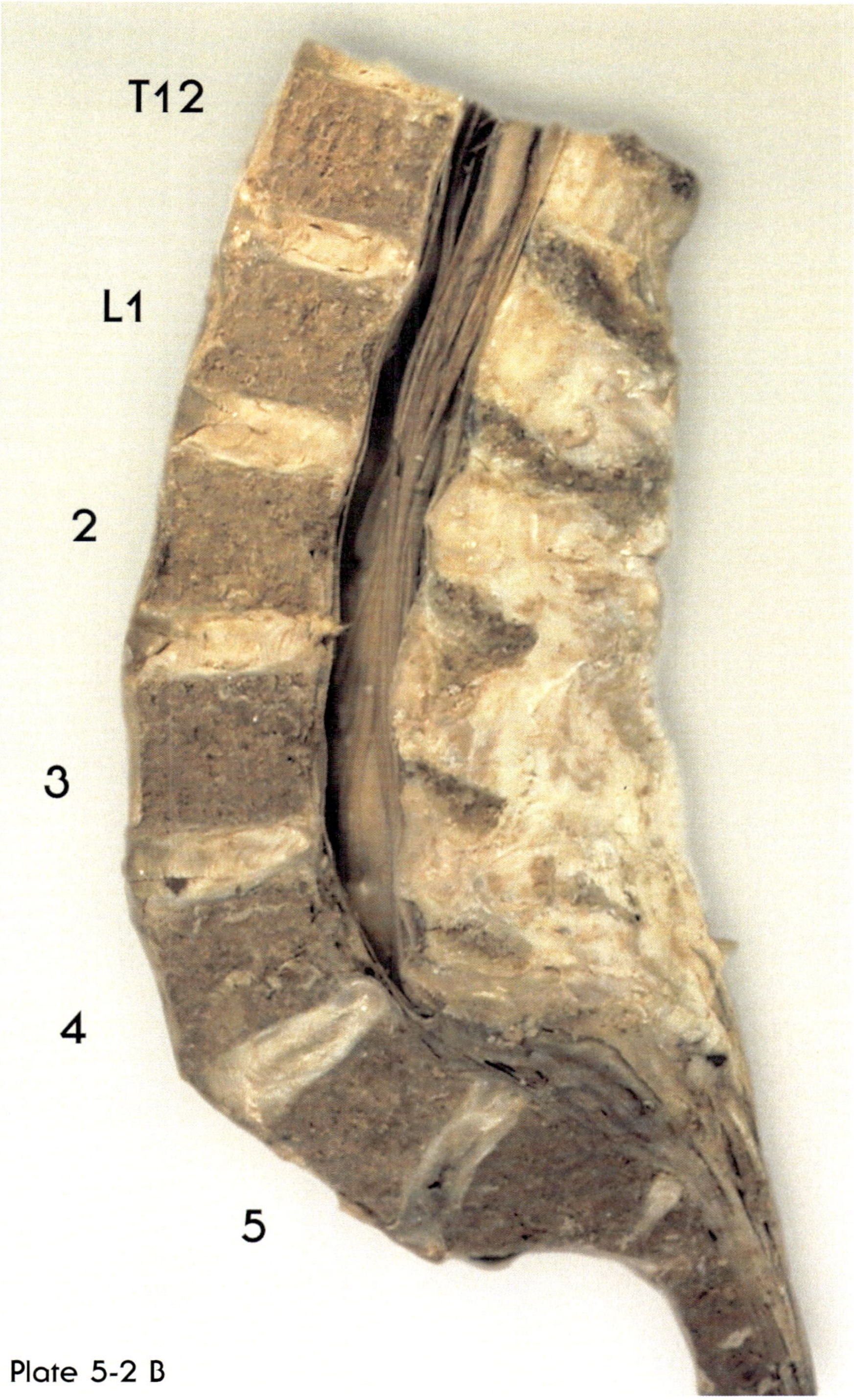

Plate 5-2 B

brown degeneration. L3 is antero to L4 with anterior brown degeneration and tearing. L4 is slightly antero to L3 with brown degeneration, tearing. L4 is slightly antero to L5 with brown degeneration, tearing, and wedging. The sacrum is retro to L5 with significant tearing, cavitation, and some loss of disc height.

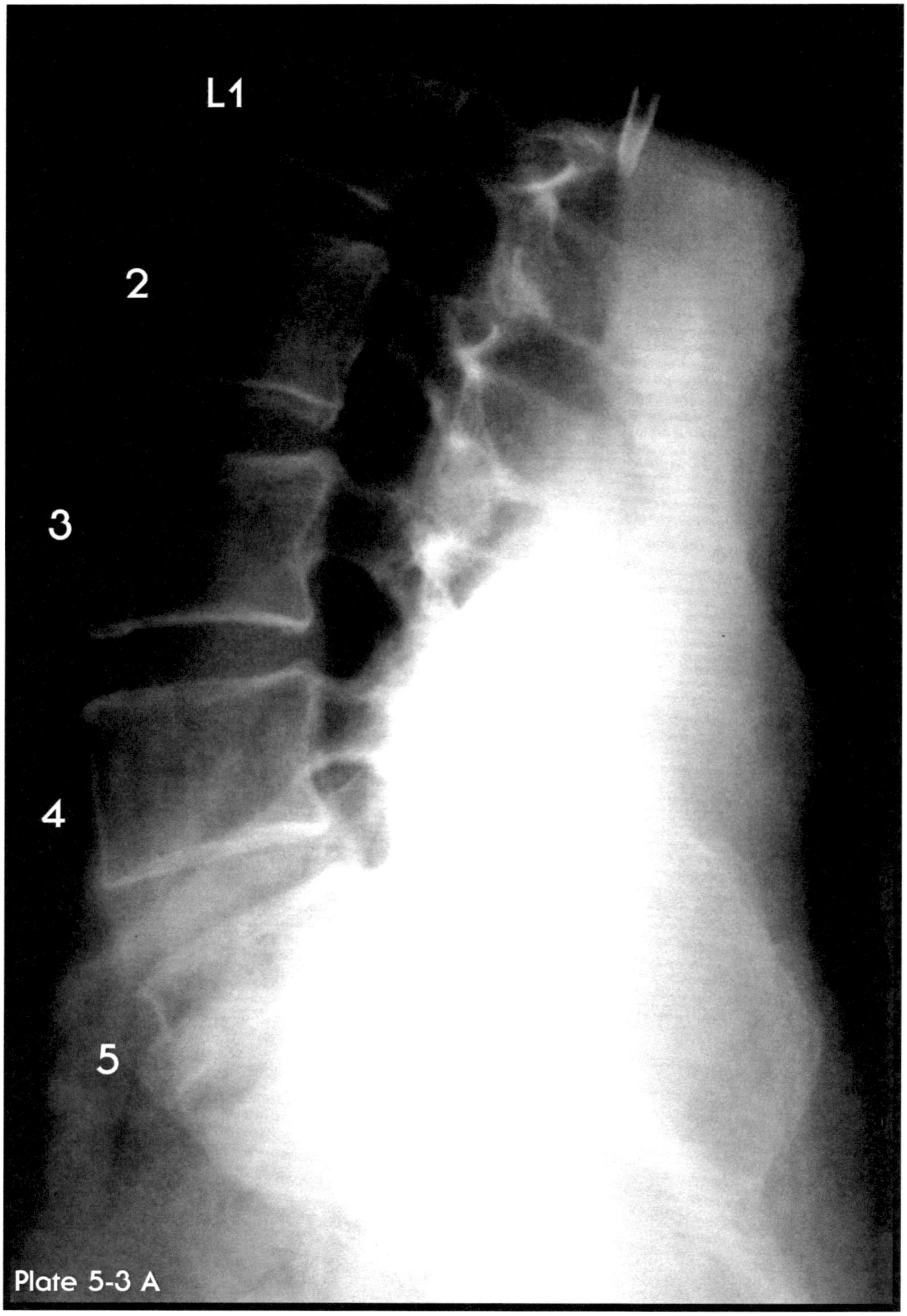

Plate 5-3 A

Plates 5-3 A & B

LUMBAR SPINE - L5 has a compression fracture with sclerosis and healthy discs. This specimen has suffered a trauma with a resulting compression fracture of the L5 vertebral body. This fracture repaired and the L4-L5 and L5-S1 discs have filled-in the lost volume of the L5 vertebral body. L1-L4 look nearly aligned with slight anterior disc brown

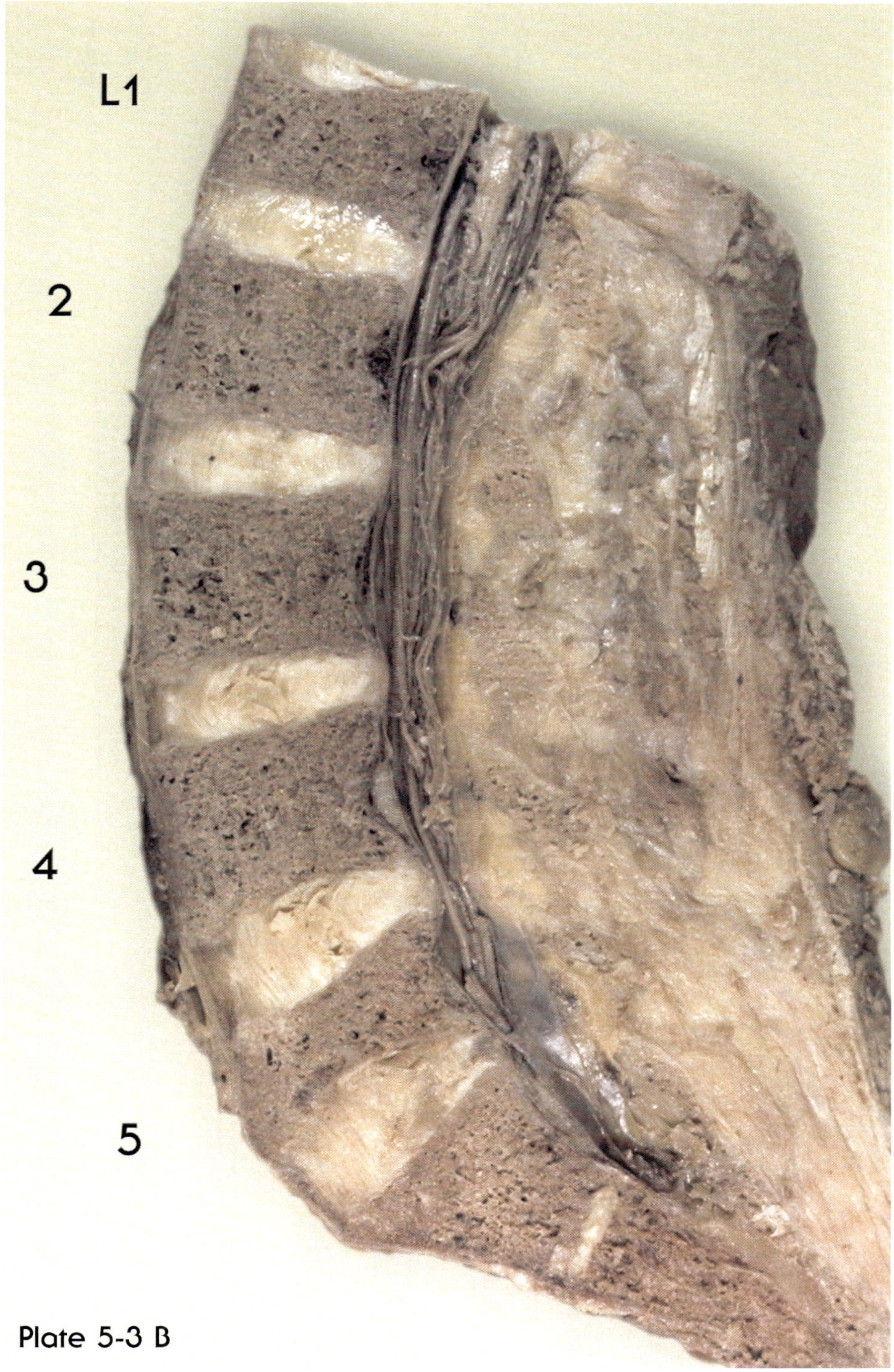

Plate 5-3 B

degeneration; L4-L5 and L5-S1 have wedging accompanying compression fracture of L5. There is a slight, but complete retro of L5 with a L4-L5 posterior disc bulge. This specimen has only minor signs of degeneration because the curve is maintained. This is another example of the vertebral body absorbing the shock.

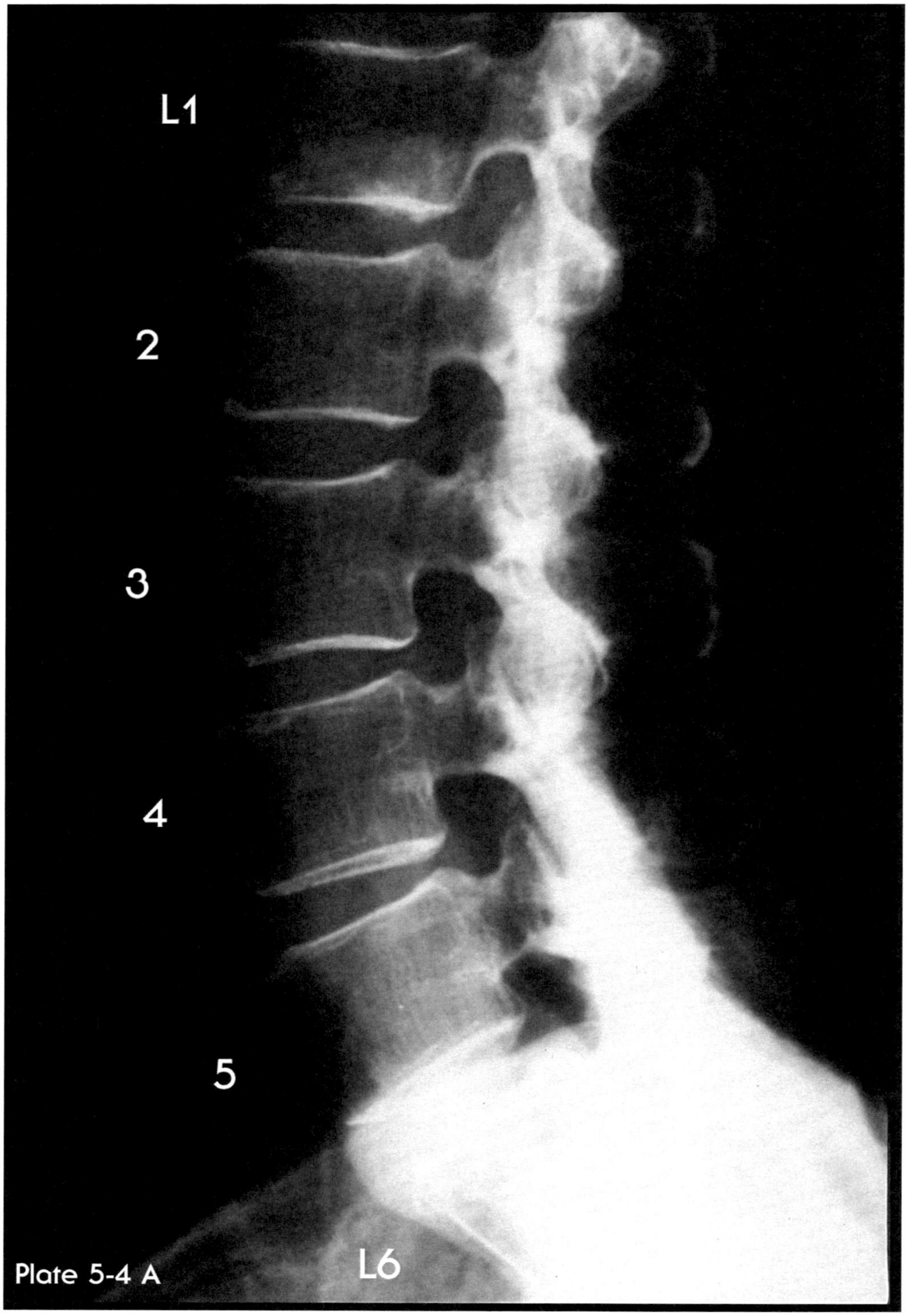

Plates 5-4 A & B

LUMBAR SPINE - Variations in the normal lumbar curve

This specimen has a lordotic curve with six lumbar vertebrae with disc degeneration that corresponds to the degree of subluxation. L1 is slightly retro to L2 with slight disc bulging.

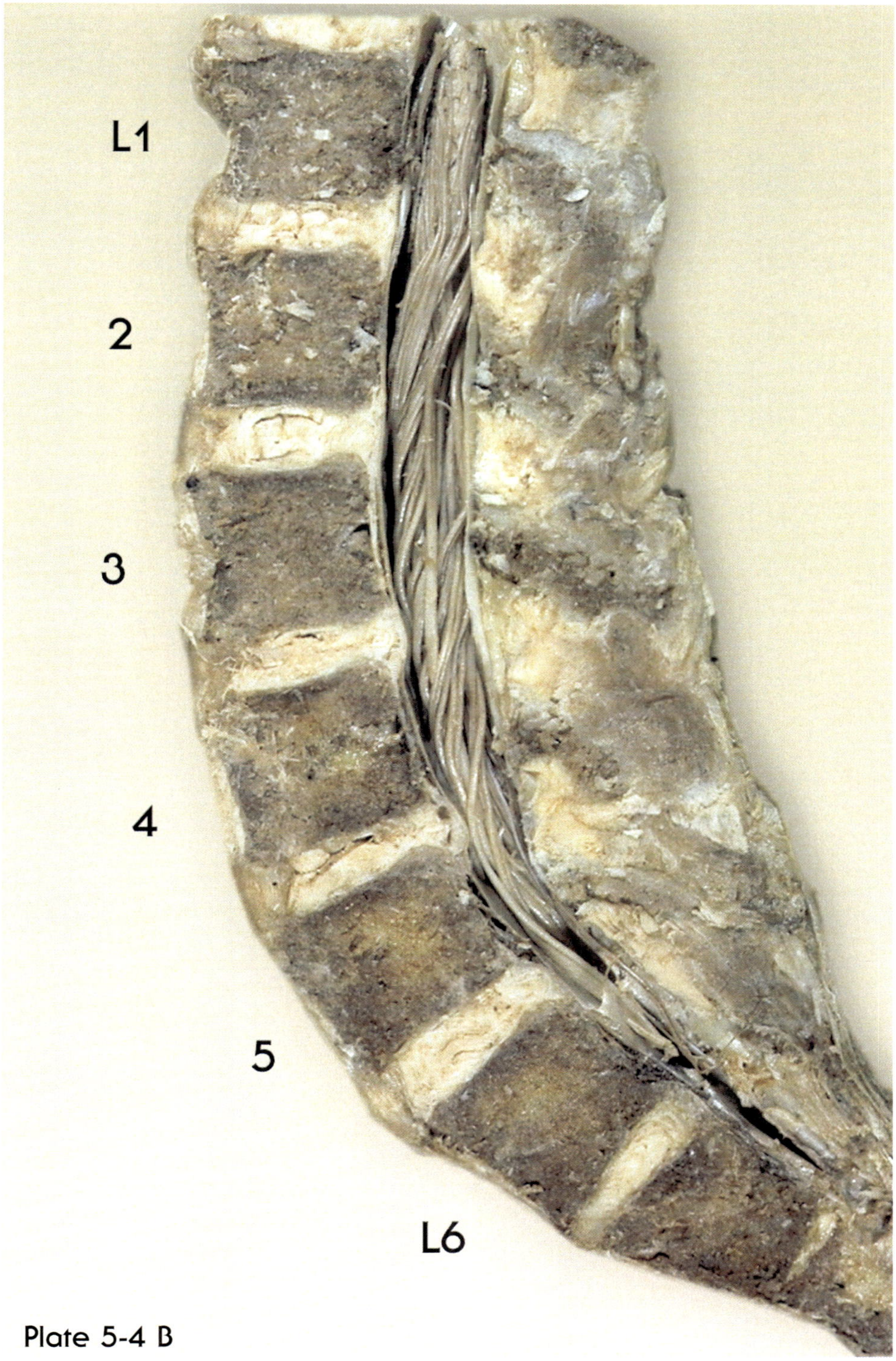

Plate 5-4 B

L2 is retro to L3 with slight disc tearing. L3 is retro to L4 with slight tearing and bulging. L4 is retro to L5 with disc tearing, wedging, and bulging. L5 is slightly antero to L6 with moderate wedging and slight tearing. L6-S1 look aligned.

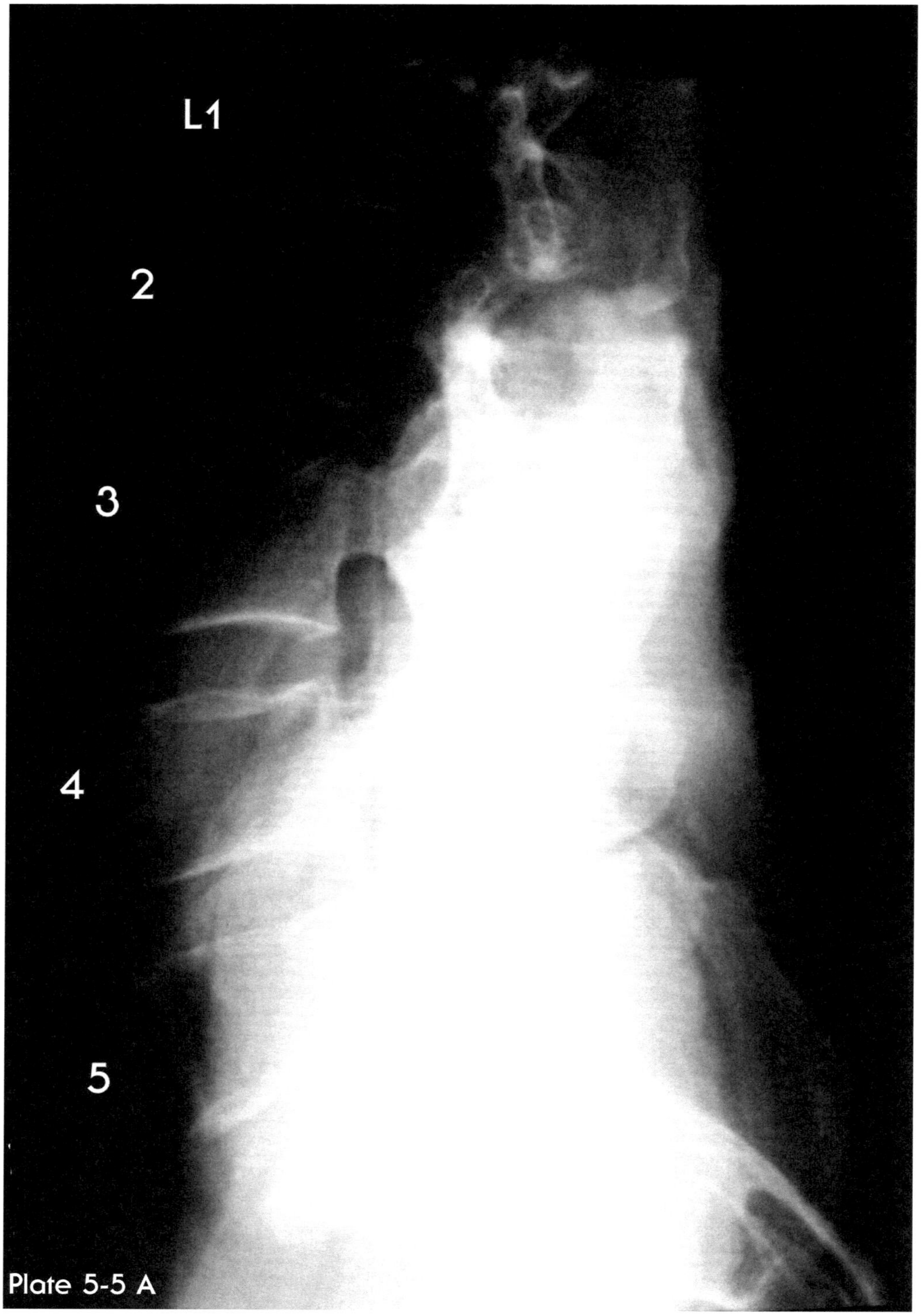

Plates 5-5 A & B

LUMBAR SPINE - A near normal lordotic curve with L5-sacral wedging

This person had a near normal alignment with the sacrum angled or subluxated posteriorly. The contracture of the thoracolumbar fascia can make permanent this "sacral base posterior" subluxation. L1 is retro to L2 with disc tearing, and anterior and posterior bulging; L2-L3 are aligned with slight wedging; L3-L4 is normal; the L4-L5 alignment is near normal, while the

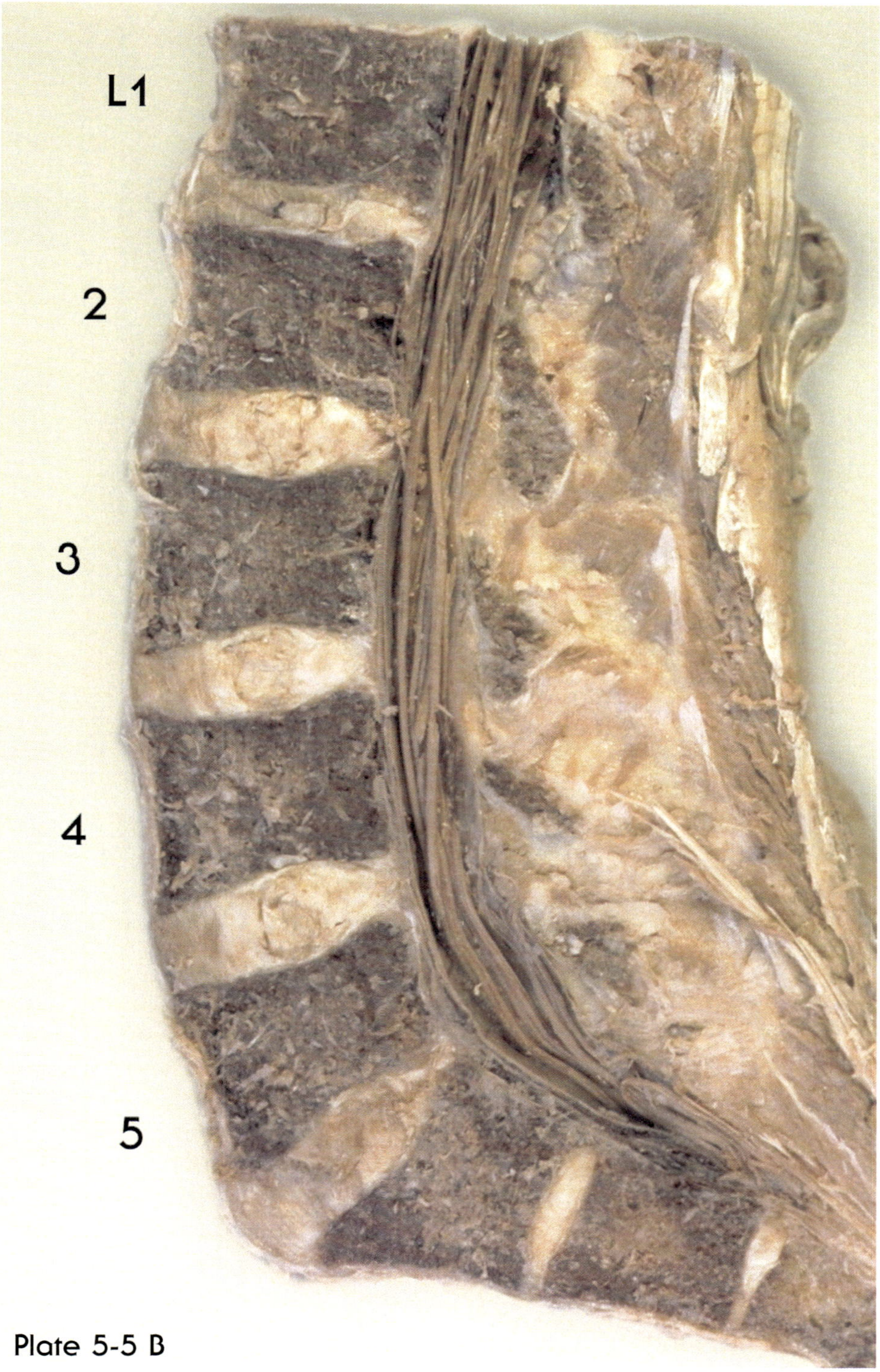

Plate 5-5 B

sacrum is only slightly retro to L5 with significant posterior disc height loss, anterior and posterior bulging, and tearing. Lack of A to P subluxation results in less DJD (degenerative joint disease).

Note: The sacral discs show that sacral motion was persistent. This lumbar spine is a good example of DJD associated with subluxation and normal discs associated with alignment and a normal curve.

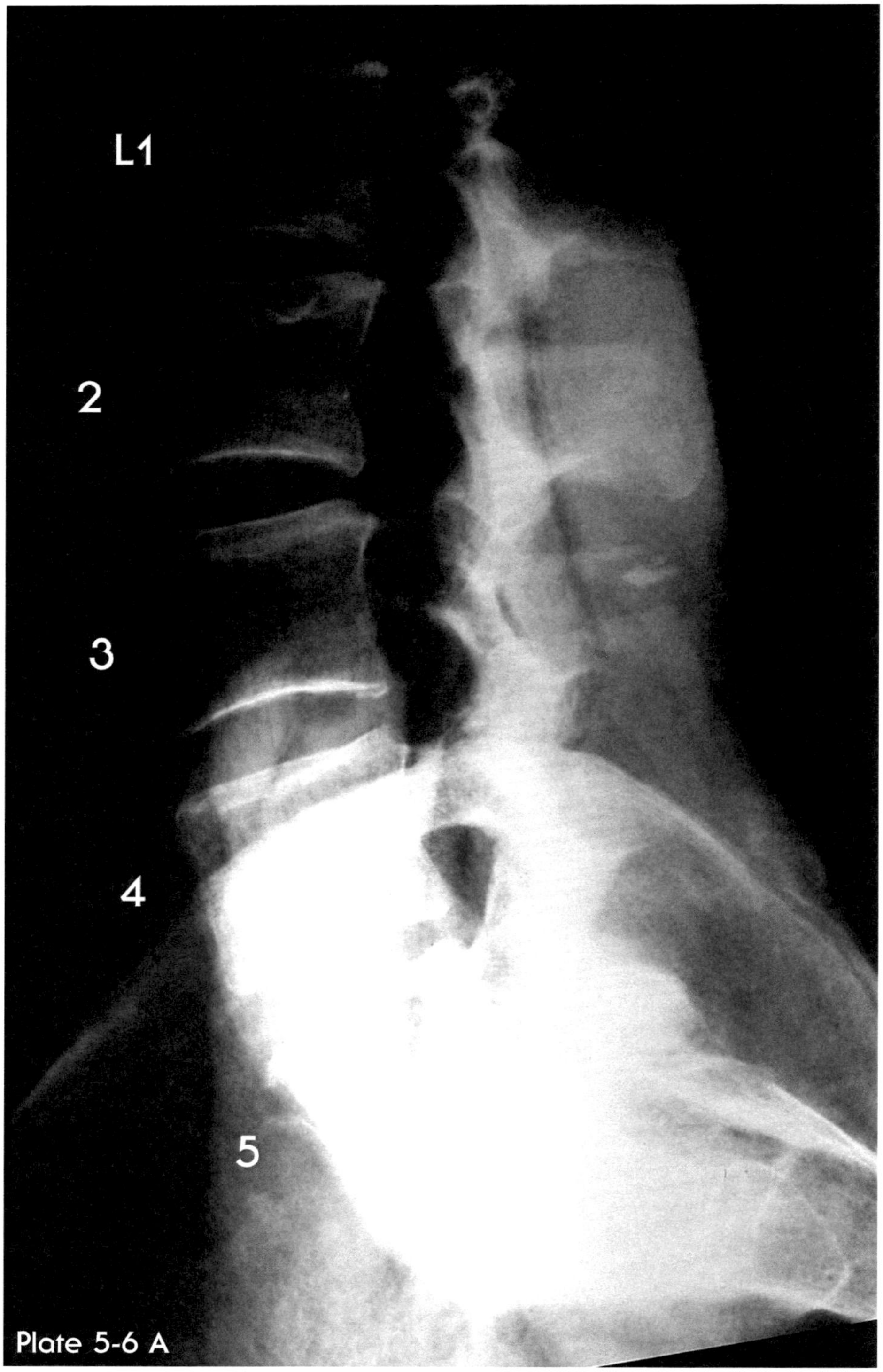

Plates 5-6 A & B

LUMBAR SPINE - This shows variations in a normal lumbar curve

L1-L2 look aligned but the endplates appear damaged and repaired, with a Schmorl's node of the superior L2 endplate, and with some disc tearing. L3 is aligned with L2 but has endplate damage with repair to both.

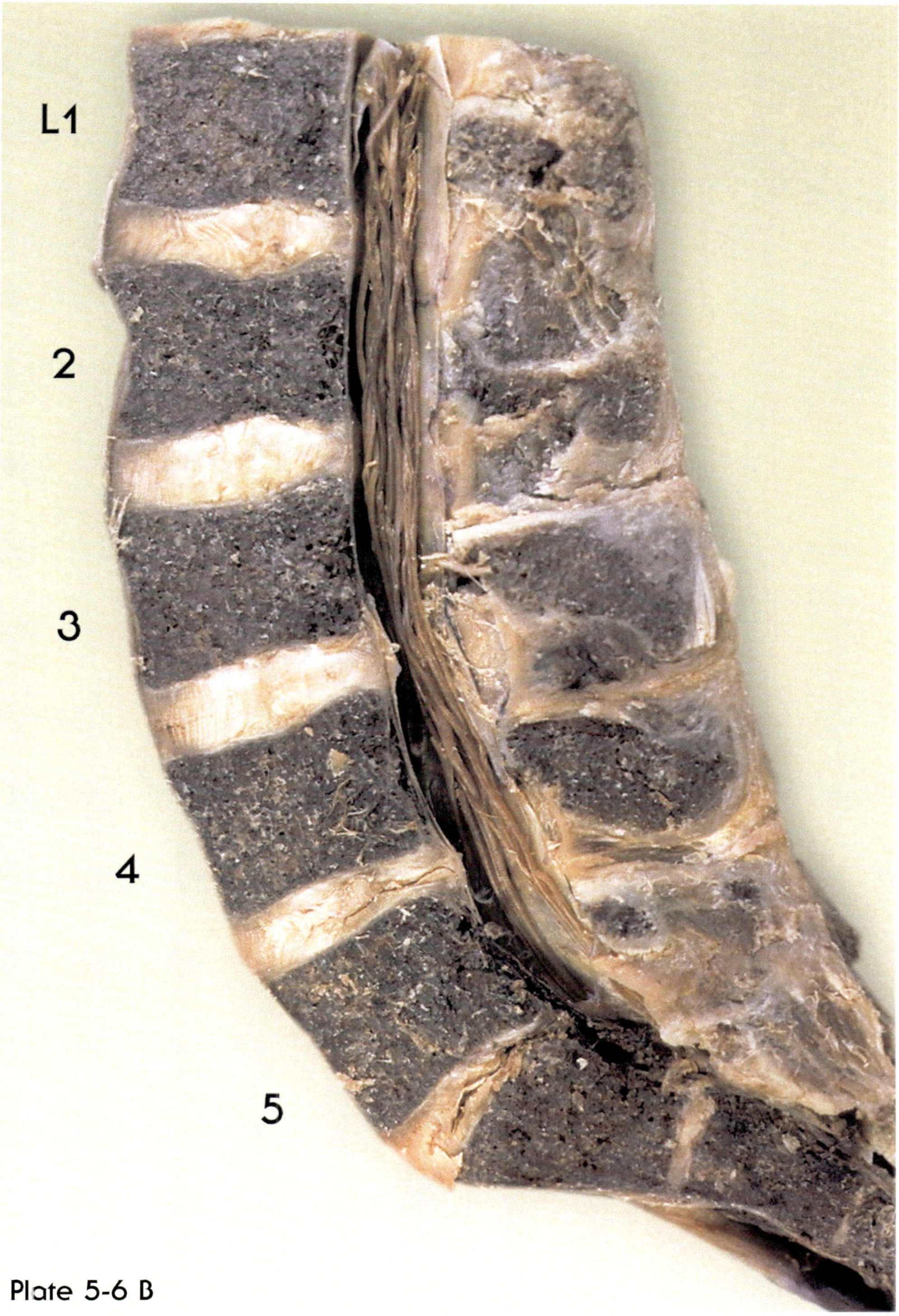

Plate 5-6 B

NOTE: The nucleus has expanded into the body of both L2 and L3 with near normal disc. L4 looks aligned with L3 with some endplate damage, repair, posterior disc bulging, and slight tearing. L4 is retro to L5 with disc tearing, posterior bulging, and loss of disc height. The L5 is retro to the sacrum with significant disc tearing, wedging, and loss of disc height.

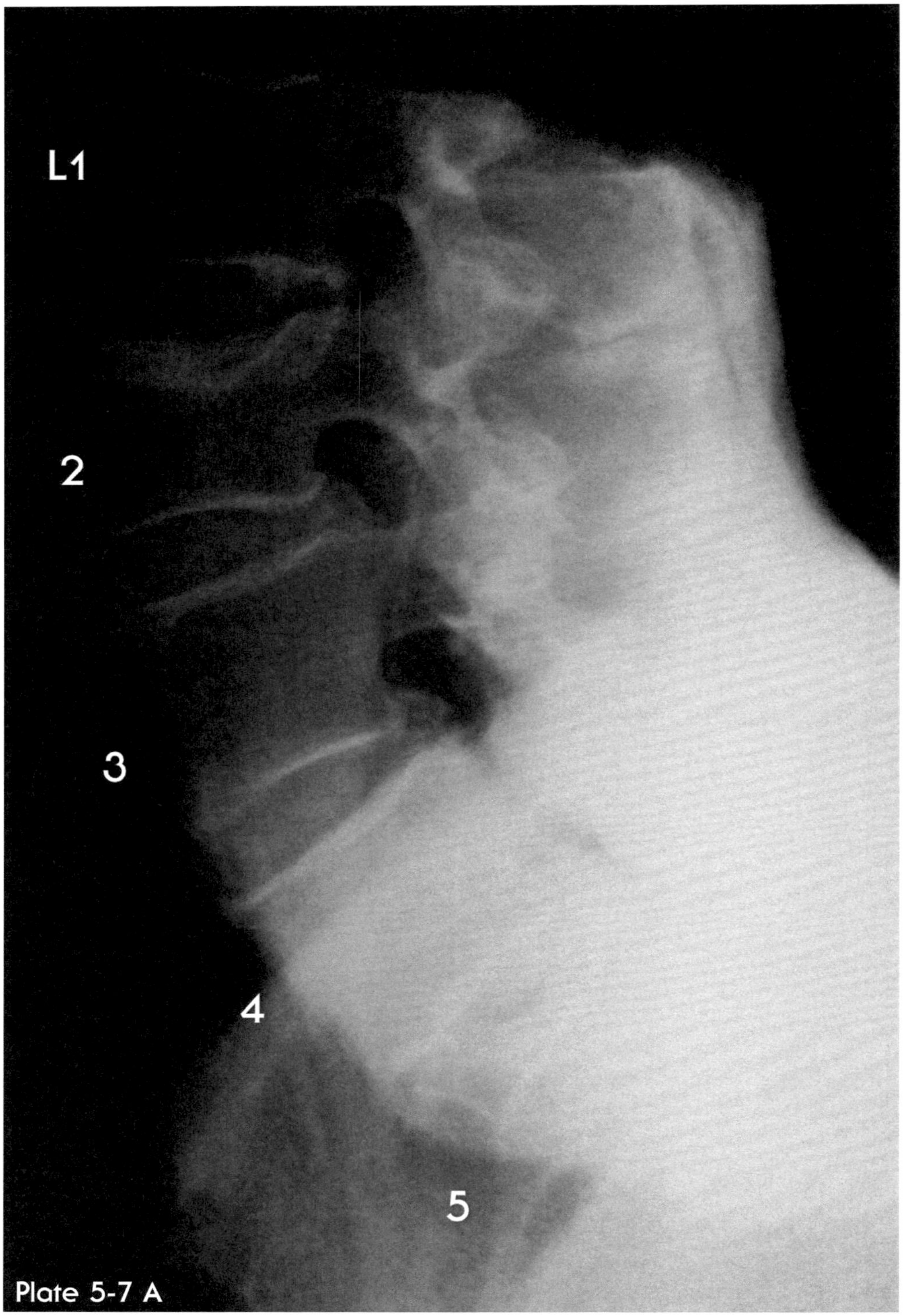

Plates 5-7 A & B

LUMBAR SPINE - This specimen has subluxated segments with the curve maintained

This shows there are signs of trauma with repair in the vertebral bodies. There is minor to moderate A to P subluxations but the normal lordotic curve is present. L1-L2 look aligned with compression fracture of L2. There is disc wedging and expansion of nucleus pulposus into vertebral body of L2. L2 is antero to L3 with disc tearing, wedging, and slight posterior bulging.

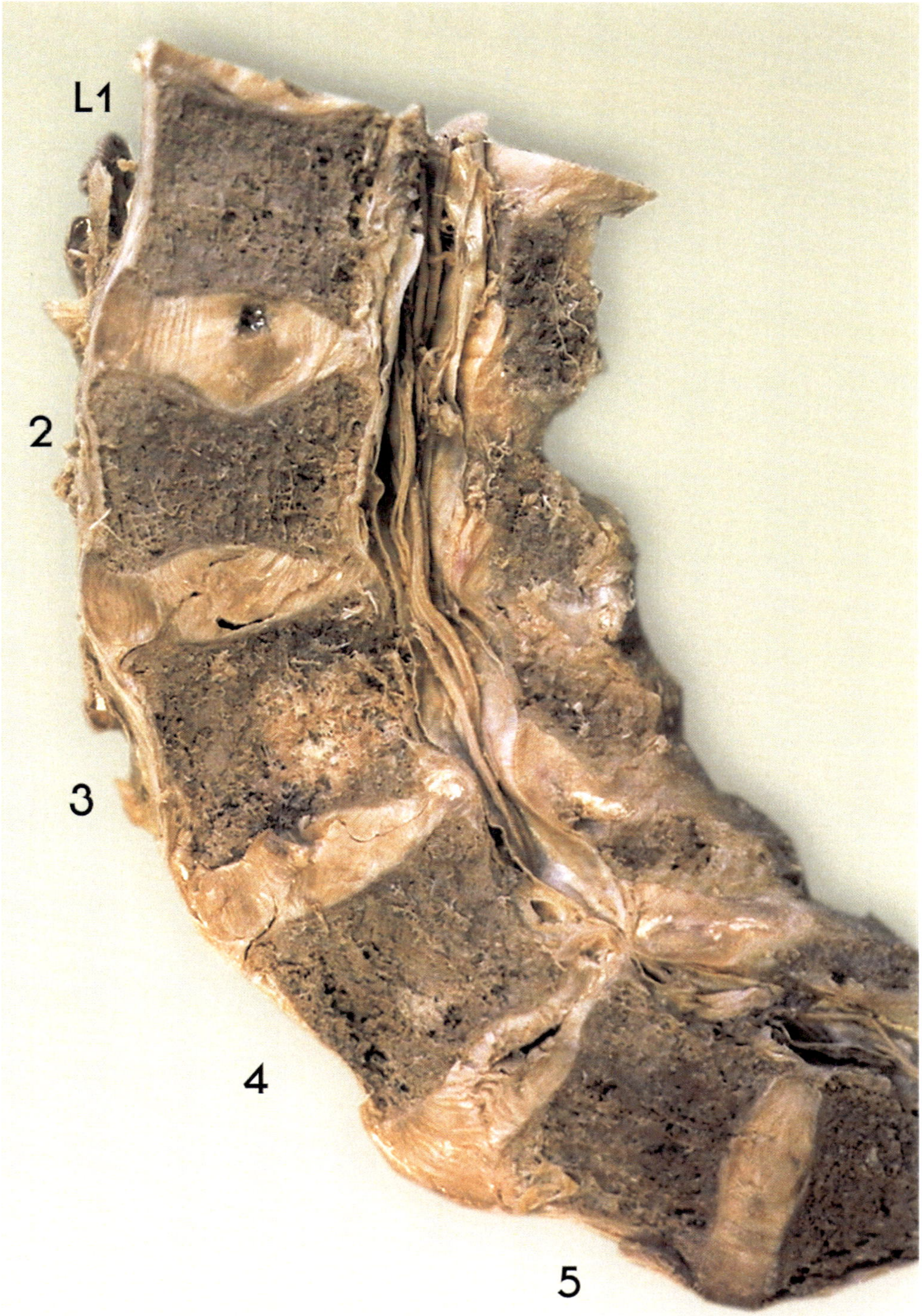

Plate 5-7 B

L3 is antero to L4 with disc tearing, wedging, and posterior bulging. L4 is antero to L5 with disc tearing, slight cavitation, wedging, and bulging. The L5-sacrum alignment looks normal. Note: The L2 vertebral body deformation with compressive force indicates it took the absorption of the shock, not the disc.

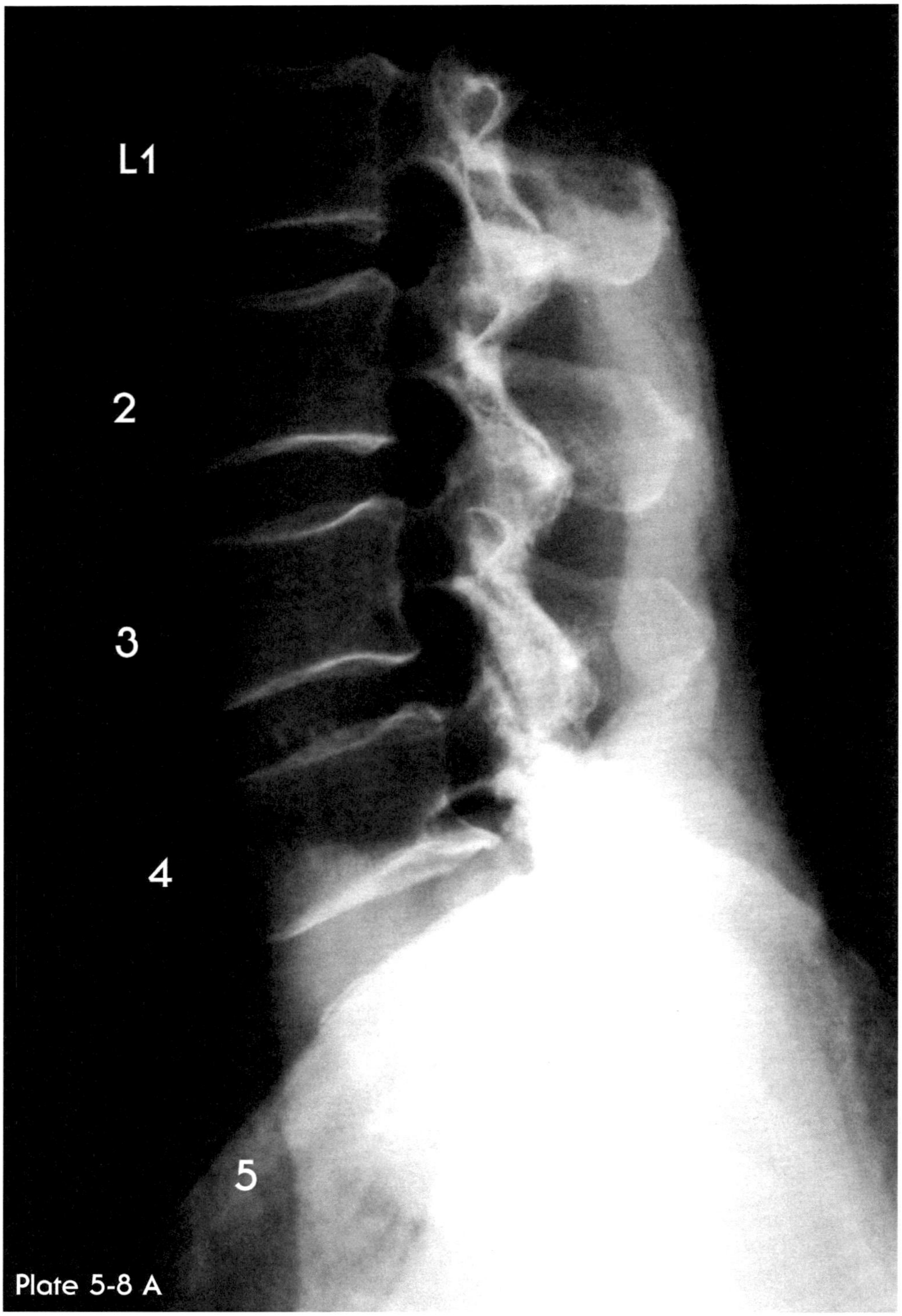

Plate 5-8 A

Plates 5-8 A & B

LUMBAR SPINE - variations in normal lumbar curve

In this specimen L1-L4 has good alignment with slight anterior brown degeneration. L4 is slightly antero to L5 and L5 is retro to the sacrum, making L5 a retrolisthesis.

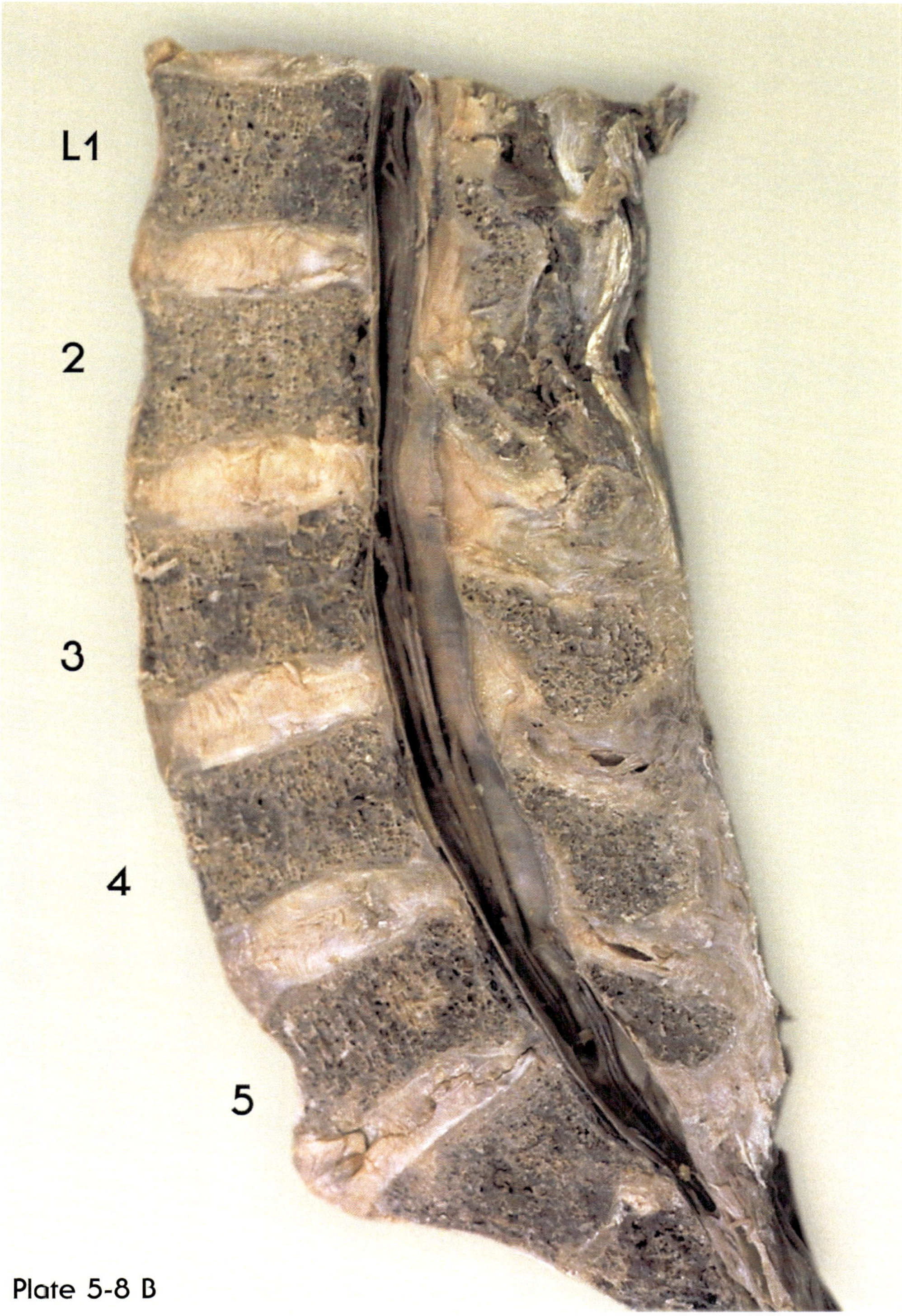

Plate 5-8 B

The L5-S1 disc is wedged, bulging anteriorly, and with disc tearing.
Note the presence of a slight lordotic curve.

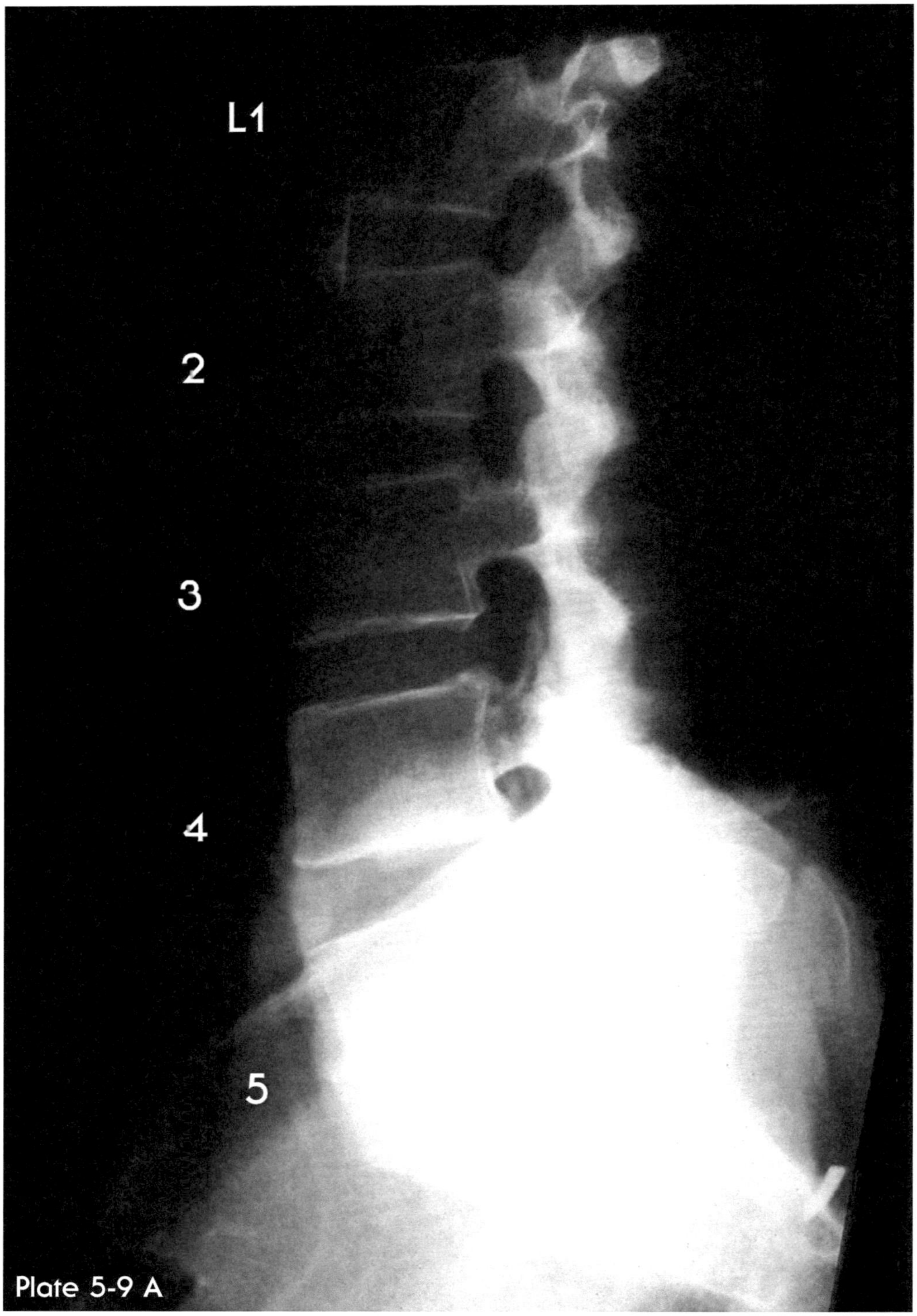

Plates 5-9 A & B

LUMBAR SPINE - Normal discs above a major subluxation with damaged discs

This specimen has maintained a moderate lordotic curve and the subluxation of L5 and the sacrum did not generate major osteophytic changes. L1 through L4 have normal alignment. L4 is slightly retro to L5 with nucleus desiccation, tearing and cavitation.

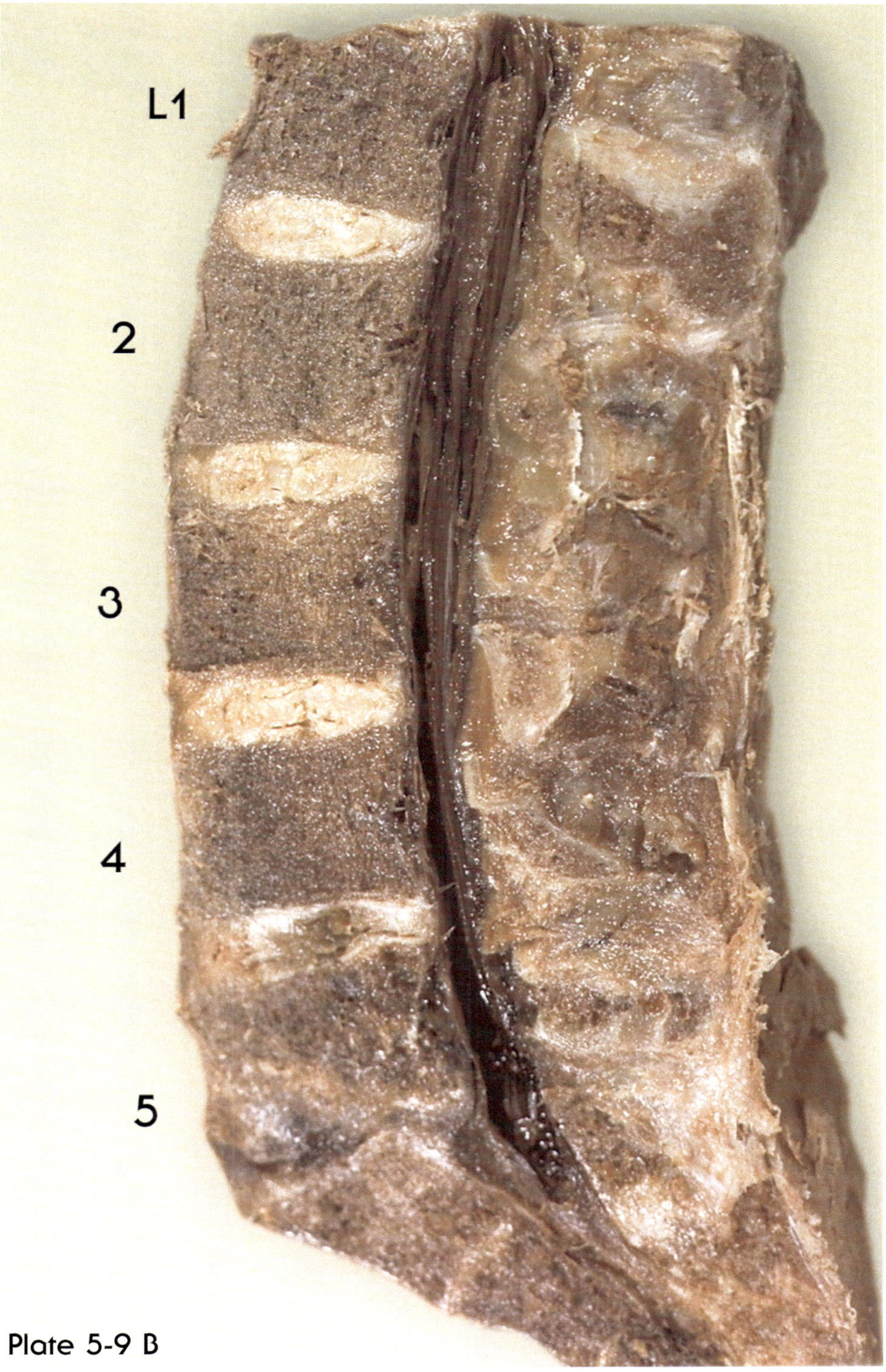

Plate 5-9 B

L5 is significantly retro to the sacrum with major degenerative changes, desiccation of the disc, and near fusion

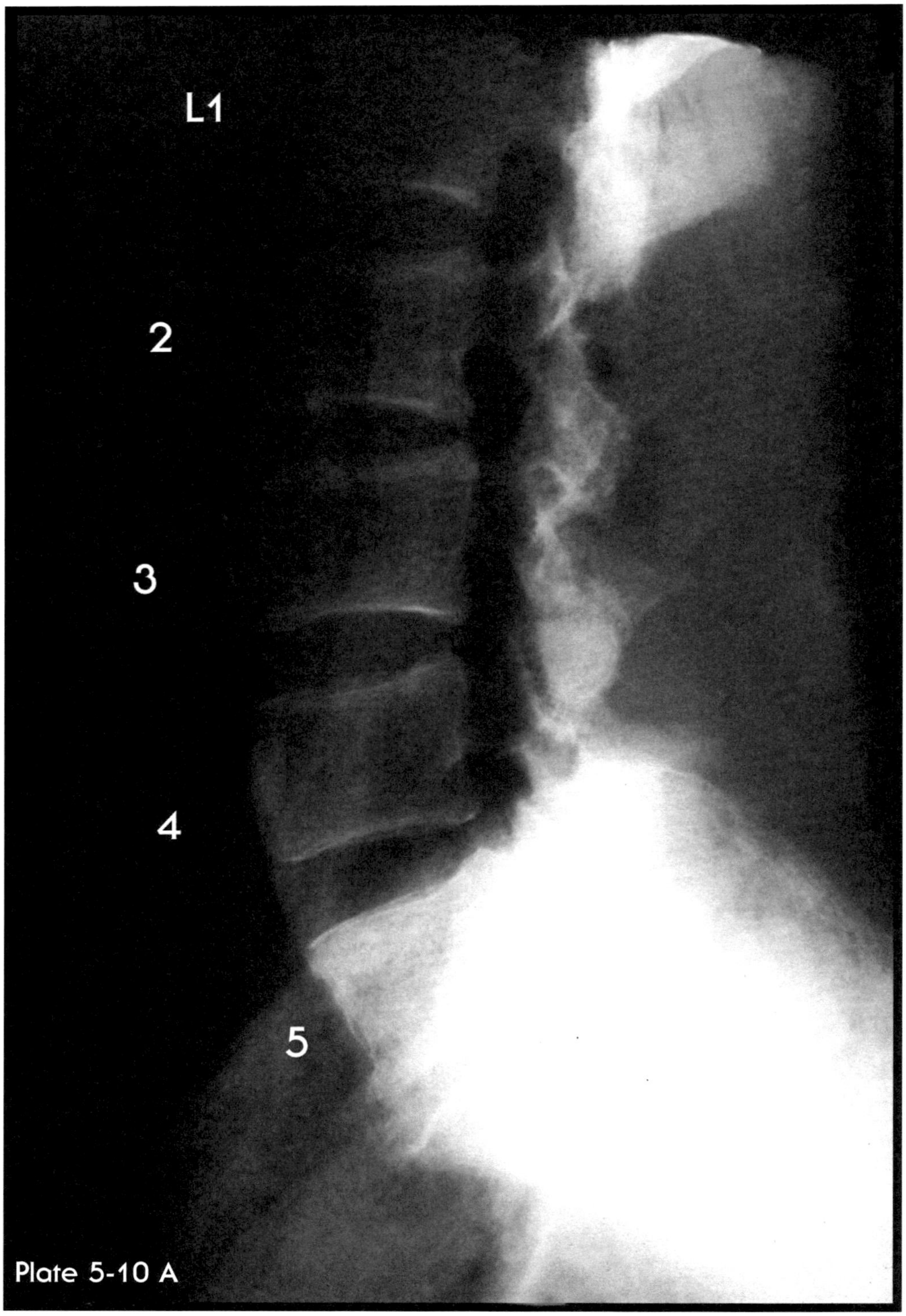

Plates 5-10 A & B
LUMBAR SPINE - This demonstrates L5-sacrum wedging with anterior displacement of the sacrum

This specimen has significant disc degeneration in the presence of normal and near normal discs. L1-L2 are near normal with the beginnings of brown degeneration. L2 is antero to L3 which is slightly retro to L4 with L2-L3 disc tearing and loss of height. L4-L5 looks good with

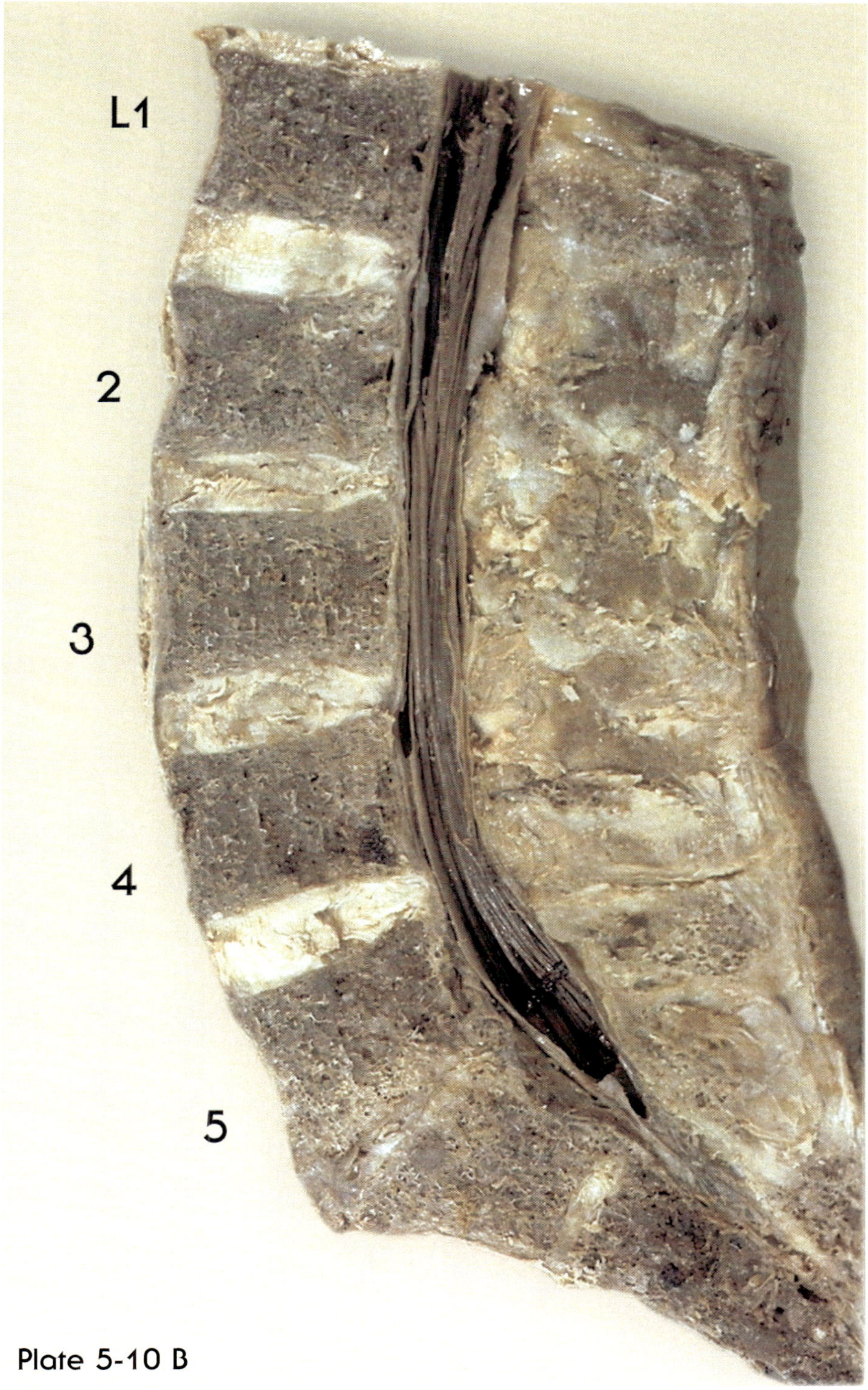

Plate 5-10 B

slight wedging and tearing, the sacrum is antero to L5 with fusion of posterior aspect of both segments. The disc has anterior bulging, tearing, and cavitation indicating an injury years earlier. The degree of A to P subluxation of the sacrum stopped normal motion and doomed the disc. Contracture of the thoracolumbar fascia reinforces the subluxation.

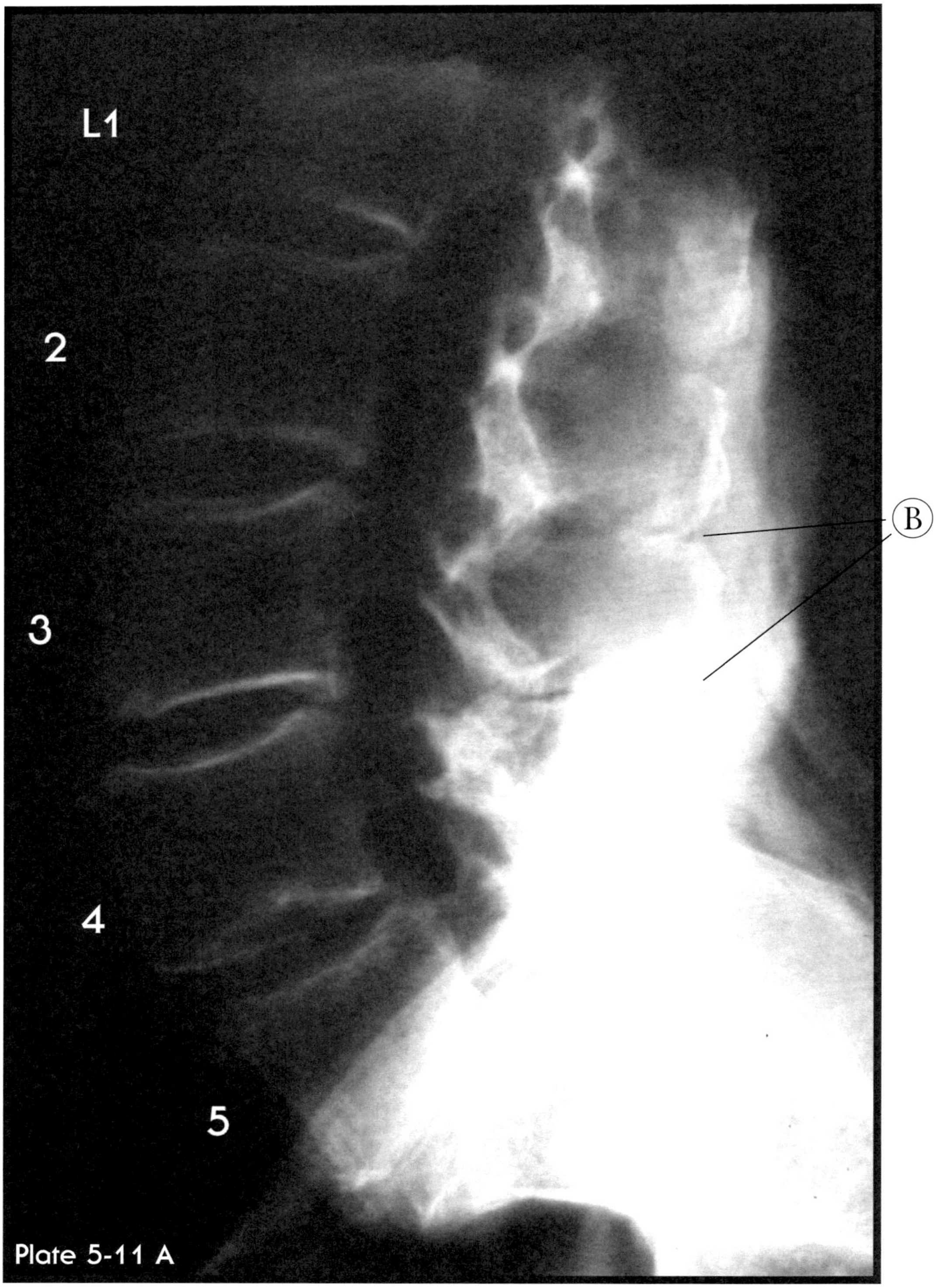

Plates 5-11 A & B
LUMBAR SPINE - This shows complete anterolisthesis of L4 and partially of L5 and S1 with end stage fusion

This is a specimen that has every segment subluxated with the lordotic curve maintained. An L1 compression fracture with repair has occurred. L1 is retro to L2 with disc wedging, tearing, and posterior bulging. L2 is retro to L3 with slight wedging, tearing, and bulging. L3 is retro to

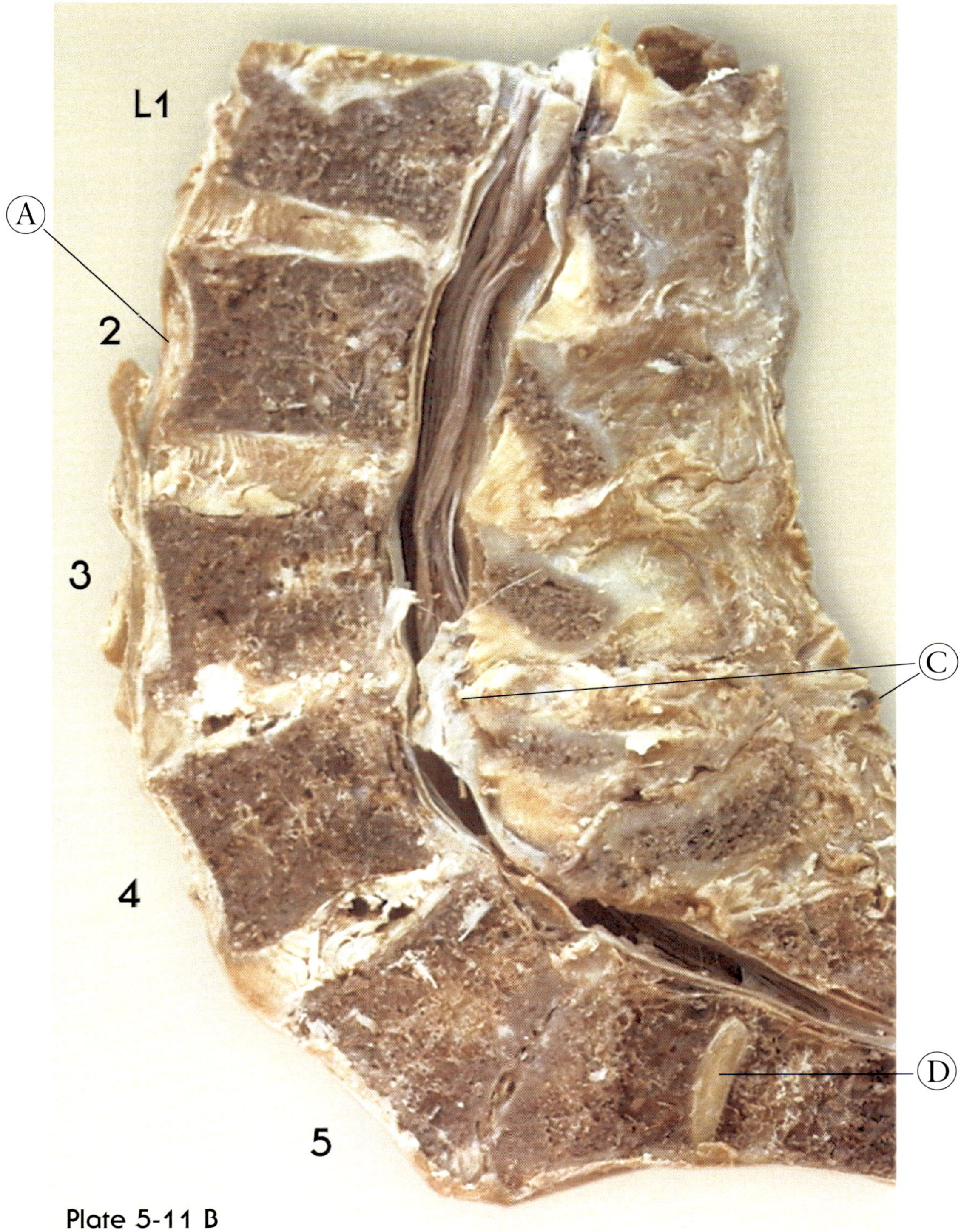

Plate 5-11 B

L4 with disc tearing, cavitation, slight bulging, and significant posterior disc height loss. L4 is antero to L5 with disc tearing, cavitation, anterior and posterior bulging. L5 is significantly antero to the sacrum with fusion.

(A) A.L.L. hypertrophy
(B) L1-L5 spinous process proximity
(C) Dissection of specimen diverges from mid-sagittal plane at L3
(D) Sacral disc

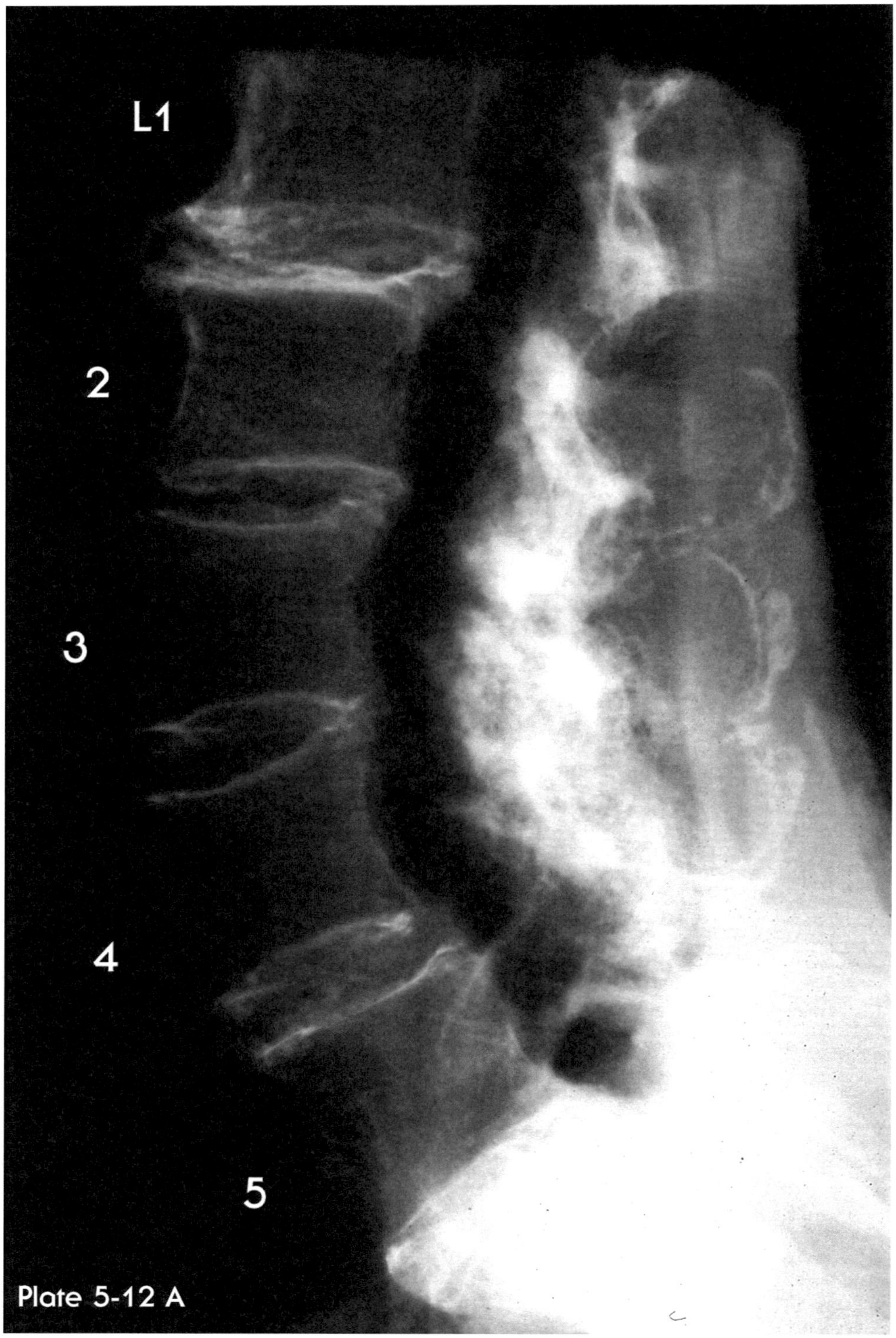

Plate 5-12 A

Plates 5-12 A & B
LUMBAR SPINE - This illustrates normal discs below damaged discs with lordotic curve maintained

In this specimen there are degrees of subluxation with corresponding degenerative changes. L1 is retro to L2 with significant endplate disturbance, loss of height, and anterior and

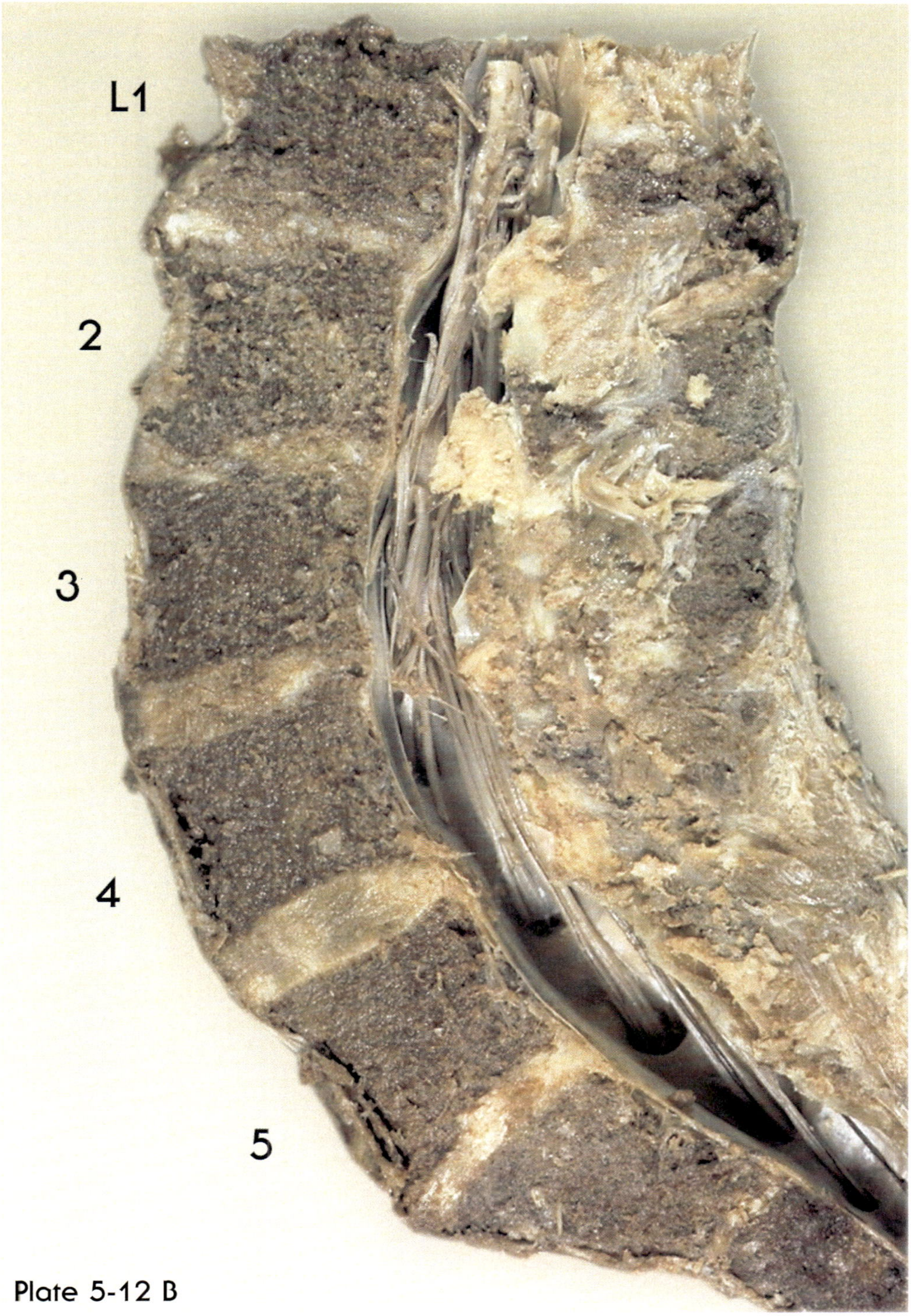

Plate 5-12 B

posterior disc bulging. L2 is retro to L3 with spurring and loss of disc height. L4 is anterior to L3 and L5 with disc wedging, bulging, and brown degeneration. The sacrum is slightly retro to L5 with loss of the disc height and calcification.

Note the lordotic curve is maintained and there is significant sclerosis of the facets and some of the spinous processes.

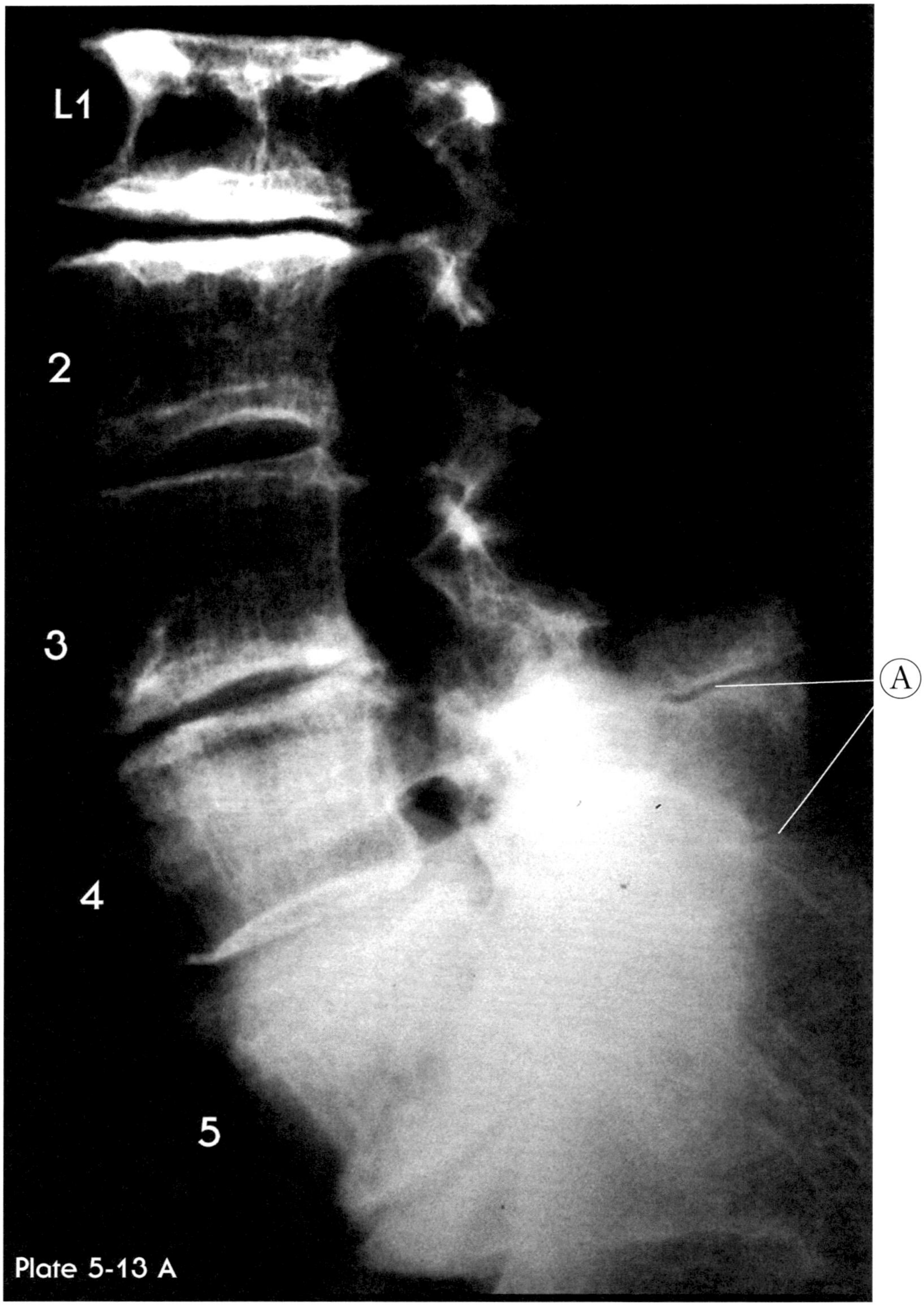

Plate 5-13 A

Plates 5-13 A & B

LUMBAR SPINE - The end stages of degeneration, post trauma

L1 has significant endplate repairs with anterior and posterior spurring. L1 is retro to L2 with significant loss of disc height, bulging anterior and posterior, tearing, and endplate repairs. L2 retro to L3 with disc tearing, bulging, loss of height, and impression into the inferior endplate of L2. L3 is retro to L4 which is antero to L5 with endplate repairs, anterior and

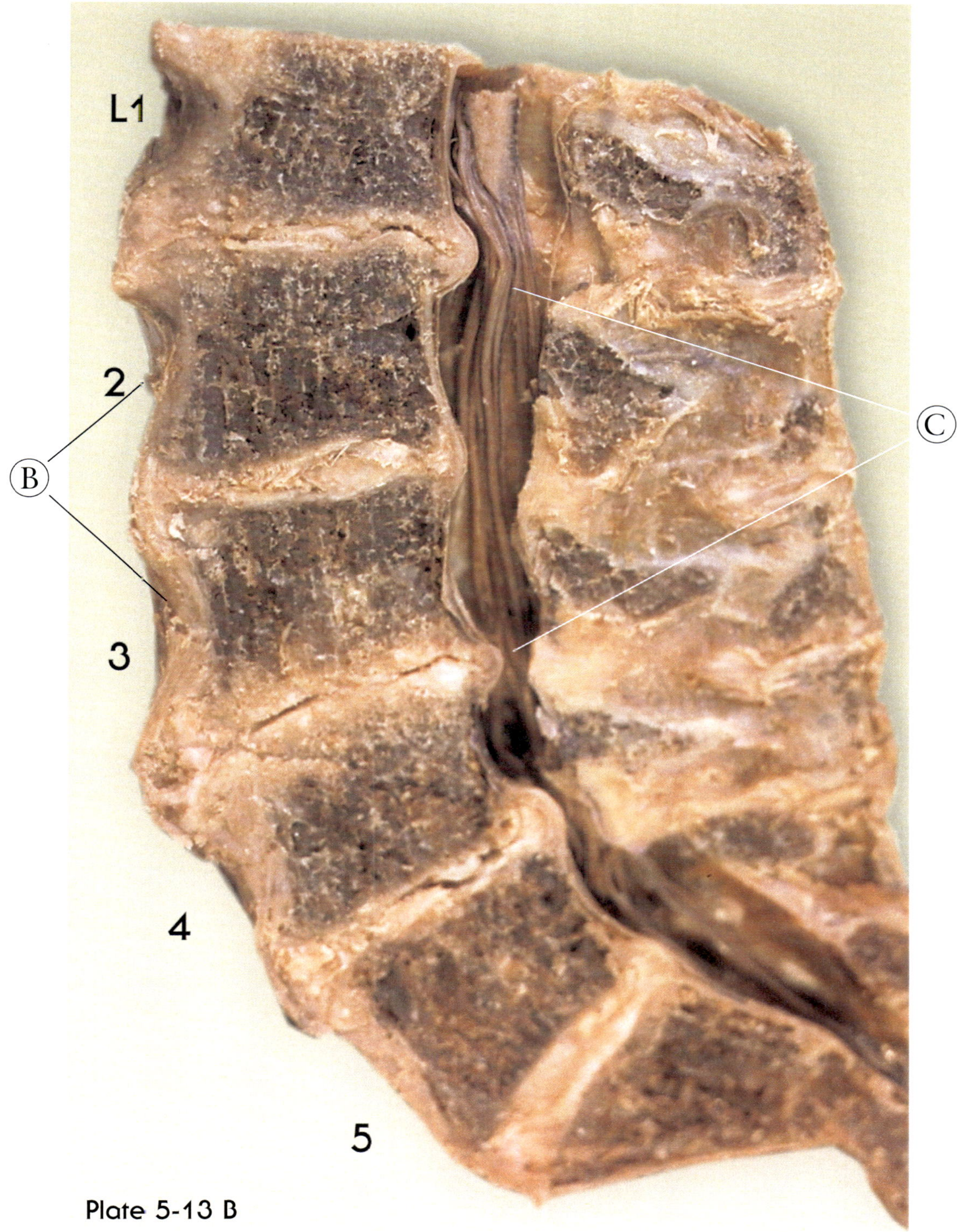

Plate 5-13 B

posterior spurring, disc tearing, and anterior and posterior bulging. L4-L5 has slight anterior and posterior spurring, disc tearing, anterior and posterior bulging, and loss of disc height. The sacrum is slightly antero to L5 with disc tearing, anterior and posterior bulging, loss of height, and anterior spurring.

(A) Spinous process contact forming pseudo-joints
(B) Hypertrophy of anterior longitudinal ligament
(C) Narrowing of spinal canal due to spurring and disc bulging

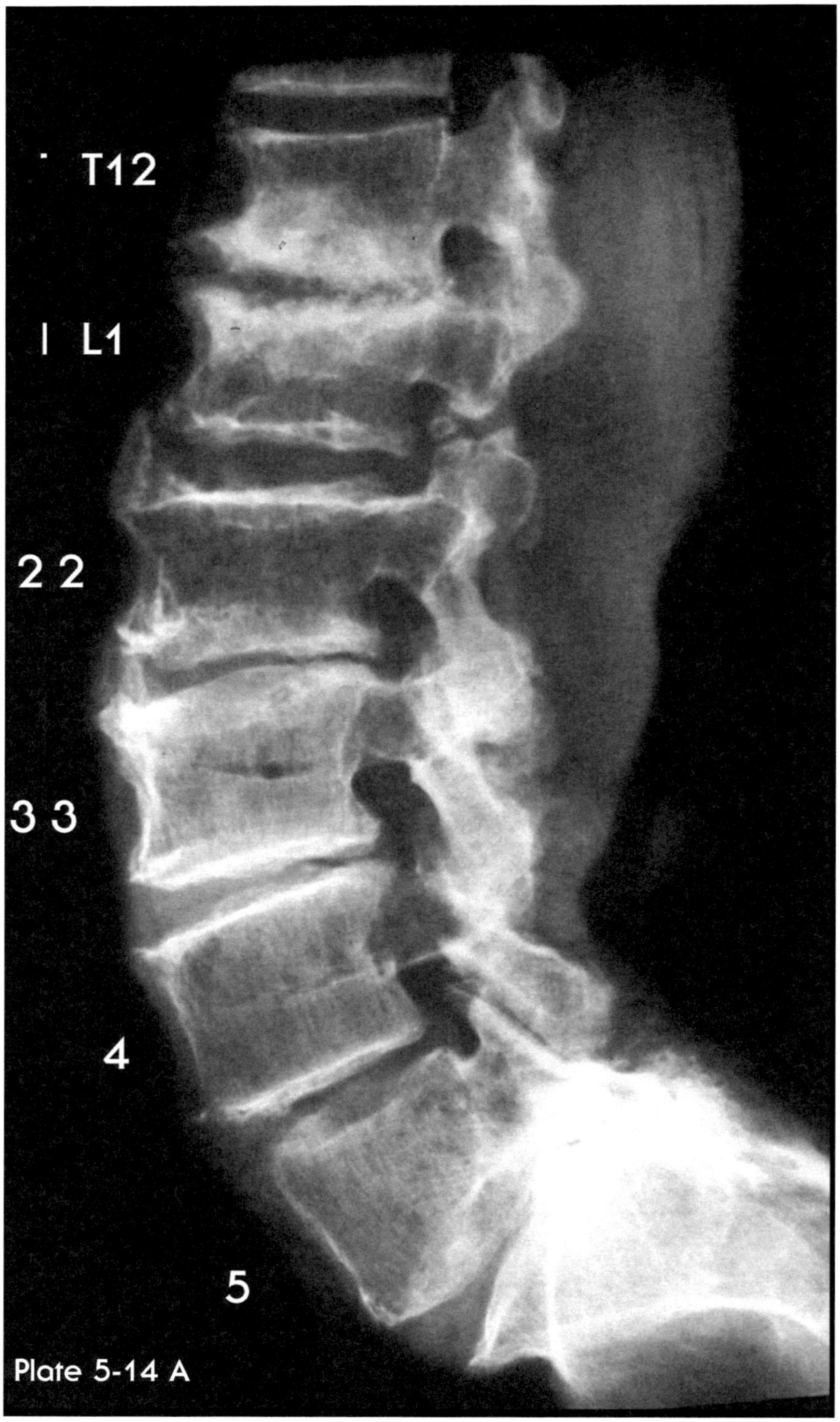

Plates 5-14 A & B

LUMBAR SPINE - This has subluxated segments with the curve maintained, sequential retrolisthesis to the segment below, or stairstepping

This specimen has a subluxation at every level. T12 is retro to L1 with spurring anterior and posterior, disc bulging, and loss of height. L1 is retro to L2 with disc tearing, calcification of disc, and the anterior longitudinal ligament.

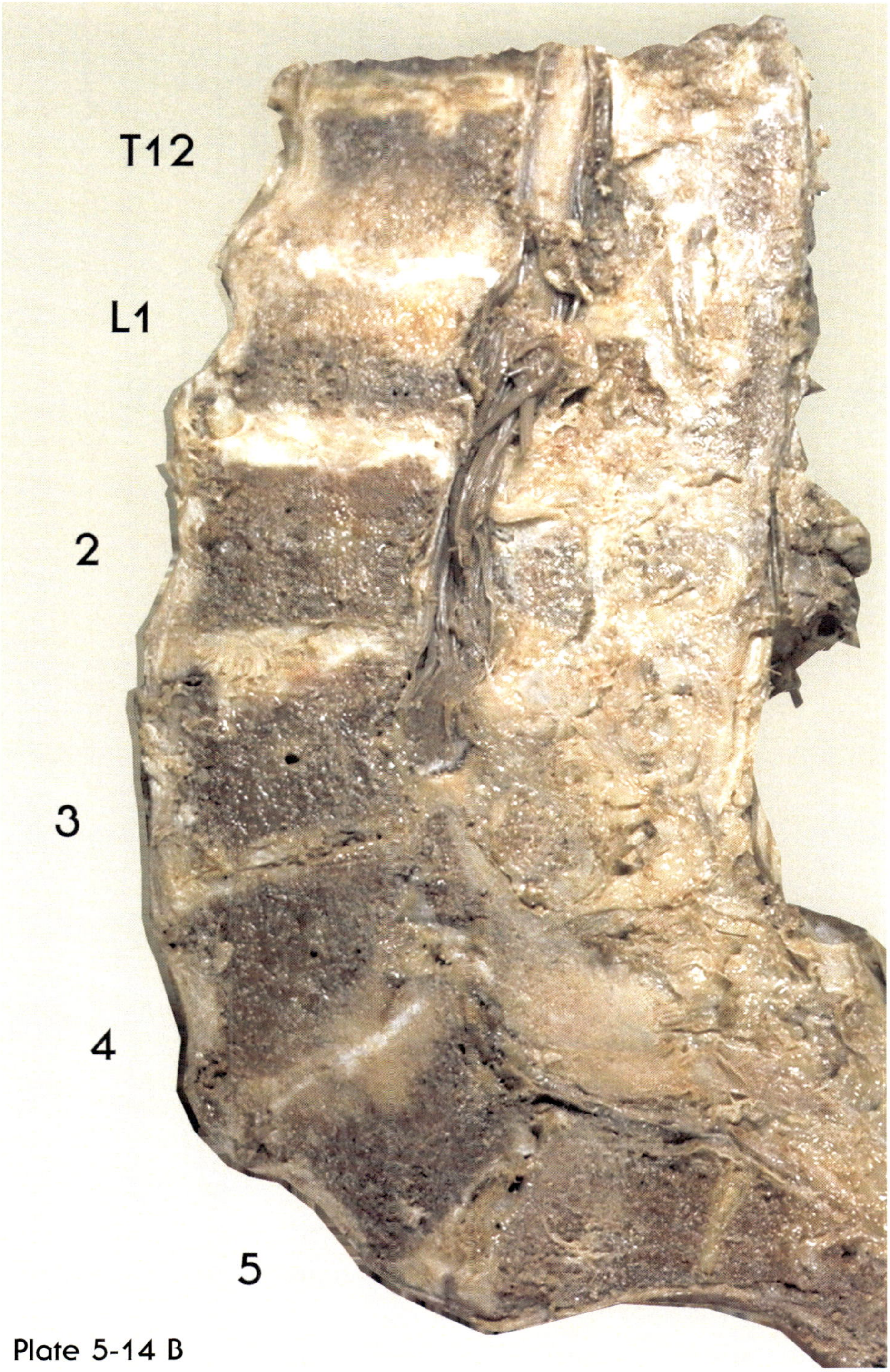

Plate 5-14 B

Note fracture of L1 inferior facet. L2 is retro to L3 with disc tearing, loss of height, calcification of anterior disc, and anterior and posterior spurring; L3 is retro to L4 with disc tearing, cavitation, and anterior and posterior spurring; L4 is antero to L5 with anterior and posterior disc bulging and loss of disc height. L5 is antero to the sacrum with disc tearing, cavitation, wedging, and near fusion of the posterior aspect of L5 and S1. Note lack of spinous processes on X-ray due to perisagittal plane of the specimen.

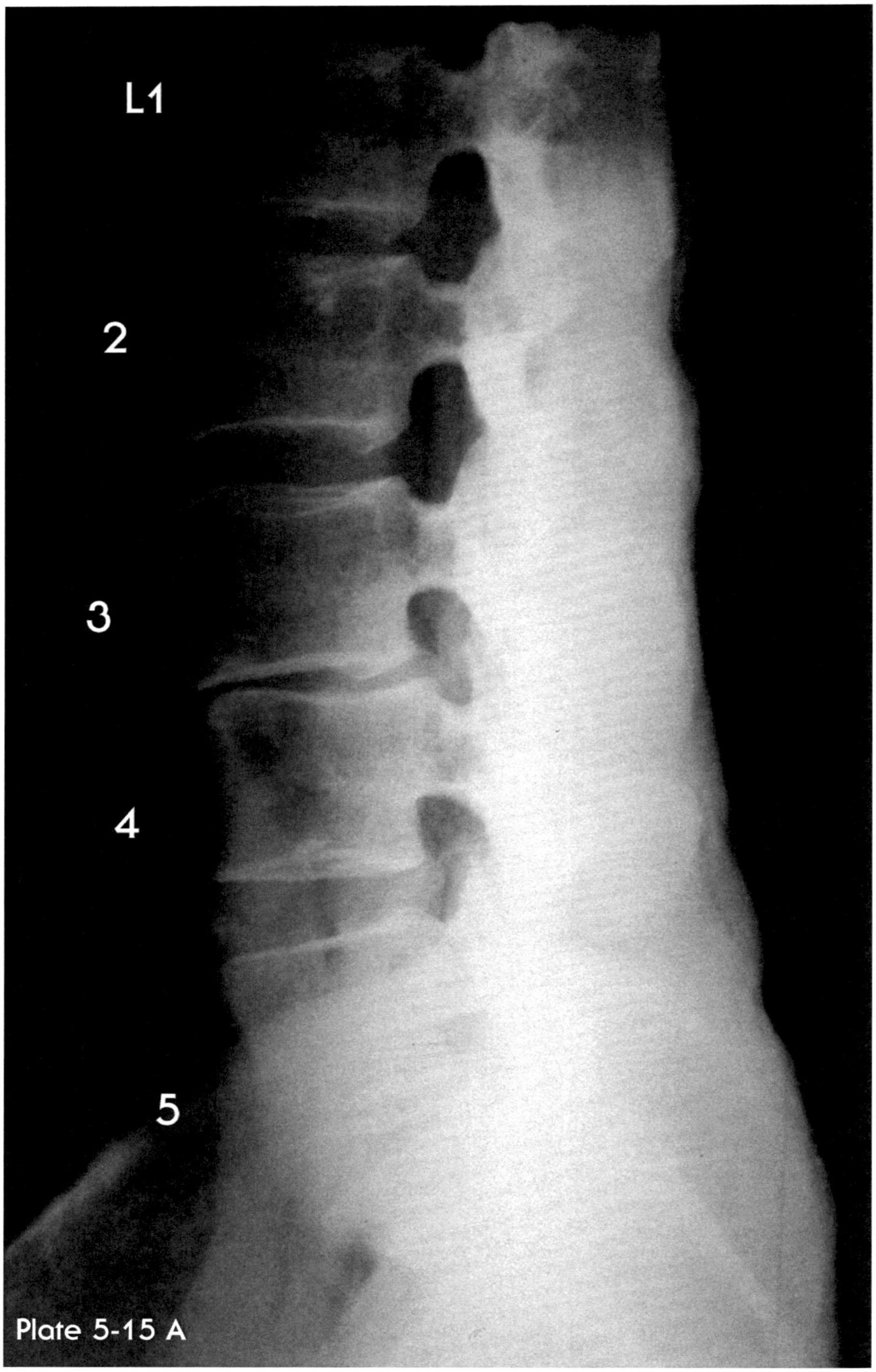

Plates 5-15 A & B

LUMBAR SPINE - This shows a hypolordotic curve with one significant subluxation

This specimen has near normal alignment and joints with the presence of one significant subluxation. L1 is slightly posterior to L2 with slight disc tearing, anterior and posterior bulging, and endplate damage. L2-L3 has good alignment with a normal disc, in an aged spine.

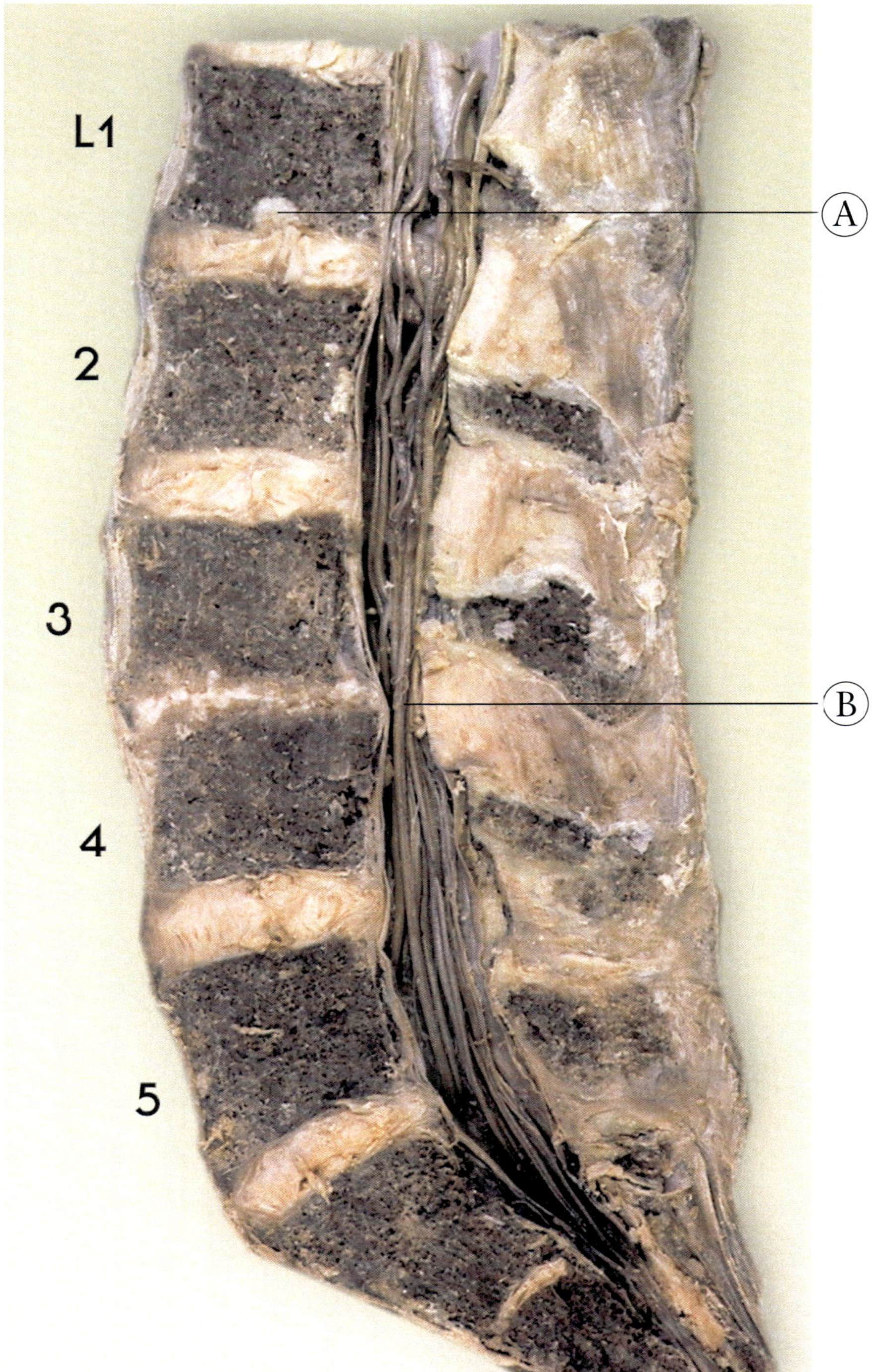

Plate 5-15 B

L3 is antero to L4 with minor disc bulge, loss of disc height, and near fusion. L4 is retro to L5 with a slight posterior disc bulge. L5 and sacrum alignment is near normal with slight anterior and posterior disc bulging.

(A) Schmorl's Node (invagination of nucleus pulposus into vertebral body) of inferior L1 endplate

(B) Canal stenosis at L3-L4

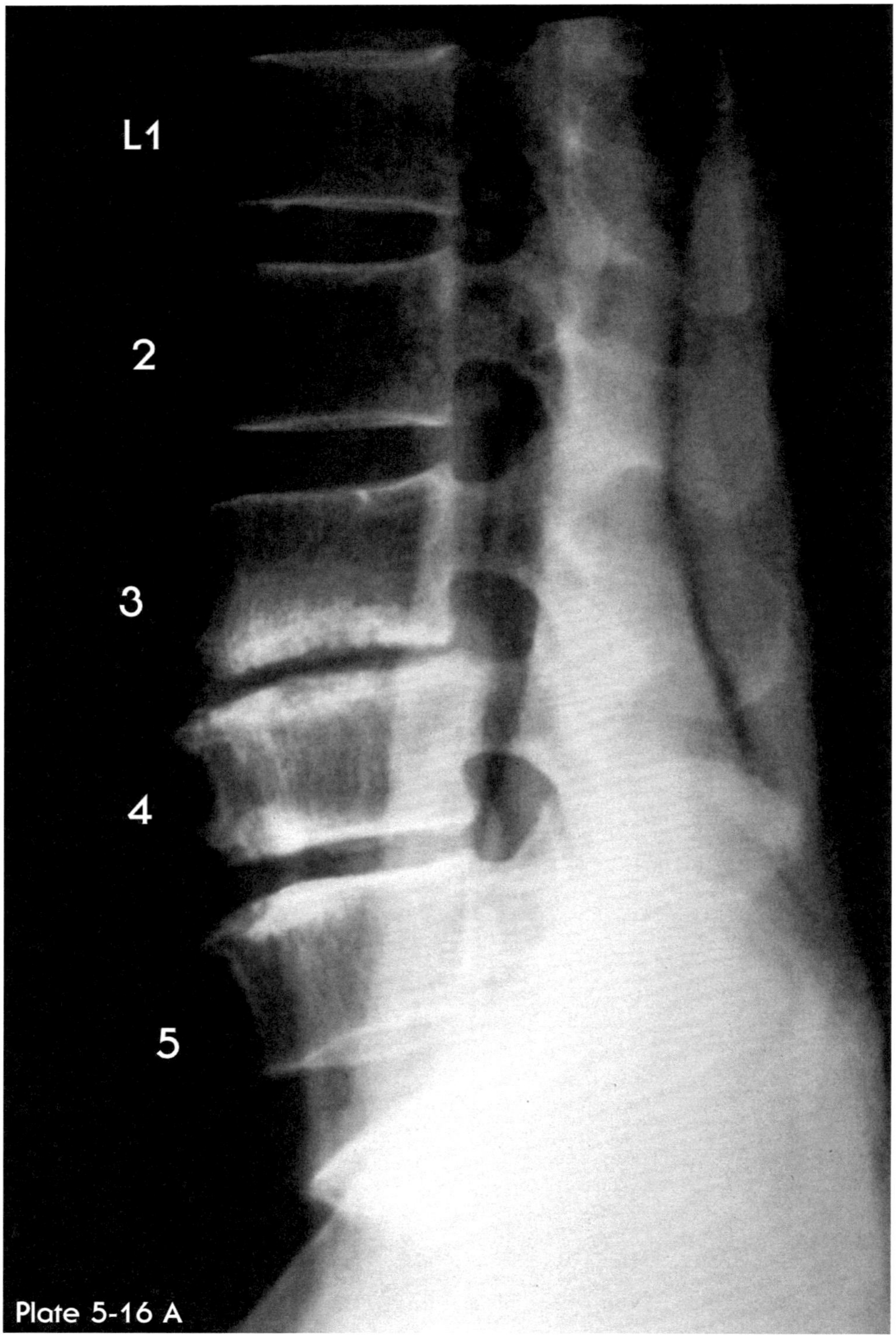

Plates 5-16 A & B

LUMBAR SPINE - This illustrates subluxations with a loss of lordotic curve and various stages of disc degeneration

The loss of lordotic curve has resulted in the increase in the vertebral body width in these subluxated segments. L1-L2 and L2-L3 look nearly normal with the beginning of brown degeneration. L3 is antero to L4 with signs of a compression fracture, anterior and posterior spurring, disc tearing, and anterior and posterior bulging. L4 is a retrolisthesis to L5. L5 is

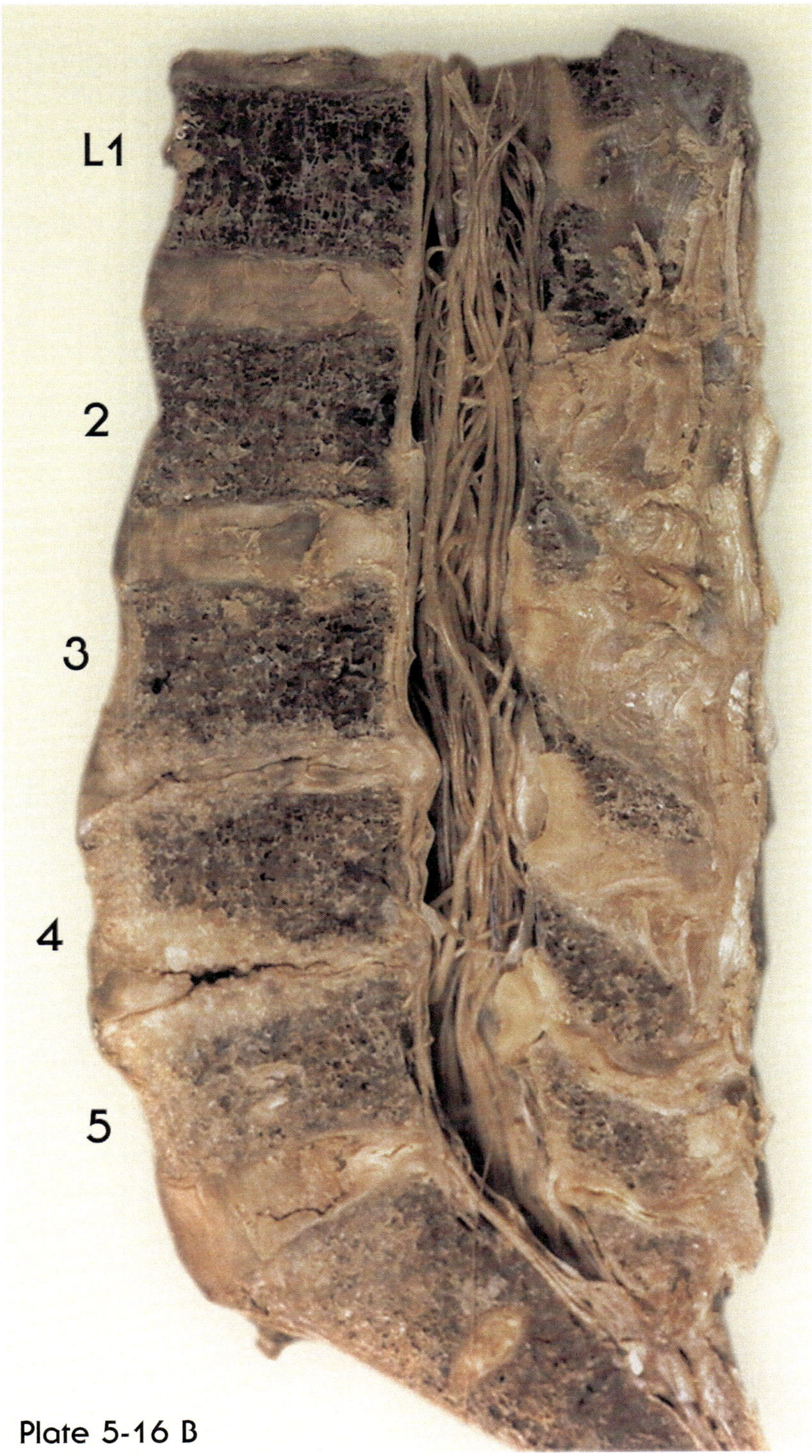

Plate 5-16 B

posterior to the sacrum, with anterior spurs. The L4-L5 disc has tearing, cavitation (vacuum), and separation of the posterior longitudinal ligament from L5 because of the posterior disc migration. The L5-S1 disc has wedging, tearing, and posterior bulging over the back of the sacral base. The endplates of L3, L4, and L5 indicate trauma with repair and L4 has loss of anterior body height.

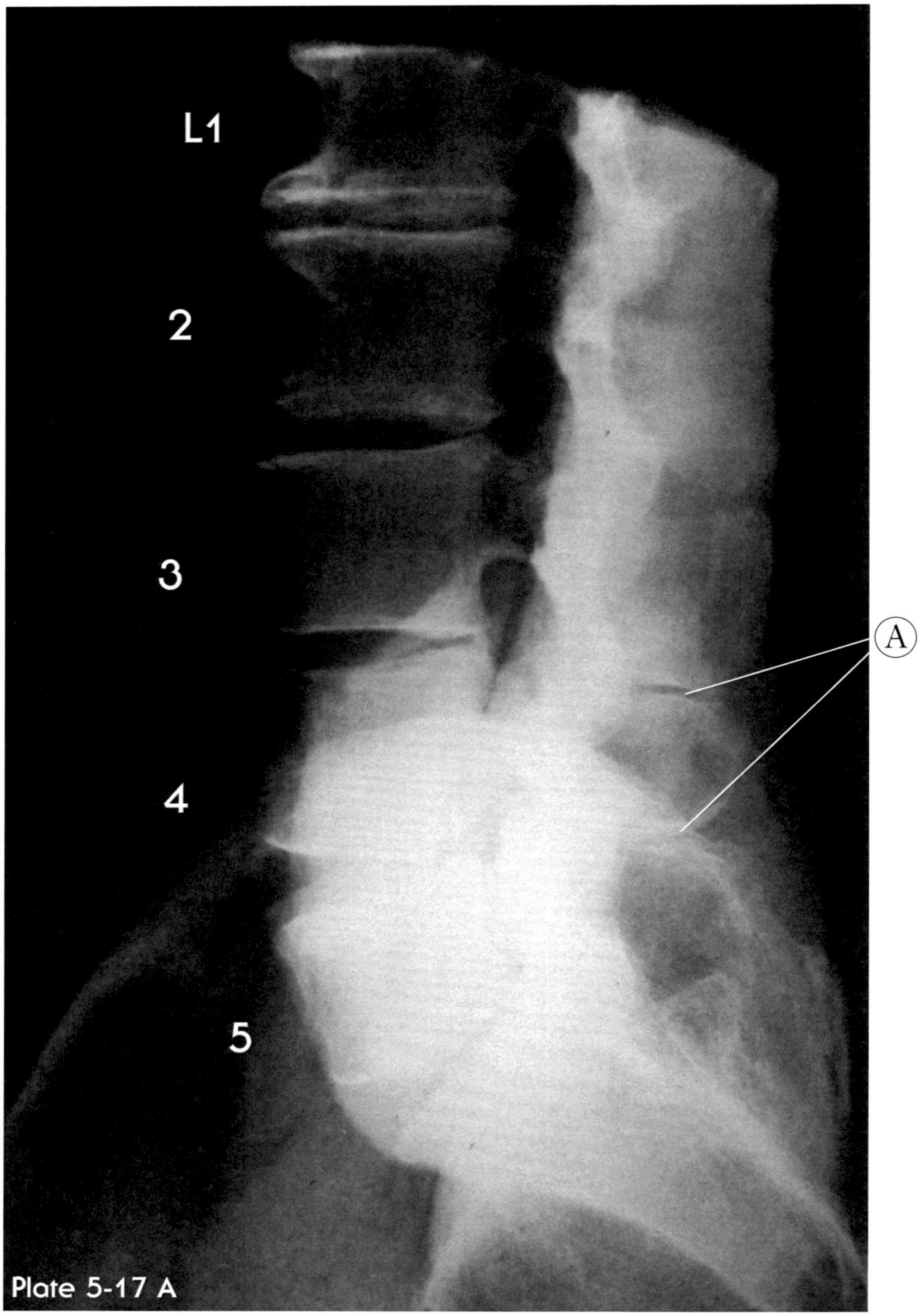

Plates 5-17 A & B
LUMBAR SPINE - The subluxation complex of this specimen involves the entire lumbar spine

There is stairstepping of each segment posteriorly to the one below. This is a common feature of the standing posture, with the pelvis being translated anteriorly to the thorax. L1 is retro to L2 and has major endplate spurring and repair processes indicating a chronic long-term condition. L2 is retro to L3 with significant spurring, tearing, loss of

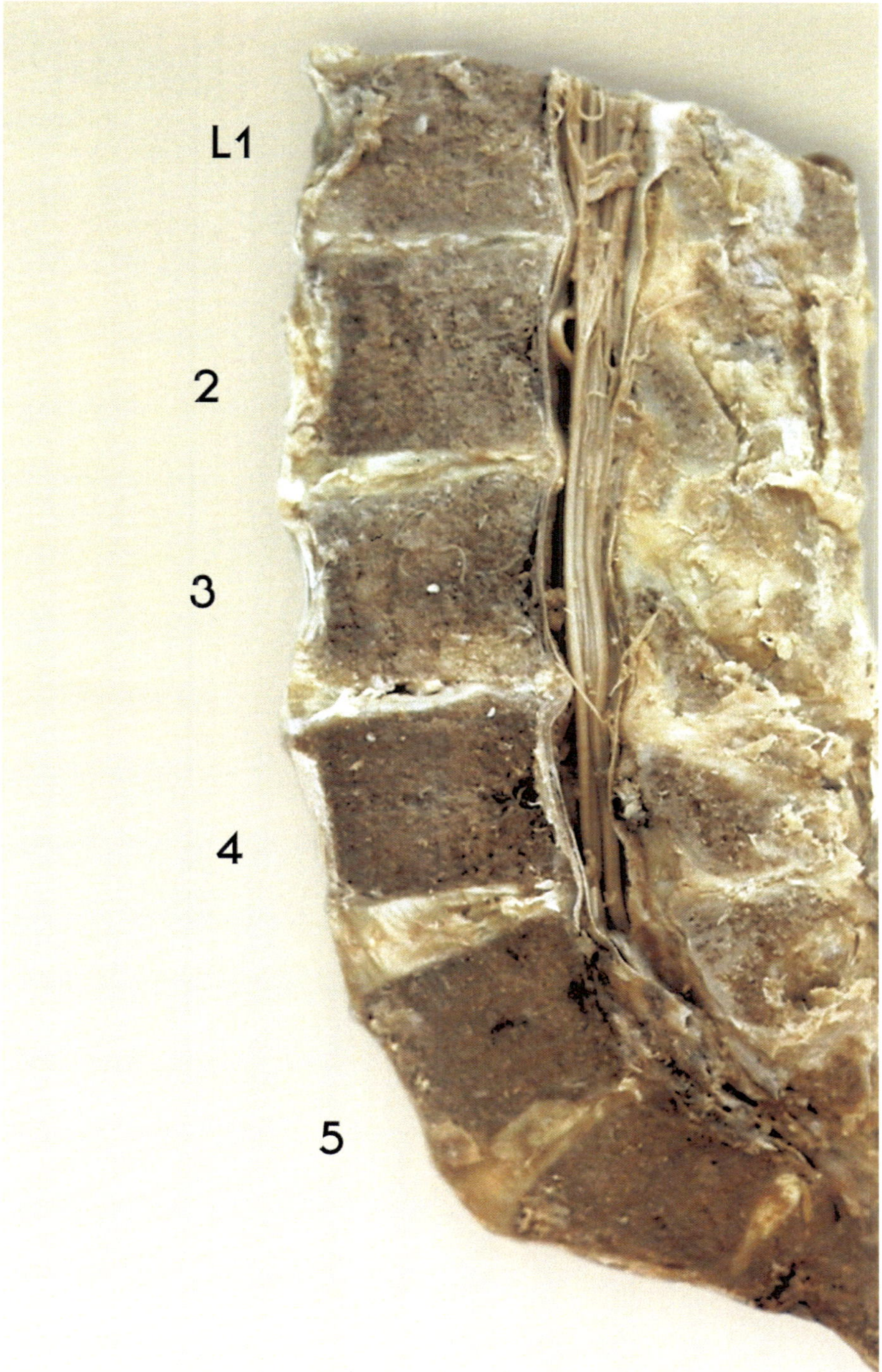

Plate 5-17 B

height and endplate changes. L3 is retro to L4 with disc tearing, minor anterior bulging, and loss of height. There is anterior longitudinal ligament hypertrophy. L4 is retro to L5 or L5 is antero to L4 and the sacrum with disc tearing, wedging, slight cavitation, and bulging. L5-S1 has disc wedging, loss of disc height, and near fusion. The sacral disc S1-S2 has wedging, slight posterior bulging, and angulation of S1-S2 segments.

(A) Spinous process pseudo-joint formation due to loss of disc height

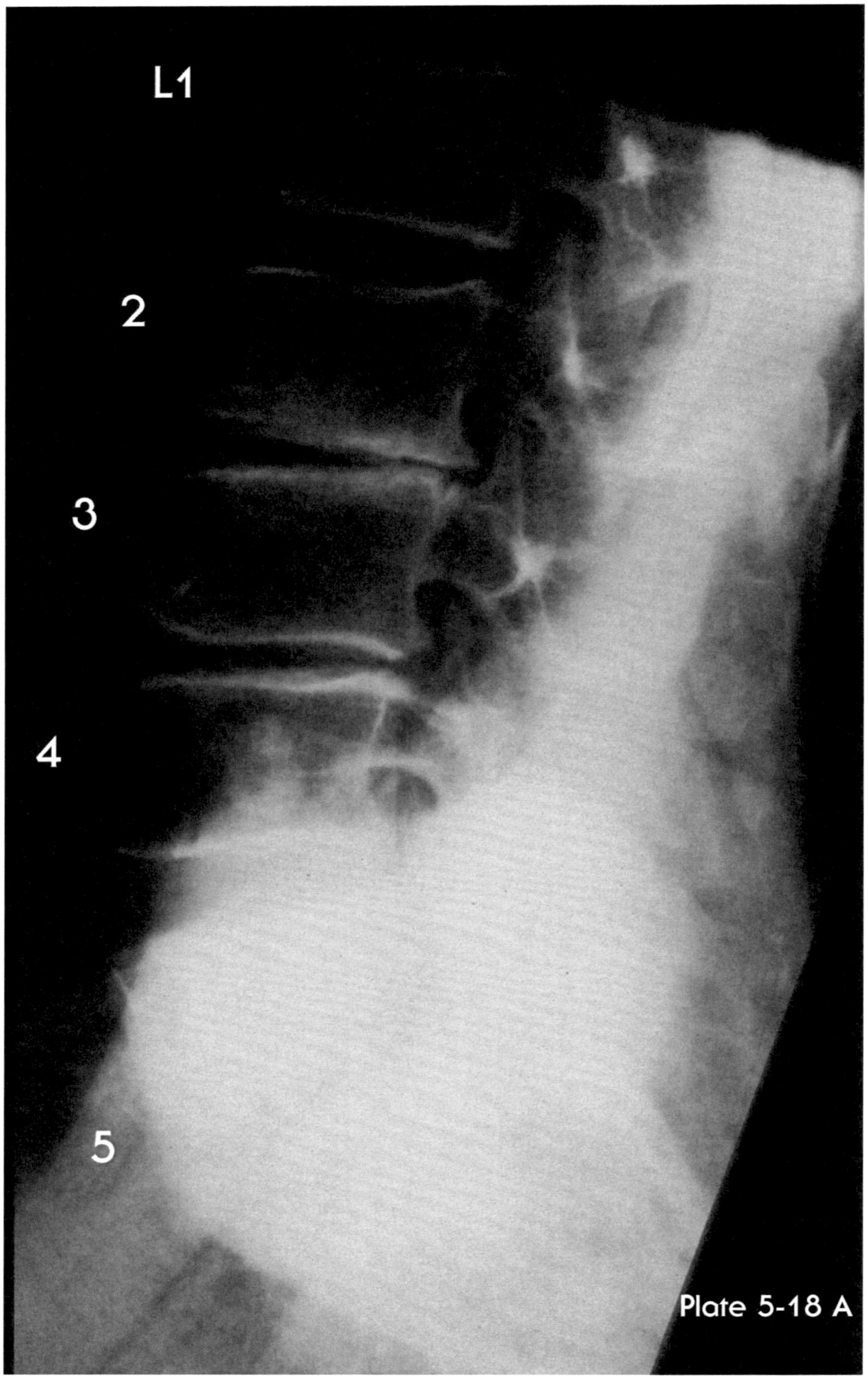

Plates 5-18 A & B

LUMBAR SPINE - This shows multiple subluxations with loss of lordotic curve

This specimen has chronic posterior stairstepping of vertebrae L2-L4 to the segment above. L1 is retro to L2 with disc tearing, cavitation, and endplate repair, and has a slight compression fracture. L2 is retro to L3 with posterior spurring, endplate repair, disc wedging, tearing, anterior and posterior bulging, and loss of disc height. L3 is

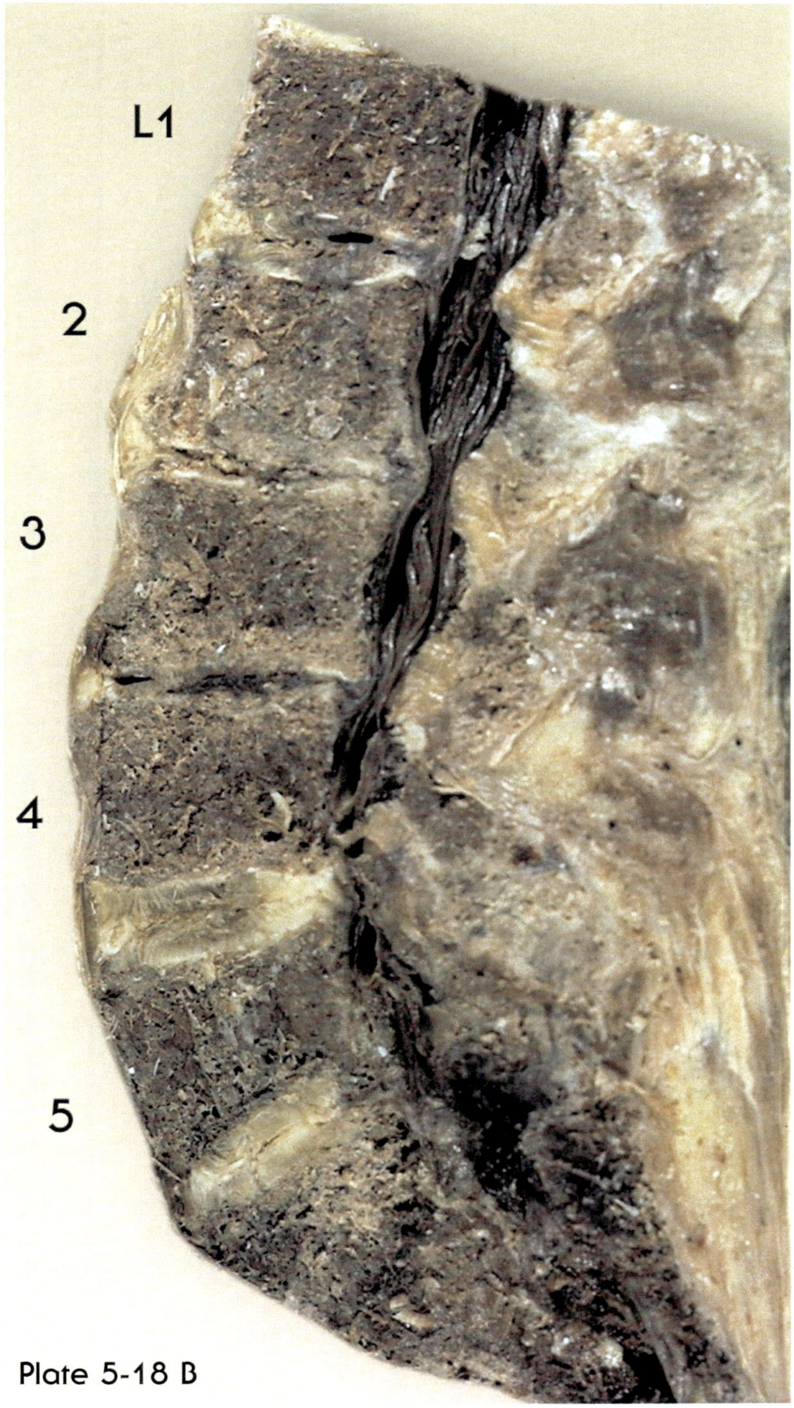

Plate 5-18 B

retro to L4 with disc tearing, cavitation (vacuum), loss of disc height, slight wedging, and spurring. L4-L5 are aligned with slight tearing, wedging, and inferior endplate repair, with the L5 compression fracture indicating trauma to these joints. L5 and sacrum are fairly well aligned with a persistent disc, with disc expansion into the L5 vertebral body, disc wedging, loss of disc height.

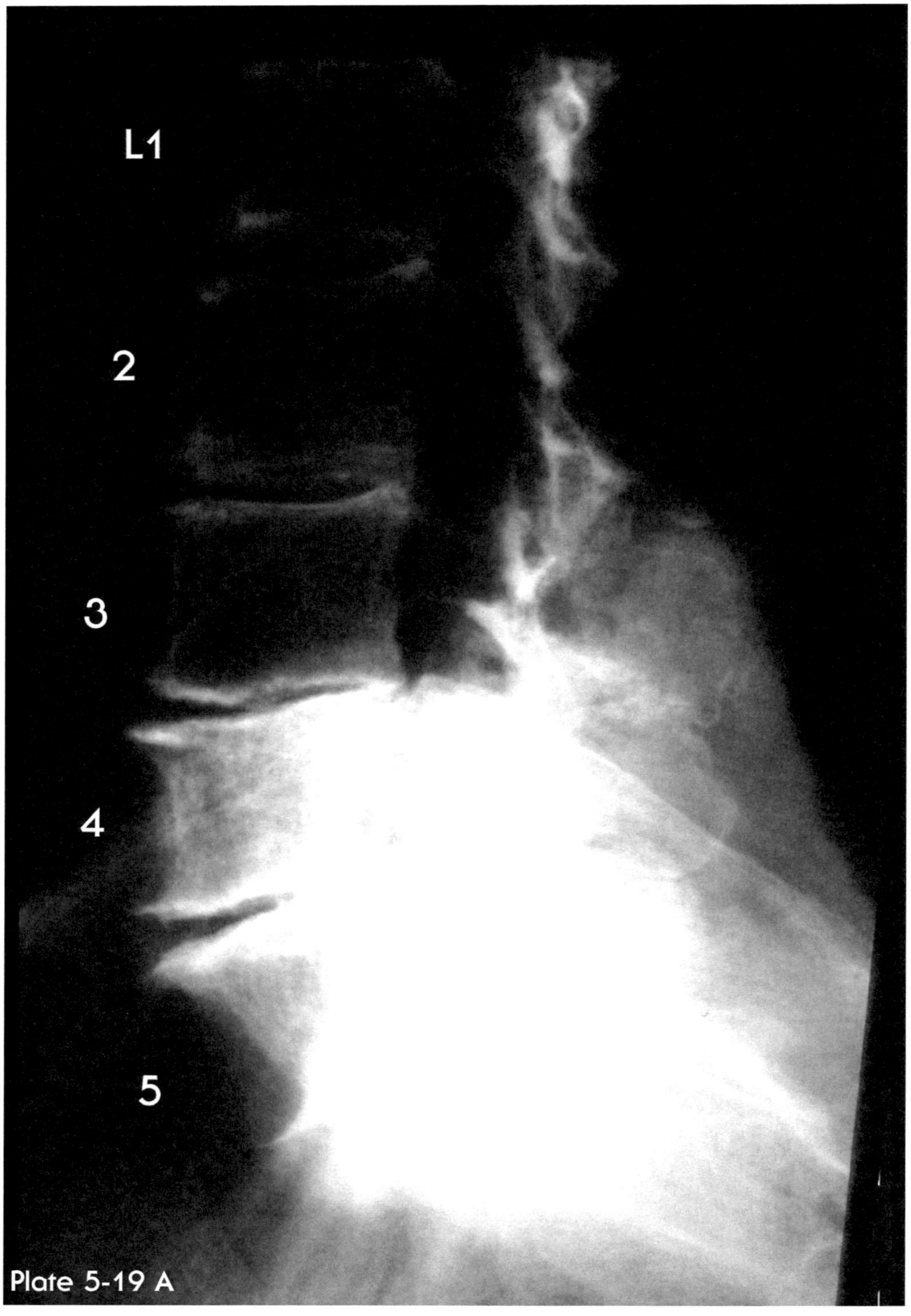

Plate 5-19 A

Plates 5-19 A & B
LUMBAR SPINE - This illustrates subluxations in end stages of degeneration with a loss of lordotic curve

L1 is retro to L2 and has inferior endplate damage anteriorly, and repairs with anterior spurring, disc tearing, and both anterior and posterior bulging. L2 is retro to L3 with anterior and posterior spurring, near fusion with anterior and posterior disc bulging, and loss of

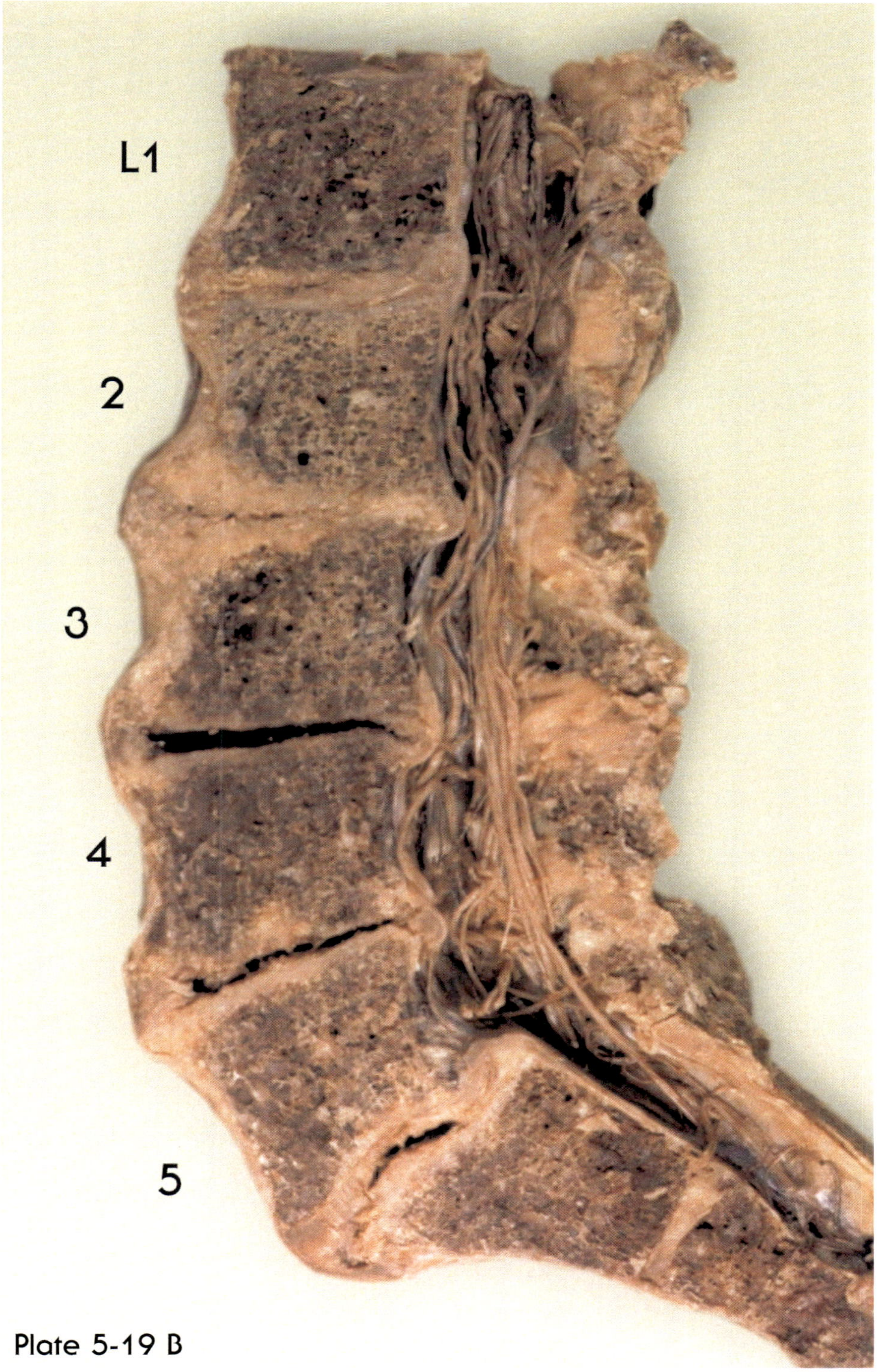

Plate 5-19 B

height. L3 is retro to L4 with anterior and posterior spurring, significant cavitation, total loss of disc matrix, and wedging of the space; L4 is retro to L5 with some anterior disc annulus remaining with cavitation, anterior and posterior spurring, loss disc height and matrix. L5 is antero to the sacrum with disc tearing, cavitation (vacuum), anterior and posterior bulging, and loss of height. This subluxation pattern of L5 and the sacrum can be described as a "sacral base posterior."

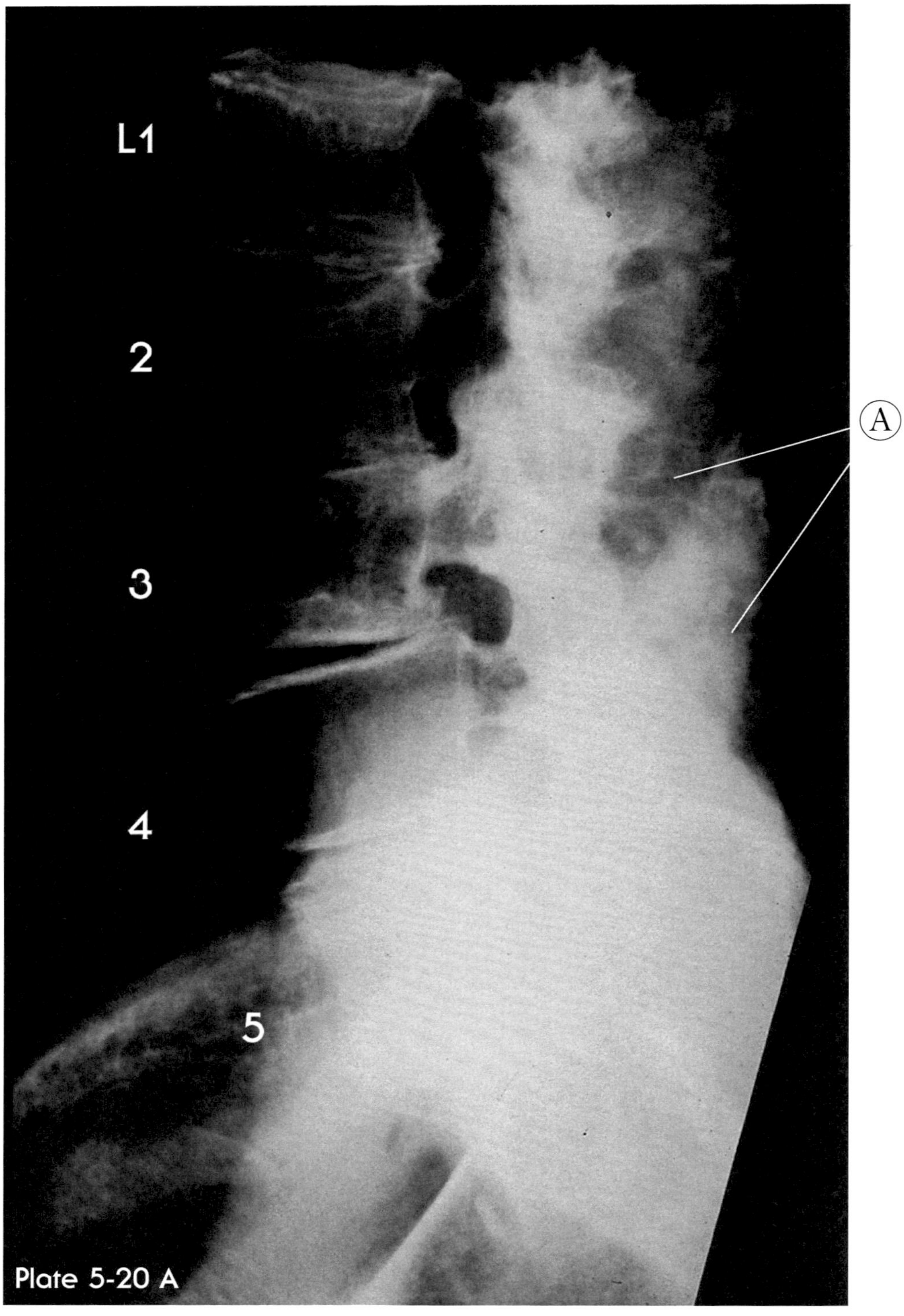

Plates 5-20 A & B
LUMBAR SPINE - This specimen has multiple subluxations and the end stages of degeneration

It has a reduced lordotic curve with chronic loss of joint integrity from L1 to L4. Note the increased vertebral body width due to the altered weight bearing produced by the subluxations. L1 is retro to L2 and has inferior and superior endplate damage, and spurring with disc tearing, anterior and posterior bulging, and loss of disc height.

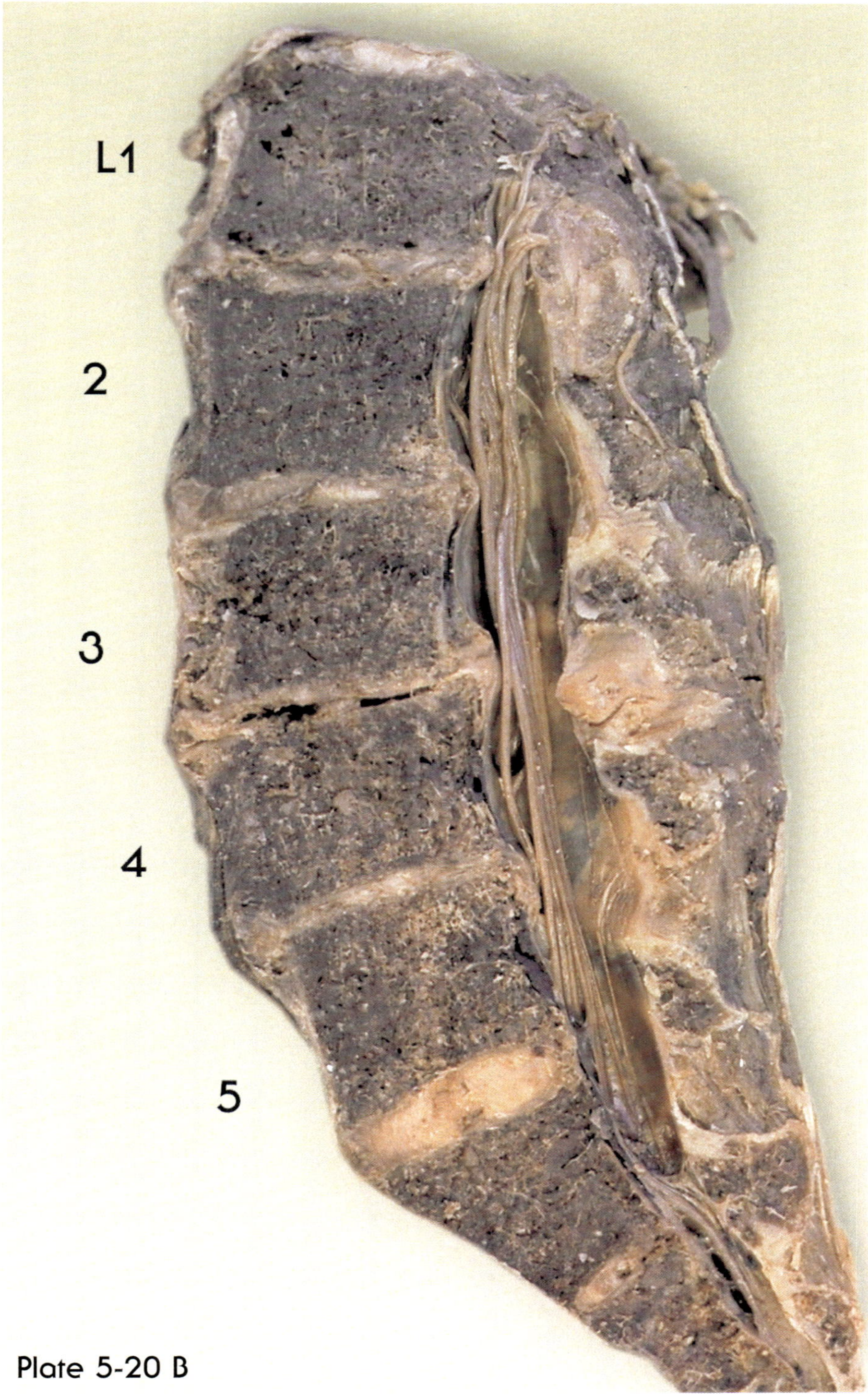

Plate 5-20 B

L2 is antero to L3 with posterior spurring, disc tearing, bulging, wedging, and loss of disc height. L3 is antero to L4 with disc cavitation, anterior and posterior bulging, near fusion, and anterior and posterior spurring. L4 is antero to L5 with disc tearing, loss of height, and anterior bulging. The sacrum-L5 segments are aligned with a near normal disc, in an aged spine This illustrates how subluxation results in chronic degenerative changes of the involved vertebrae.

(A) Spinous process contact from loss of disc height

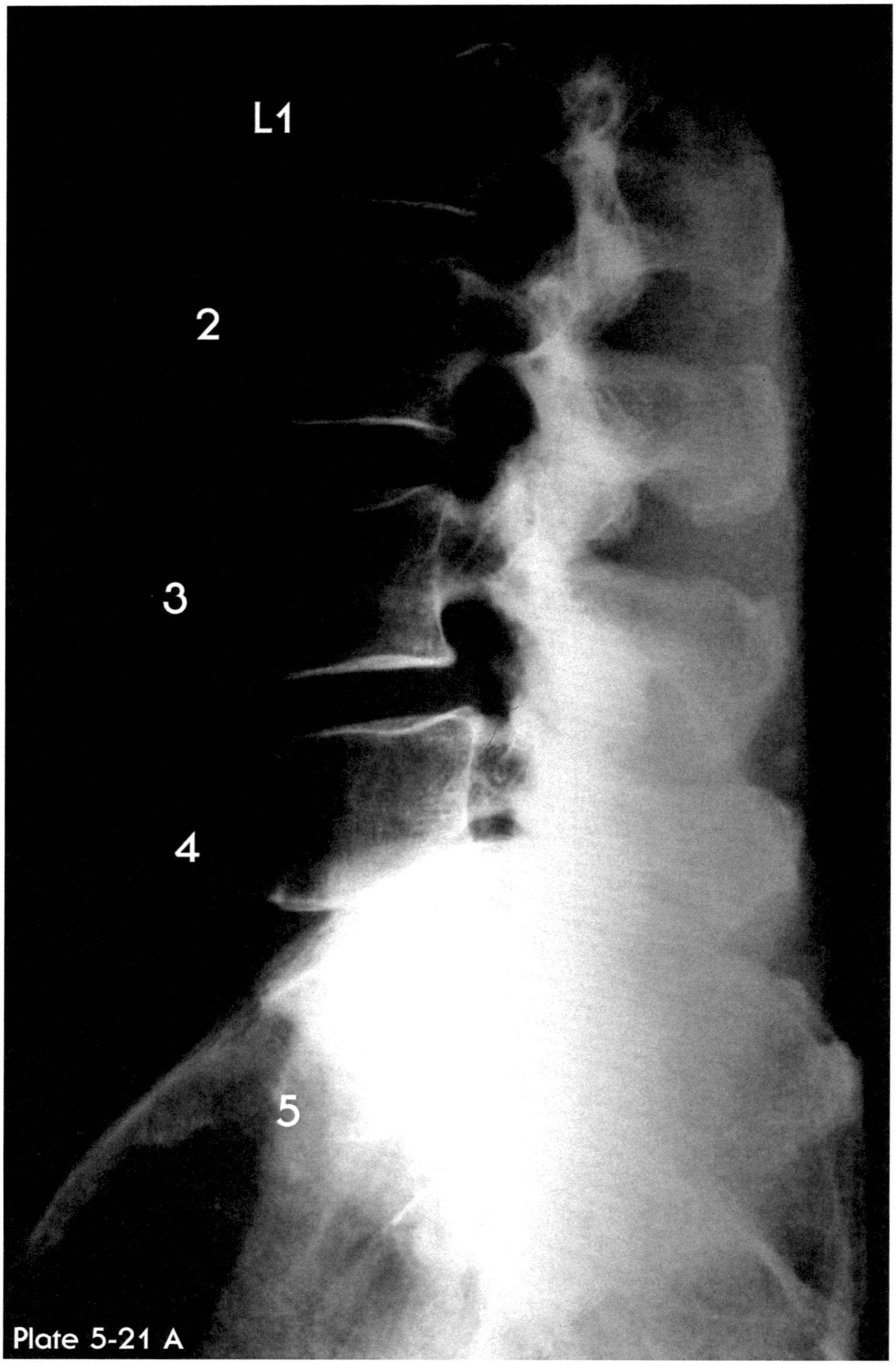

Plates 5-21 A & B
LUMBAR SPINE - This individual has a reversed lumbar lordotic curve with complete retrolisthesis of L4

This specimen has significant posterior displacement of L4 which causes loss of curvature. L1 and L2 have near normal alignment. L3 is antero to L4 which is retro to L5

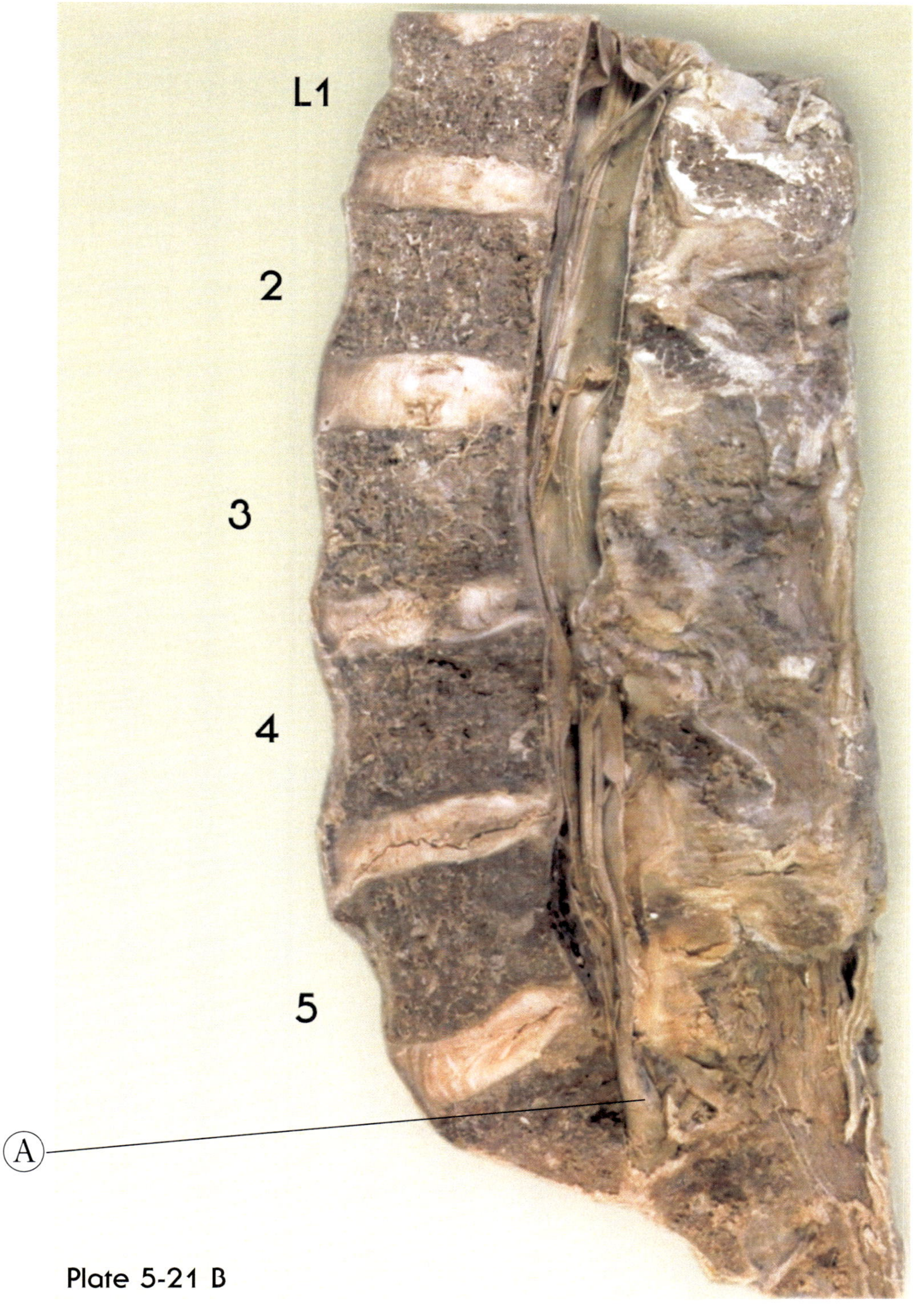

Plate 5-21 B

with tearing and loss of normal disc height and anterior and posterior spurring of the L5 superior endplate. The L5-sacral alignment is normal.

(A) The sacrum view is perisagittal with the first sacral nerve descending from the caudae equinae

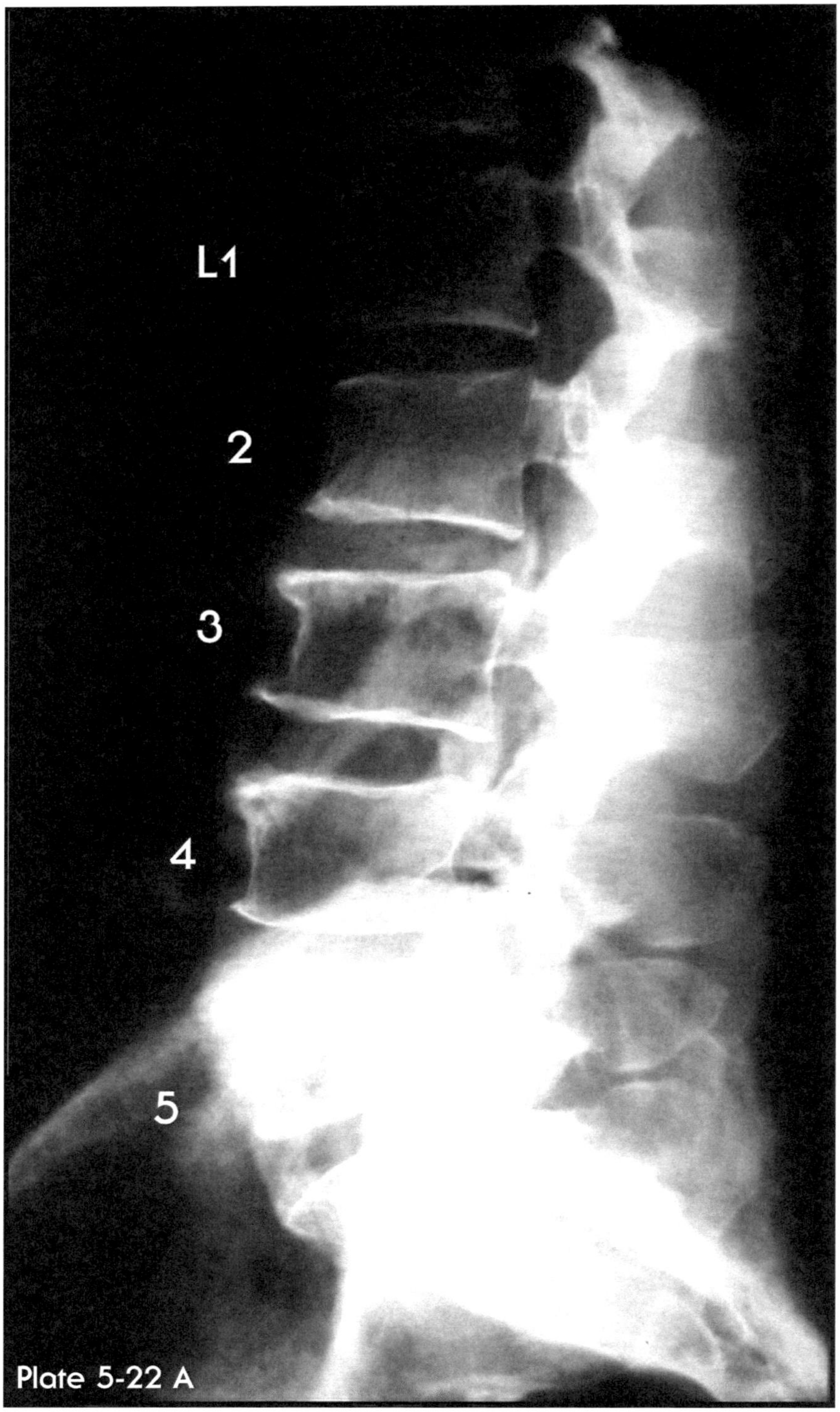

Plates 5-22 A & B

LUMBAR SPINE - Sequential retrolisthesis forming a "stairstepping" of L1-L5 into a reversed lordotic curve

L1 is slightly retro to L2 with anterior L1 spurring, disc tearing, and anterior and posterior disc bulging. L2 is retro to L3 with anterior spurring. There is hypertrophy of the anterior longitudinal ligament and wedging of the vertebral

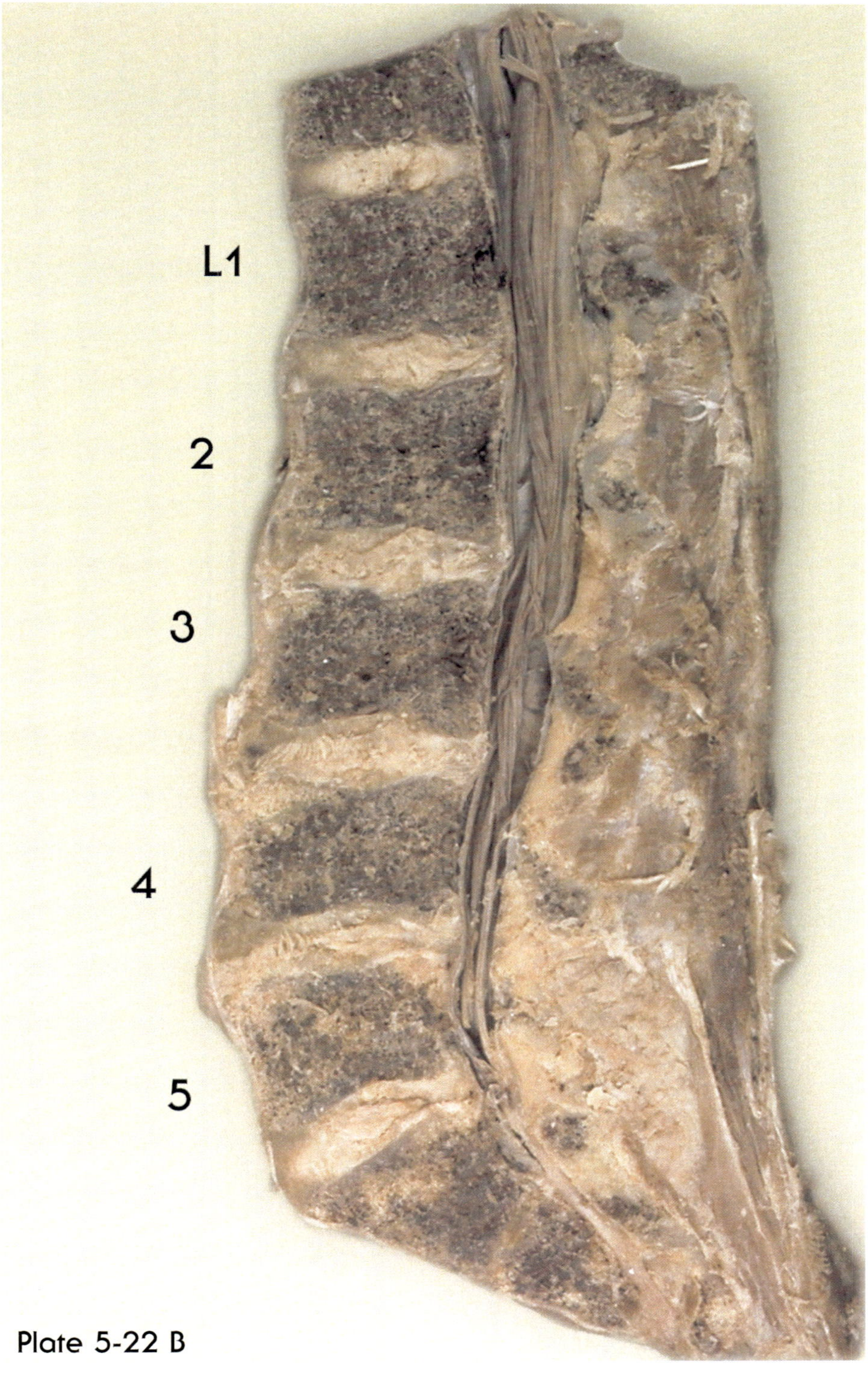

Plate 5-22 B

body of L3, with signs of endplate repair, and anterior and posterior disc bulging. L3 is retro to L4 with anterior spurring and wedging of disc, tearing, anterior and slight posterior bulging. L4 is retro to L5 with disc tearing and slight posterior bulging, anterior spurring, loss of disc height, and spinous process approximation. The sacrum and L5 have minor disc tearing and slight bulging and wedging.

Note the increase in the length of the spinal canal and stretching of the caudae equinae.

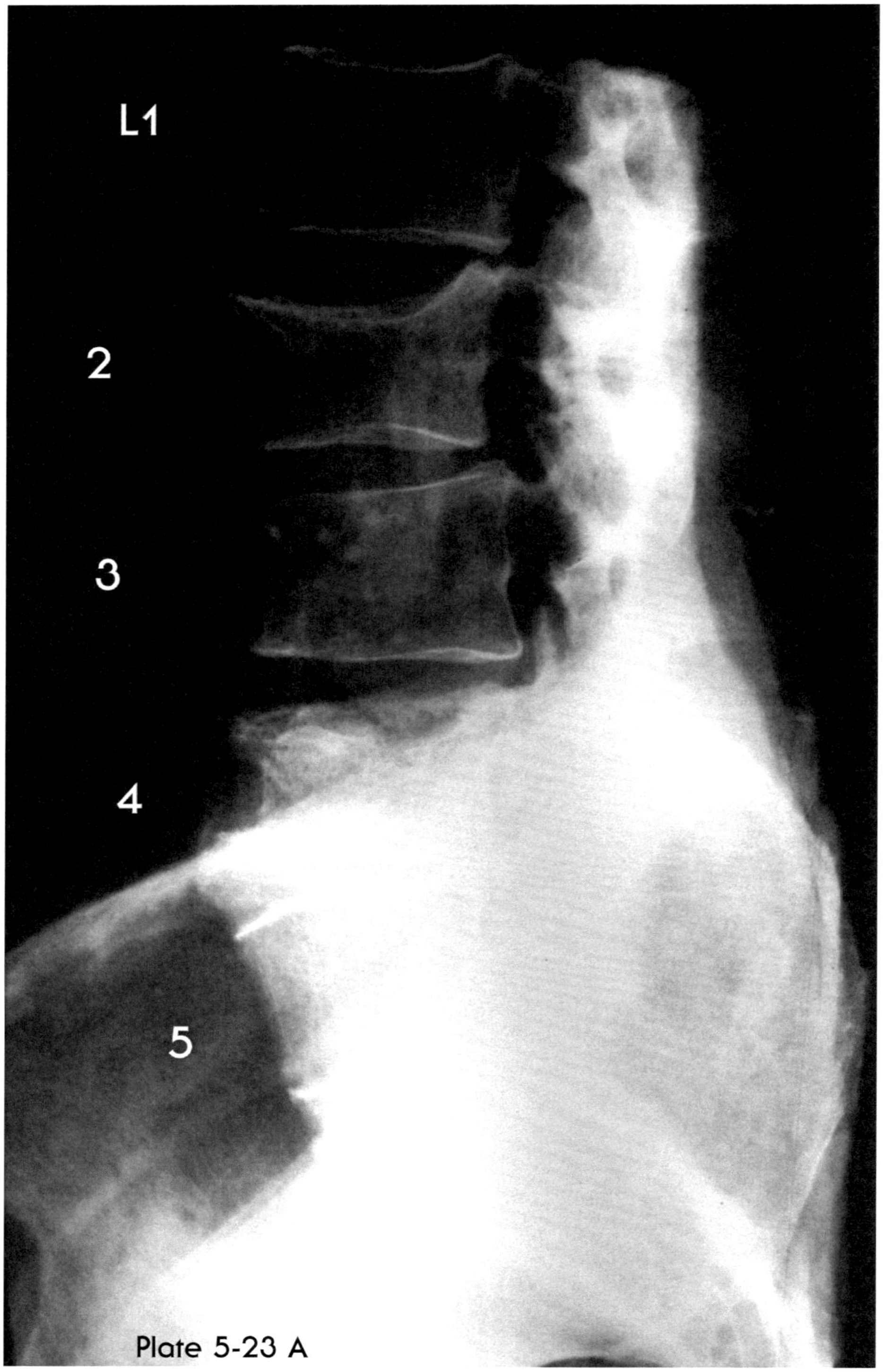

Plates 5-23 A & B
LUMBAR SPINE - L3 is a complete retrolisthesis creating a reversed lordotic curve

This specimen has suffered an injury that subluxated and damaged L2 through L4. Notice the altered length and width of the spinal canal. L2 is slightly retro to L1 with significant endplate destruction indicating a compression fracture of L2 with anterior and posterior disc bulging, tearing, wedging, and anterior and posterior spurring.

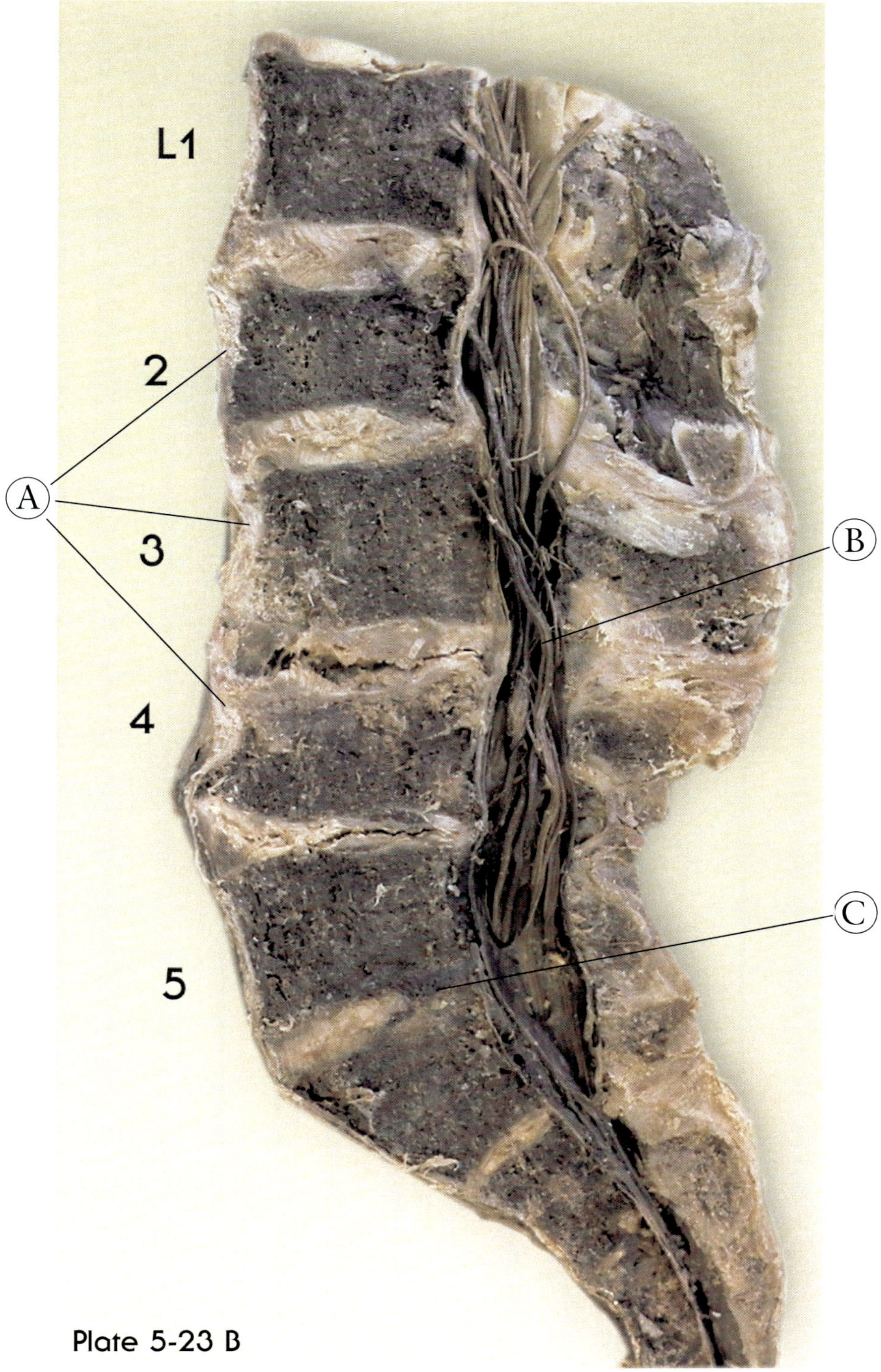

Plate 5-23 B

L3 is retro to L2 with disc tearing and wedging. L3 is retro to L4 with disc tearing, cavitation, wedging, bulging with compression fracture of L4, and anterior spurring. L4 is retro to L5 with disc tearing and significant loss of height. The sacrum is slightly antero to L5 with near fusion of segments.

(A) Thickening of A.L.L. over L2-L4
(B) Spinal canal narrowing
(C) End stage wedging of L5-S1

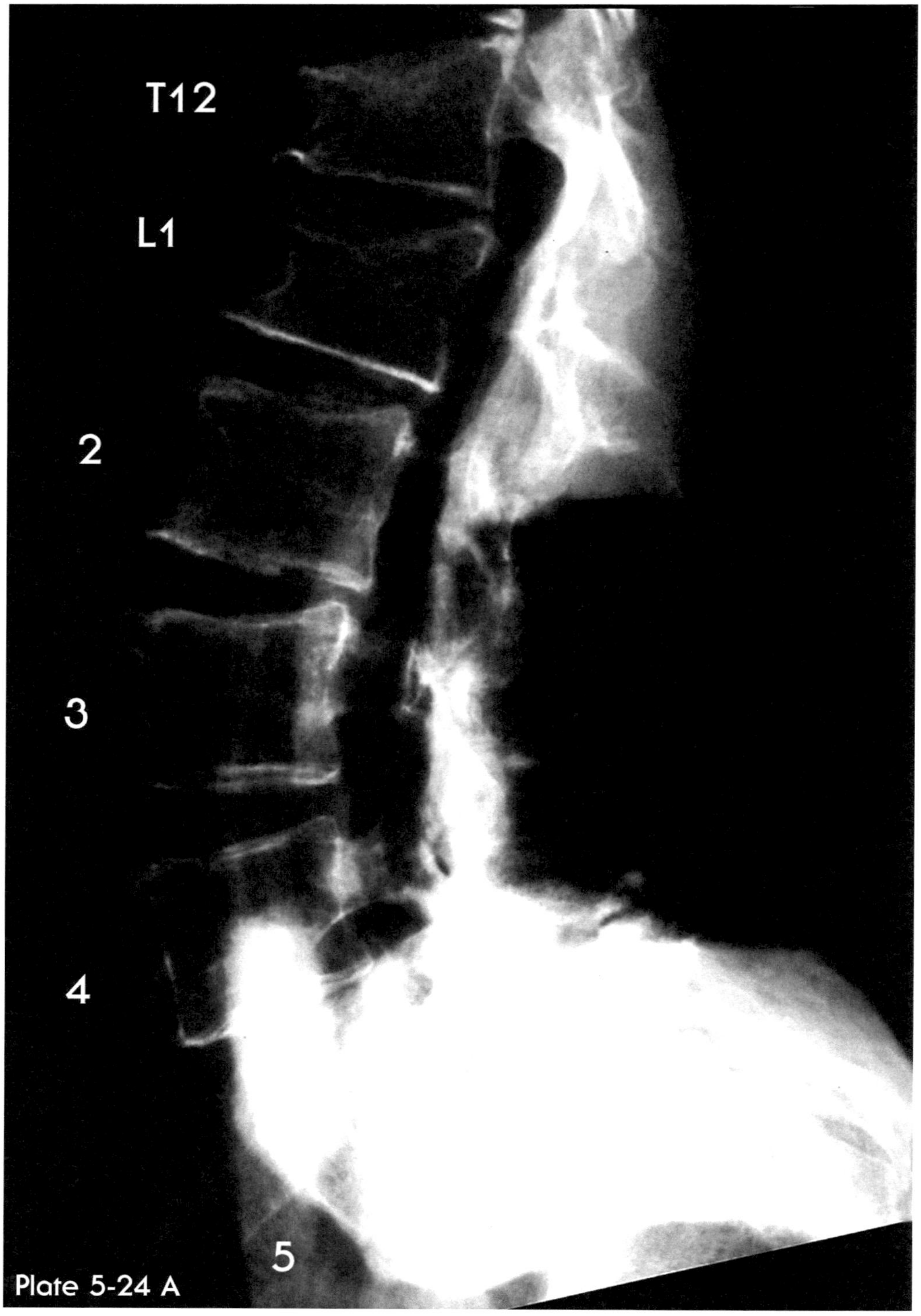

Plates 5-24 A & B
LUMBAR SPINE - This shows a reversed lordotic curve in the upper lumbar spine

This specimen has suffered compressive force causing anterior vertebral damage of T12 and L1. L1 is a complete retrolisthesis. T12 has an anterior compression fracture with loss of the anterior vertebral body height. L1 is retro to T12 with disc wedging, tearing, anterior and posterior bulging, and an anterior compression fracture with loss of vertebral body height. L1 is retro to L2 with disc tearing, bulging, and anterior spurring. L2 is retro to L3 with disc

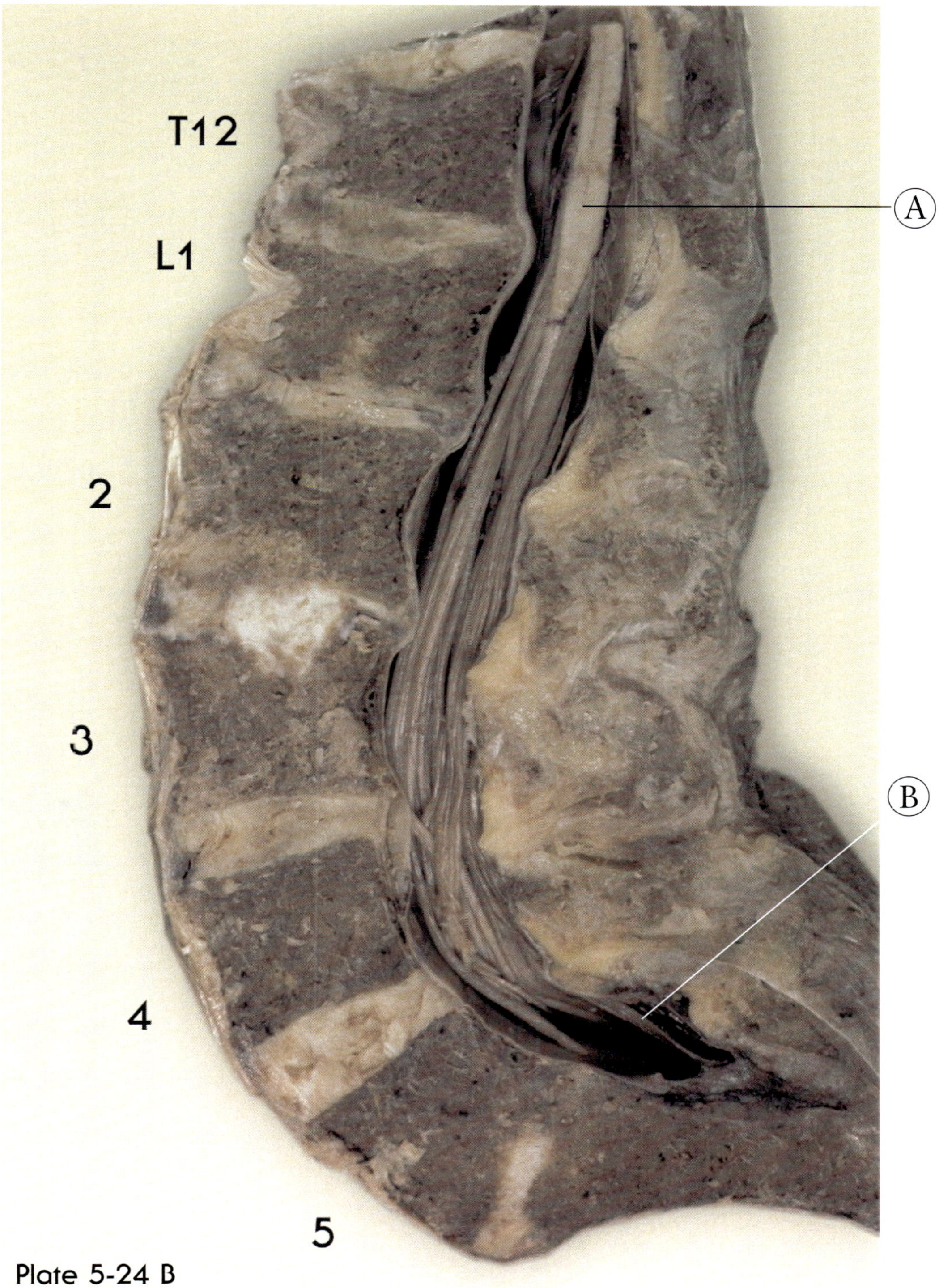

Plate 5-24 B

wedging and anterior spurring and bulging posteriorly (with some kind of change in the L2-L3 disc that is not radiographic). L3 is retro to L4 with tearing of the disc and posterior bulging and some endplate damage. L4-L5 look aligned with slight tearing and wedging. L5 is slightly antero to sacrum with near fusion.

(A) Sagittal section of conus medularis and caudae equinae

(B) Note how caudae equinae components are pulled around posterior canal to the sacrum. Cervical flexion can make this worse.

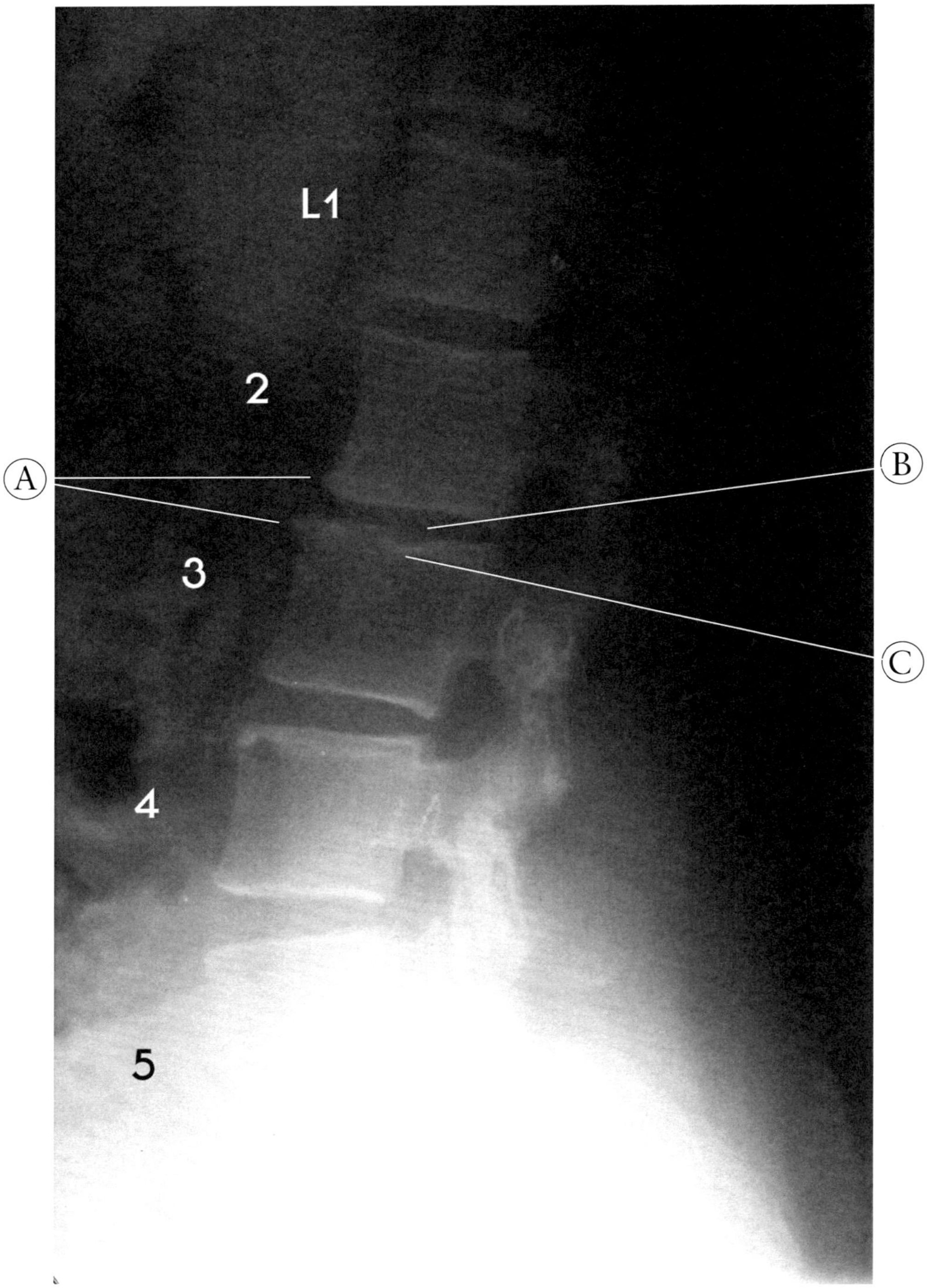

Plate 5-25 A

Plates 5-25 A & B
LUMBAR SPINE WITH A LOSS OF LORDOTIC CURVE
An X-ray and MRI comparison

This individual has suffered a subluxation of L2: a complete retrolisthesis to L1 and L3. L3, L4, and L5 are all posterior to the segment below. This loss of lordotic curve has a significantly damaged disc at its apex. The vertebrae with the most A to P displacement have degenerative changes. Note the osteophyte formation at

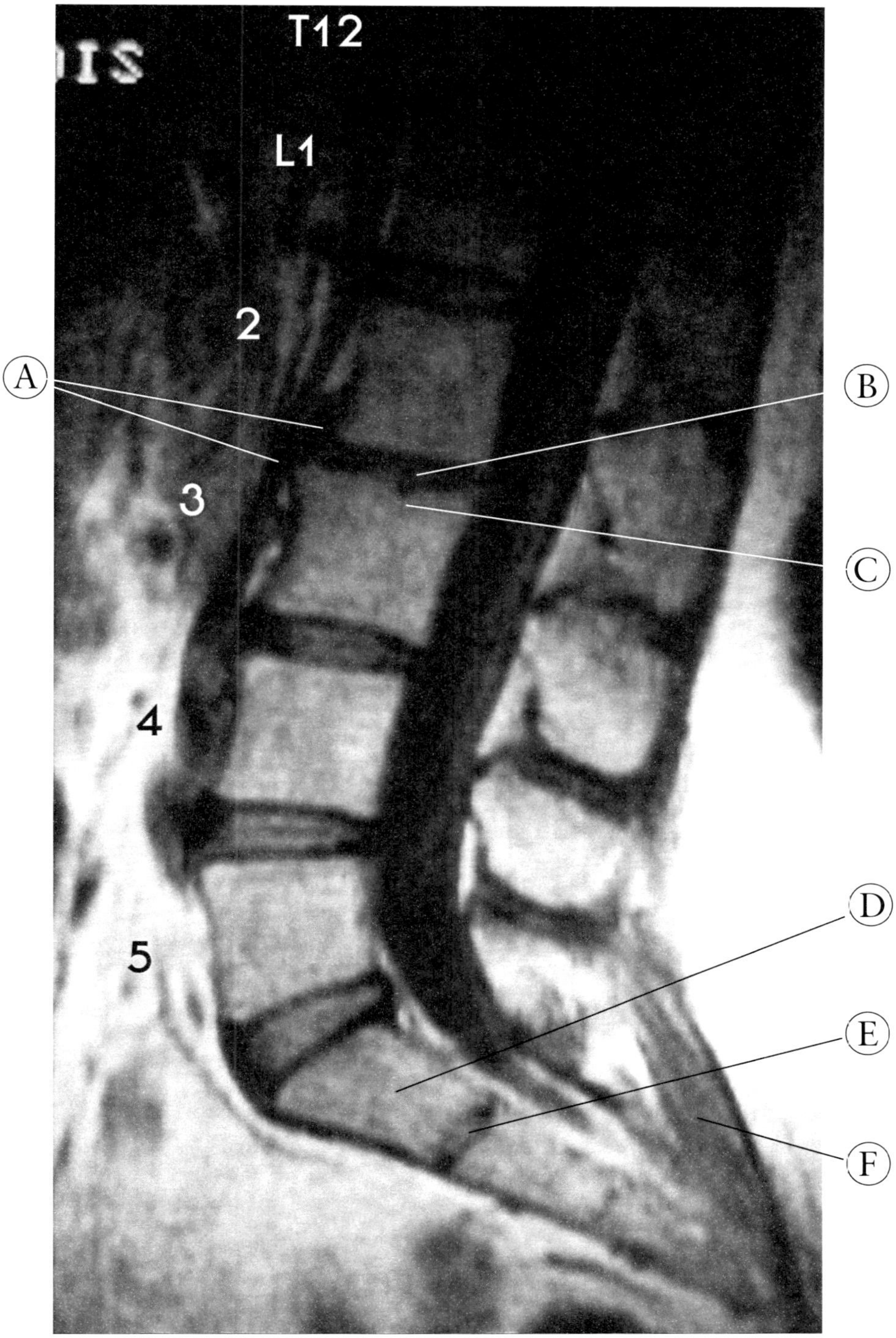

Plate 5-25 B

only L2 and L3. The endplate damage indicates old trauma. L5 is posterior to the sacrum and there is a sacral disc at the S1-S2 level. The sacrum has lost its kyphotic shape and the lower sacral discs are gone. The trauma to the sacrum with compression injuries to the spine in the upper lumbar region I find are common.

(A) Osteophytes
(B) Degenerating disc
(C) Endplate
(D) Sacrum
(E) S1-S2 disc
(F) Erector spinae

CHAPTER SIX

Subluxations Of The Pelvic Girdle

Discussion

In the adult, the pelvic girdle is a three-bone complex including the sacrum and the right and left innominates. ("Innominate" is from Latin, a word meaning "no-name," referring to its embryonic origin as three separate bones; the ilium, ischium, and pubis.) Three joints unite the bones of the pelvic girdle; the two sacro-iliac joints and the pubic symphysis. The sacrum is the base of the spine and the pelvic girdle, as a whole, is the anchor for quite a substantial part of the muscular system of the spine, legs, thorax, and abdomen. All of the abdominal, hip, and thigh muscles originate from the pelvic girdle, as do the two large back muscles, the erector spinae and the latissimus dorsi (see **Figure 6-1**). So it is not difficult to see how subluxations of the pelvic girdle can affect any or all of these muscle groups, causing them to contract, become hypertonic, or go into spasm. In my clinical experience the key to understanding the etiology of many cases of "low back pain" is the integrity and function of the three pelvic joints.

In **Figure 6-1** some of the muscles directly involved with sacroiliac joint and pubic symphysis motion and integrity are illustrated. The abdominal wall musculature has its inferior attachment from the pubic symphysis, medially, to the posterior aspect of the iliac crest. Innominate subluxation involving the SI joint and pubic symphysis will adversely affect the rectus and transverse abdominus, and internal and external abdominal oblique muscles. The psoas and iliacus muscles will be recruited neurologically to guard and protect the injured joints by limiting their range of motion. The posterior muscles will be in the same altered

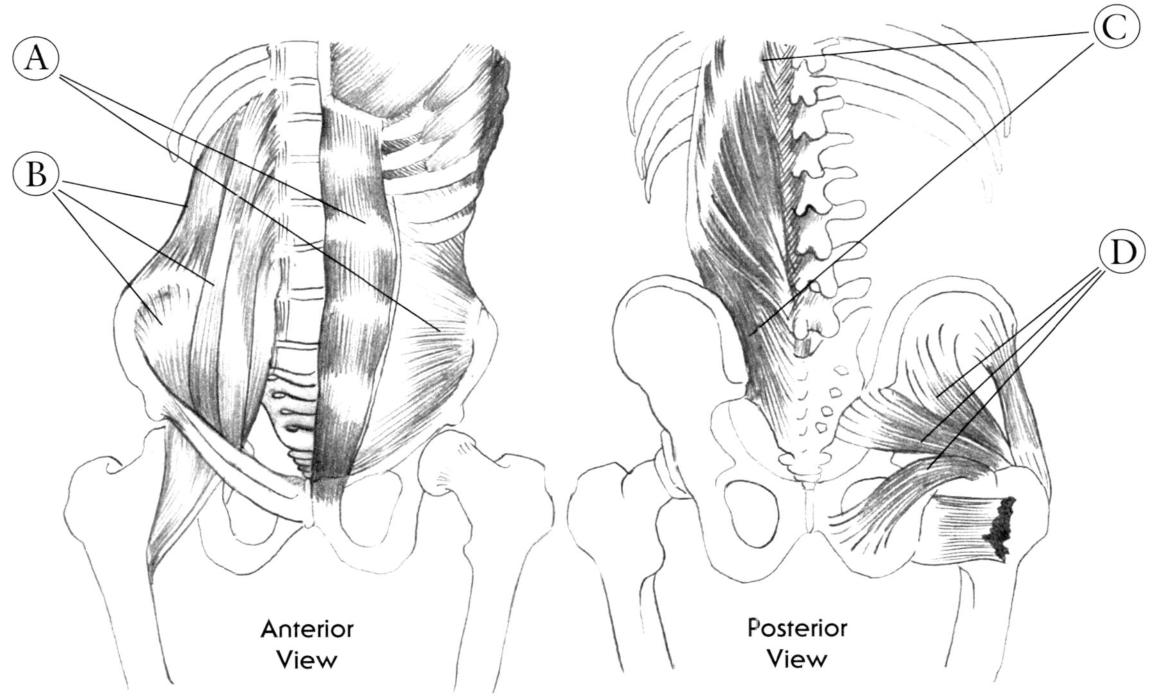

Figure 6-1

These illustrations are anterior and posterior views of the pelvis and the major muscle groups of the back, hip and abdomen. All the muscles depicted have proprioceptive links to the sacroiliac joints or pubic symphysis.

(A) The abdominal wall which include rectus and transverse abdominus, internal and external oblique muscles.
(B) The major hip flexors: psoas, iliacus and quadratus lumborum.
(C) The erector spinae muscles.
(D) The deep hip muscles include gluteus minimus and medius, piriformis, gemellus inferior and superior, obturator internus and quadratus femoris. (Note: the gluteus maximus is not shown in this illustration.)

state. These muscles are the erector spinae, latissimus dorsi and the deep hip muscles. The deep hip muscles, as well as others, experience distress when pelvic subluxation causes the acetabulum to shift relative to the femoral head, trochanter and shaft. As the hip joint alters these relationships, the bottom of the foot must still contact the ground. Analysis of these problems is complicated by the variety of pelvic tilts encountered (**see Figure 6-15**). Muscular distress, pain and limited range of motion will be only some of the clinical symptoms. The loss of motion, normal joint space and fluid exchange initiates degenerative processes.

The neurology involved is very complex and will be discussed only in general terms. All the tissues are embedded with neurological sensors of various types. However, it is extremely important to understand that the guarding (spasmed) muscles around the symphysis pubis can, like any other muscles, be relieved only by correcting the subluxation and removing the noxious proprioceptive input into the central nervous system. The nervous system may never adapt to neurological input arising from joint distress (subluxation). This neurological phenomenon is present in all the studied mammalian neuromusculoskeletal systems. The sacrum gives rise to the sacral nerves and the internal iliac arteries contribute the arteries to the pelvic organs. They are retroperitoneal and are adhesed to the back or dorsal surface of the abdominal lining. Mechanical distress can displace abdominal tissues away from the origins of their nerves and arteries.

Visceral Implications of Pelvic Subluxations.

A variety of complaints can result from subluxations of the pelvic joints, including urogenital and intestinal problems.[1] In a normal female pelvis, the broad ligament stretches between the two ilia, suspending the ovaries and the uterus (**see Figure 6-2b**). When the pelvic girdle subluxates, the broad ligament skews as the ilia displace with respect to one another (**see Figure 6-2c**). This changes the position of the ovaries and the uterus in the pelvic cavity, and can create or exacerbate any problem that might exist. The pelvic examination can reveal tight and tender musculature on one side and the uterus tractioned to one side. **See Figure 6-2a**, an X-ray of a subluxated

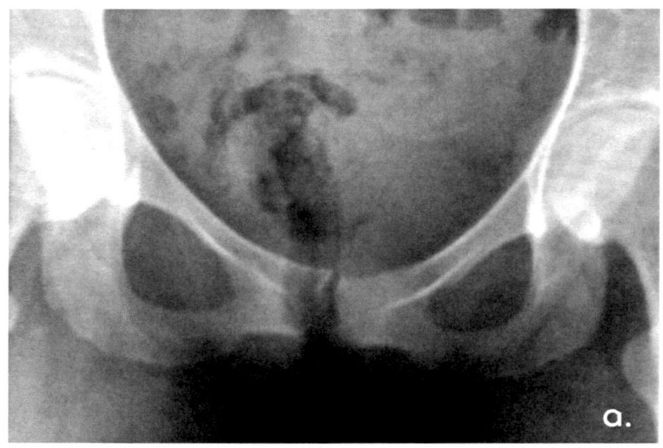

Figure 6-2 a, b & c

X-ray and illustration depicting the ovaries, fallopian tubes, uterus and broad ligament in the pelvic girdle.

These gynecological structures are suspended in the pelvic girdle by the broad ligament. When the pelvis subluxates the normal relationship is altered.

(A) Ovary
(B) Fallopian tube
(C) Broad ligament
(D) Uterus
(E) Pubic symphysis

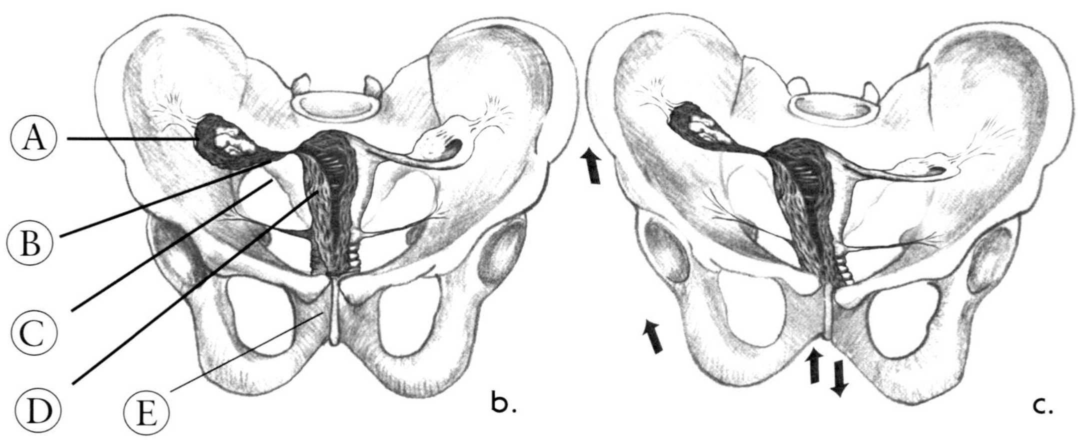

pelvis, with air introduced to the vagina and uterus. Note the right lateral shift of the gynecological structures and the pelvic subluxaton. In late stage pregnancy, this shift, with a fetus in the uterus, will cause the fetus to press or "lay" on the Psoas. This will make walking difficult or impossible. This shift is responsible for some of the breech positions that occur. I think that a large percentage of gynecological pathology may be the result of unresolved pelvic trauma. Correction of the subluxation complexes of the pelvic girdle has been shown clinically to relieve or reverse these conditions.[2]

I have also encountered instances of testicular pain, ensuing from subluxation of the pubic symphysis. This can be explained anatomically by the fact that the testicular nerve, artery and vein traverse the top of the pubic rami before they descend into the testicles, creating a neurovascular bundle that can become entrapped in some individuals.

The Sacrum

The sacrum is usually depicted as a solid bone, but I have found that even specimens 90-100 years old have viable discs in the sacrum between S1-S2, and S2-S3 (**see Figure 6-3**). The presence of a disc implies sacral motion because, from a physiological point of view, a fibro-cartilaginous disc requires motion for survival. These sacral discs are tied to, and biomechanically related to, the sacro-iliac joints and ligaments.

The sacrum and the sacroiliac joints are angled from top to bottom and from front to back (**see Figure 6-4**).The appearance of these structures on the variety of types of imaging and positions can be quite different. **See Figure 6-16** to see the different views in one study. To make the evaluation process more complex, the sacrum can be either parallel or nearly perpendicular to the ground (or anywhere in between (**see Figure 6-15**).

The sacrum is an inverted pyramidal structure formed by the partial fusion of sacral vertebrae. It articulates with both innominates at the sacroiliac joints and the fifth lumbar vertebrae with the intervertebral disc and articular facets. It has a canal posterior to the bodies of the segments that is contiguous with the spinal canal. The distal end of the caudae equinae occupies the canal and the anterior and posterior foramen house the exiting sacral nerve roots.

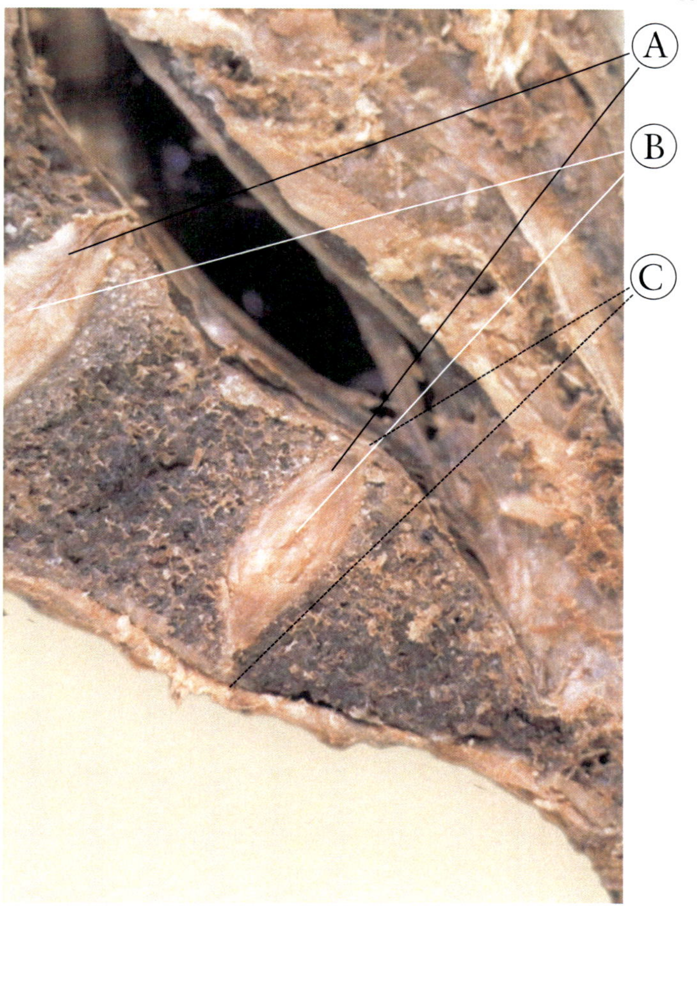

Figure 6-3

Sacral discs of an 86 year old male.

The majority of elderly specimens had persistent sacral discs. The most persistent was the S1-S2 disc. The S2-S3 disc was less often observed. The S3-S4 disc was occasionally seen, about 25%. This view was slightly off the mid-sagittal plane. Note the presence of annular rings and a nucleus pulposus. The sacral discs are oval in shape in the A to P and coronal planes (Z and X planes). Note the continuous cortical bone that must be radio dense. This is significant evidence of sacral motion front to back and side to side.Discs require motion to persist (**see Figure 1-12b**). This is the anatomical explanation of the sacrum pumping the Cerebrospinal Fluid in the spinal canal. Sacral motion is likely to be connected to central nervous system physiology and function.

(A) Annulus fibrosus
(B) Nucleus pulposus
(C) Cortex of sacrum

The sacrum has five separate segments in a child and the partial fusion of S1 to S2 and S2 to S3 remains through life. S3, S4 and S5 can be fused by age 25. The presence of the sacral discs throughout life strongly suggests sacral motion. As previously mentioned, physiological function of intervertebral discs necessitates motion as a main mechanism of nutrition and waste elimination. This is likely to be the same for the avascular intrasacral discs.

The cortex of the sacrum is a contiguous and flexible wall. The sacral discs, as well as the intervertebral discs confer flexibility. There is only one mechanism for fluid and nutrient exchange for the intervertebral disc: imbibition (hydration) through the vertebral endplates via motion.This must also be true for sacral disc physiology and function. **See Figure 6-3**, a sacrum of an 86 year old individual. It is an obviously flexible structure, with healthy intrasacral discs.

The motion of the legs rotating from the acetabulum rocks the innominates with the anterior and posterior thigh musculature. The sacrotuberous and sacrospinous ligaments connecting to the sacrum from the innominate transfer movement alternating back and forward. The femur is an enormous lever. A handle on a wrench as long as the leg would snap a 3/4 quarter inch tightened bolt in a partial turn. The joints and ligaments that hold the pelvic girdle together must withstand tremendous rotational and shearing forces. Part of the strength and stability of the pelvis is its flexibility.[3] The sacrum, forming the bottom of the spinal canal, confers motion to the entire lower central nervous system, from the sacral nerve roots to the brainstem. Motion of the spinal cord is the major mechanism for capillary bed blood flow.[4,5,6] A static spinal cord has reduced blood flow.

The sacral discs are evident to the 9th and 10th decades of life. In the limited study presented here there is evidence of intersacral subluxation (**see Figures 6-36** through **6-41** on pages 216-217). The S1-S2 disc has a dorsal and ventral cortical bone covering. This will thicken with loss of integrity between the S1 and S2 segments and the disc will dehydrate.[7,8,9,10] The S2 and S3 segments seem to have the same relationship.

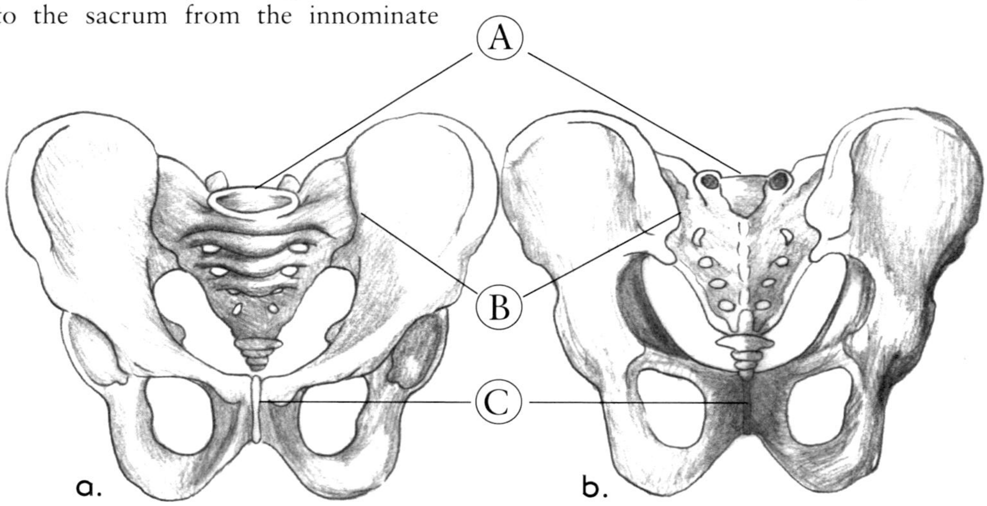

Figure 6-4

Illustration of the human pelvis from the (a) anterior and (b) posterior view.

The three joints of the pelvis, the right and left sacroiliac joints, and the pubic symphysis can all be seen.

Note the sacrum is wider at the top, this is called the sacral base, narrower at the bottom, this the sacral apex. The sacrum is also wider in the anterior aspect than the posterior.

(A) Sacrum
(B) Sacroiliac joint
(C) Pubis symphysis

The Sacroiliac Joints

Sacroiliac joints have two components; fibrous and cartilaginous ("synovial"). I have dissected more than 200 individuals' sacroiliac joints, and have found extreme variation among specimens. The main differences are in the shape, contour and size of the joint. The fibrous part is large in some specimens and small in others; the cartilaginous part shows the same variation, and there is no consistency in the ratios of one part to the other (see **Figures 6-5** and **6-6**). Such variation in a normal joint is unique among the body's joints. Other joints only show major variation from a "normal" configuration after injury or disease.

The cartilage portion of the sacroiliac joint can be smooth and flat or extremely irregular and contoured. It can be in the same plane as the fibrous portion or at almost right angles at either medial or lateral orientation. This amount of variation of this significant joint complex can explain the wide range of responses to injury and recovery. Clinically it is common to find that the sacroiliac joint, once injured, never fully recovers.

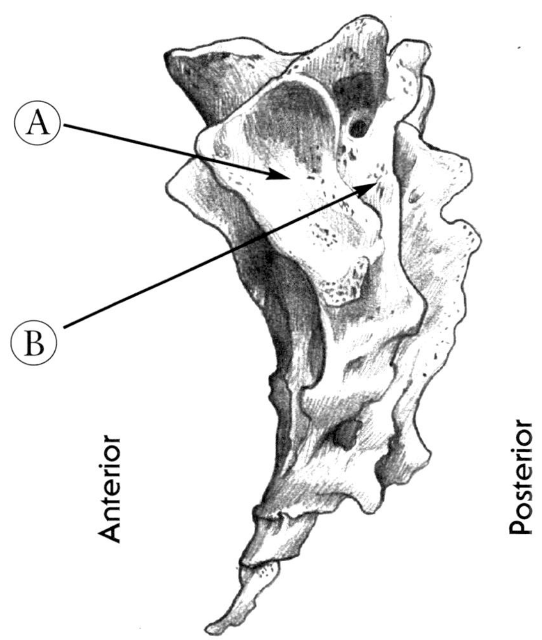

Figure 6-5
This illustration is a lateral view of the sacrum. The cartilage and synovial portion of the joint is generally anterior and inferior to the fibrous portion of the joint. These two components vary in size and contour between individuals. This is the most individually unique joint complex in the body. The sacro-iliac joint variations can explain the different responses to injury and recovery among individuals.
(A) The cartilage portion of the SI joint.
(B) The fibrous portion of the joint.

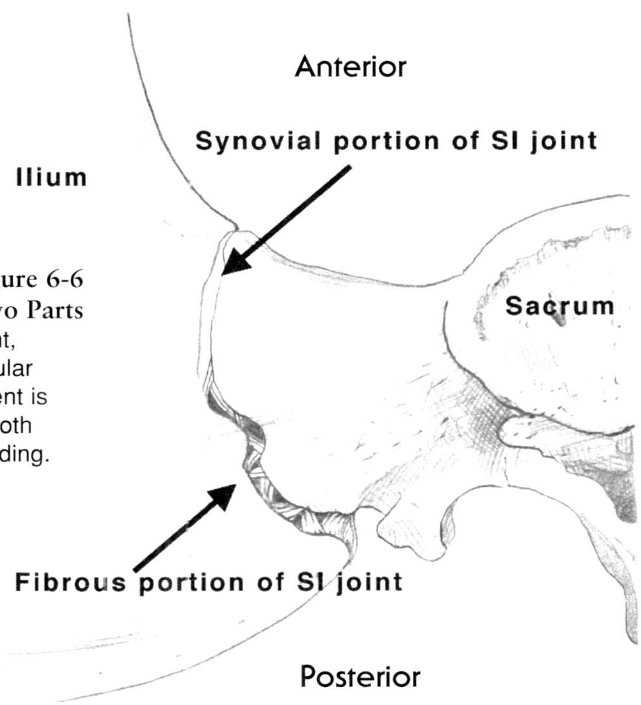

Figure 6-6
Sacroiliac Joint – Two Parts
The sacroiliac joint has a fibrous component, which is posterior and superior to the auricular surface. The auricular or cartilage component is anterior and inferior. There is cartilage on both surfaces and synovial fluid is a common finding. The auricular surfaces can be smooth or contoured, see **Figure 6-7**.

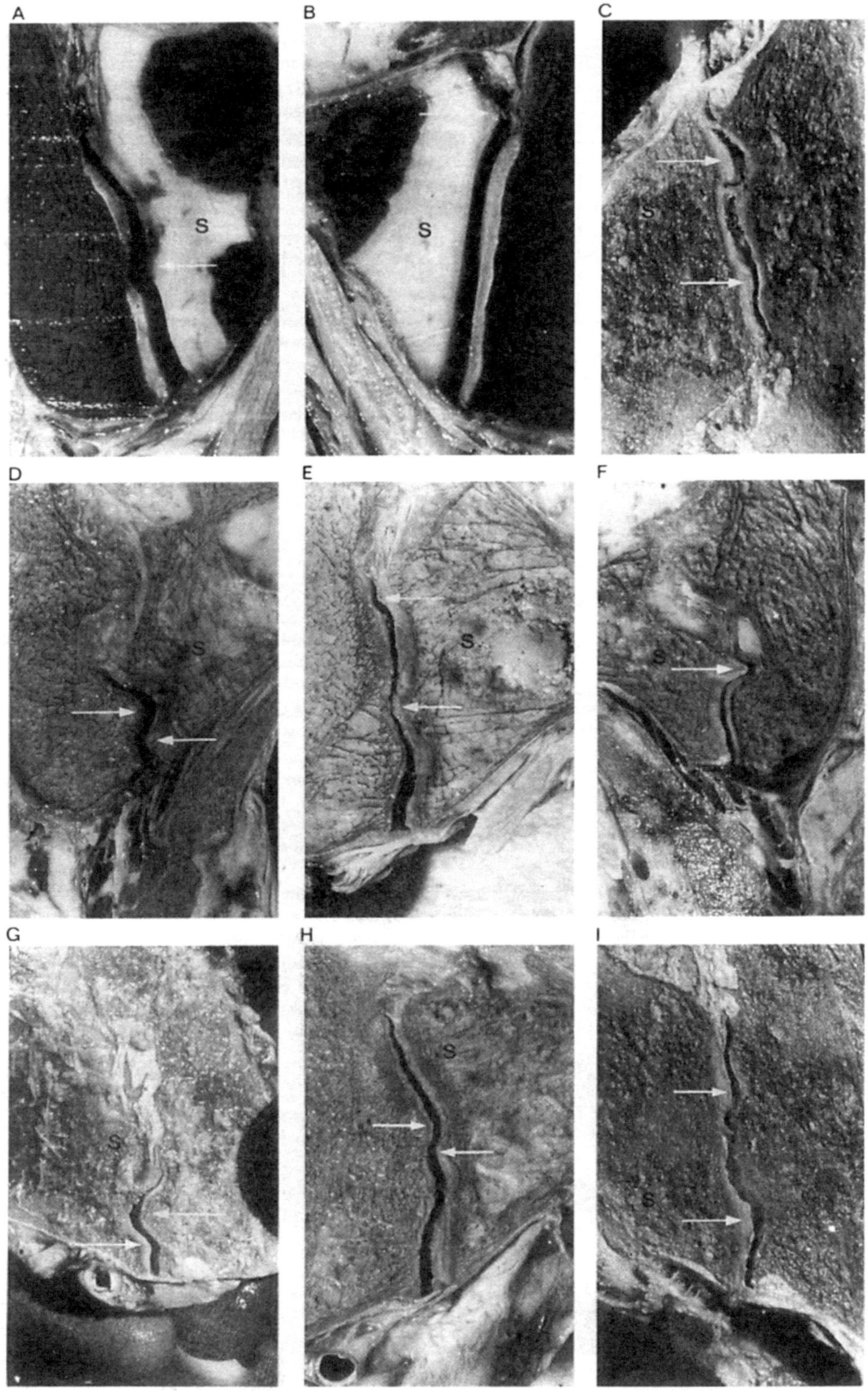

Figure 6-7
Frontal sections of the SI joints of enbalmed male specimens. S indicates the sacral side of the SI joint. **A** and **B** concern a 12-year-old boy. **C** to **I** concern male specimens older than 60 years. Arrows are directed at ridges and depressions. The ridges and depressions shown are covered by intact cartilage, which was checked by opening the joints afterwards.

With permission of Dr. A. Vleeming. Originally published in SPINE (European Ed.), 1990, 2: 130-132

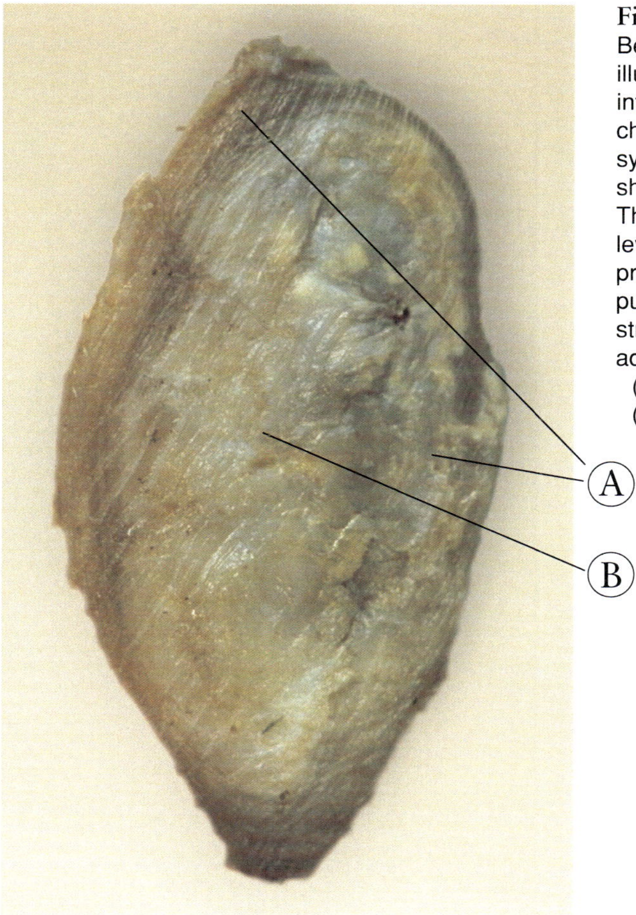

Figure 6-8
Because of the annular rings and a pulpy center, this illustrates a motion segment. Shearing or tearing of the intervertebral discs have been detailed in previous chapters. Similar disruption can occur to the pubic symphysis. Shearing of the vertebrae tear the disc; shearing of the pubic bones tear the pubic symphysis. The problem with the pubic symphysis over the IVD is leverage. The transverse processes and spinous processes are lever arms that move the vertebrae. The pubic symphysis has the legs as levers for motion. This structure must withstand the significant mechanical advantage that the legs have as levers.
(A) Annular ring
(B) Nucleus pulposus

The Pubic Symphysis

The third joint of the pelvic girdle is the pubic symphysis, an avascular fibrocartilaginous disc. The end of each pubic ramus is covered by hyaline cartilage and the fibrocartilaginous pad in between has annular rings with a pulpy, spongy center. It is very similar to an intervertebral disc, even into advanced age. Extrapolation from intervertebral disc physiology would indicate that the pubic symphysis is supposed to move (see **Figure 6-8**), or else it cannot obtain sufficient nutrients. The pubic symphysis, like any other movable joint can subluxate, and in different directions. Because of the complex ligamentous and muscular attachments that connect to the pubic rami, such subluxation can wreak physiological, proprioceptive, and painful havoc on the legs, thorax, and abdomen.[11,12]

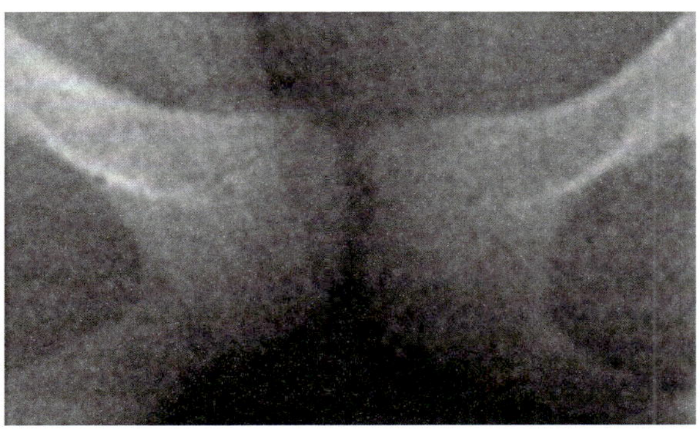

Figure 6-9
A-P pelvic X-ray with the right leg in abduction to 75 degrees. (Detail of Figure 6-11)
The pubic symphysis is showing movement with the left pubic bone superior to the right.

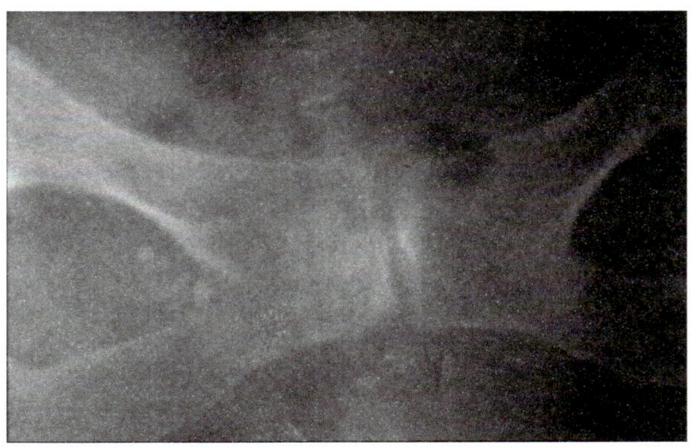

Figure 6-10
(Detail of Figure 6-12)
This subluxation of the pubic symphysis is chronic and sclerosis has occurred. This patient had a long history of groin, hip and low back pain.

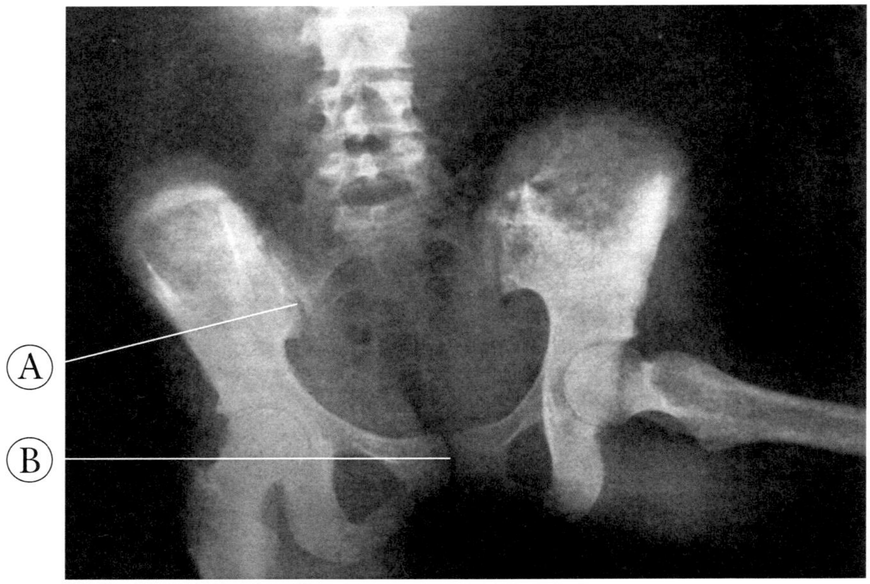

Fig.6-11
A-P pelvic X-ray with the right leg in abduction to 75 degrees. (Used with permission from the Ilford publishing company.)

The sacroiliac joints can be seen to be asymmetrical with the left SI joint separating more than the right. The pubic symphysis is also showing movement with the left pubic bone superior to the right.

(A) Left sacroiliac joint
(B) Pubis symphysis

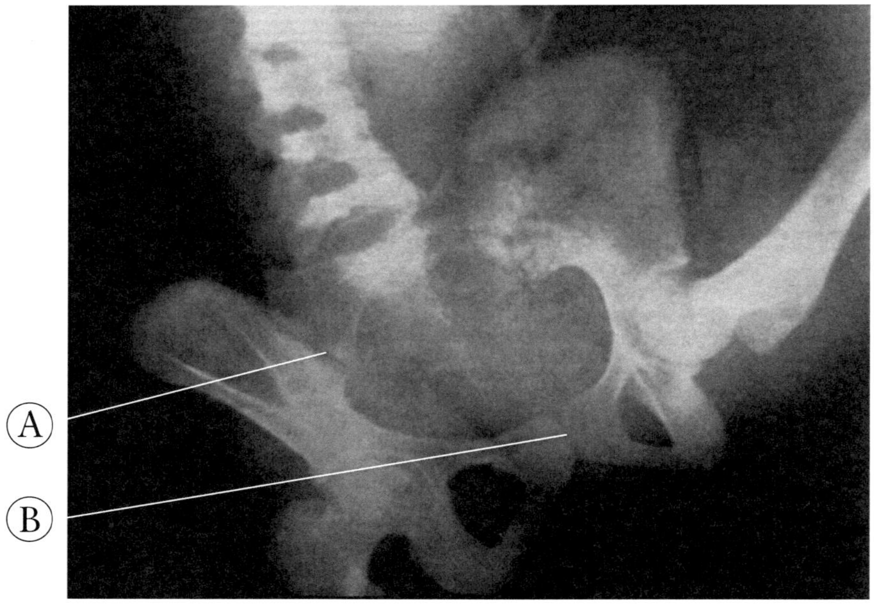

Figure 6-12
A-P pelvic X-ray with the right leg in abduction to 150 degrees. (Used with permission from the Ilford publishing company.)

The gapping of the left SI joint is more pronounced than the previous picture. The pubic symphysis has continued to show mobility in this position.

(A) Left SI joint
(B) Pubis symphysis.

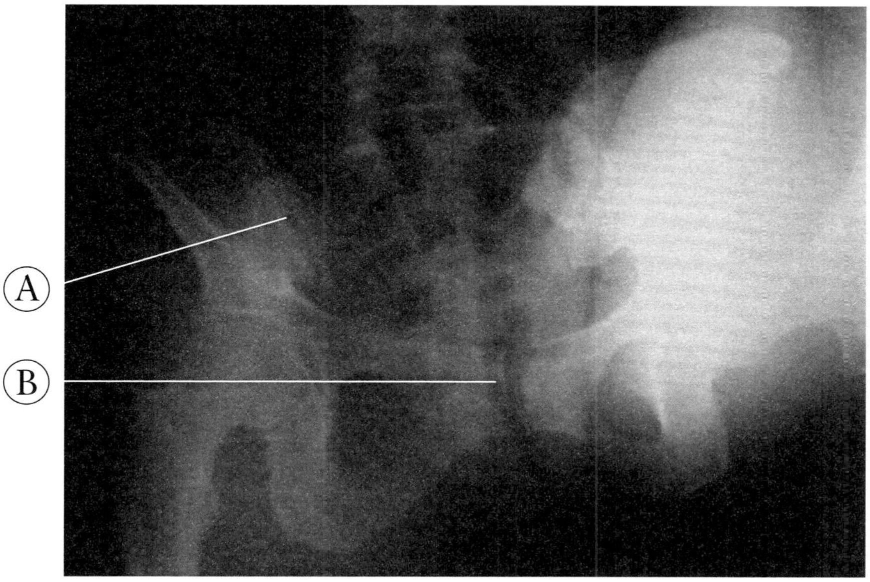

Figure 6-13
A-P pelvic X-ray with the right leg in hyperflexion.
The left SI joint has gapping similar to the previous X-rays. The pubic symphysis is showing some movement.
(A) Left SI joint
(B) Pubis symphysis.

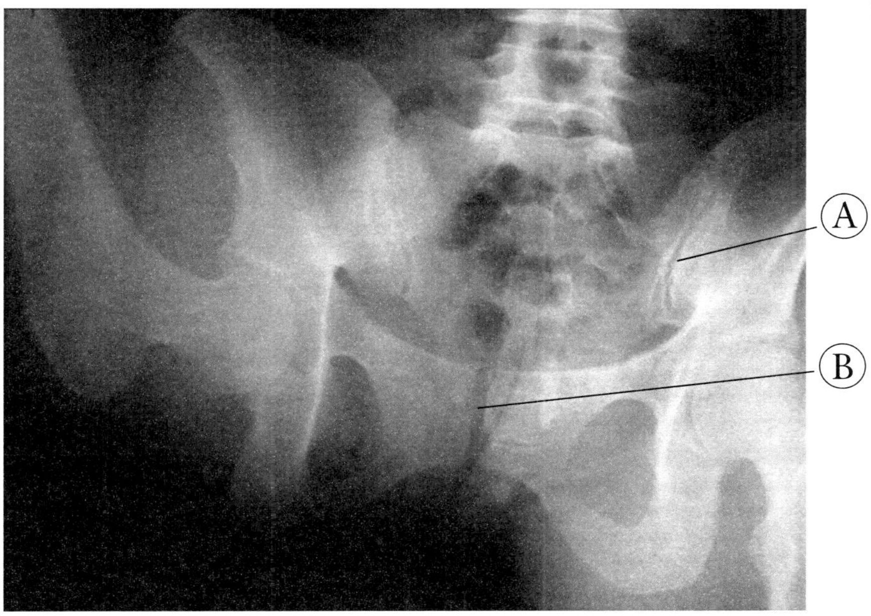

Figure 6-14
A-P pelvic X-ray with the left leg in hyperflexion.
The right SI joint is gapping and showing movement. The pubic symphysis is shifted so the right pubic bone is slightly superior.
(A) The right SI joint
(B) Pubis symphysis.

Pelvic Motion

The joints of the pelvic girdle are the strongest in the body.[13] In dynamic studies minor joint motion is seen (**see Figures 6-12** and **6-14**). The X-rays were taken weight bearing. The legs are the levers that move the pelvic joints, not lumbar motion. The last three pictures are positions of extreme motion. These are end range abduction and forward flexion of the hips and require athletic ability. The pelvic motion seen here is normal with leg motion. But the patterns of displacement seen here are commonly also seen in patients with both feet on the floor. The asymmetry of the SI joints and pubic symphysis seen with the patient in a neutral position is a sign of joint failure and a pathological condition. There are many of these "pain" patterns of the pelvic girdle.

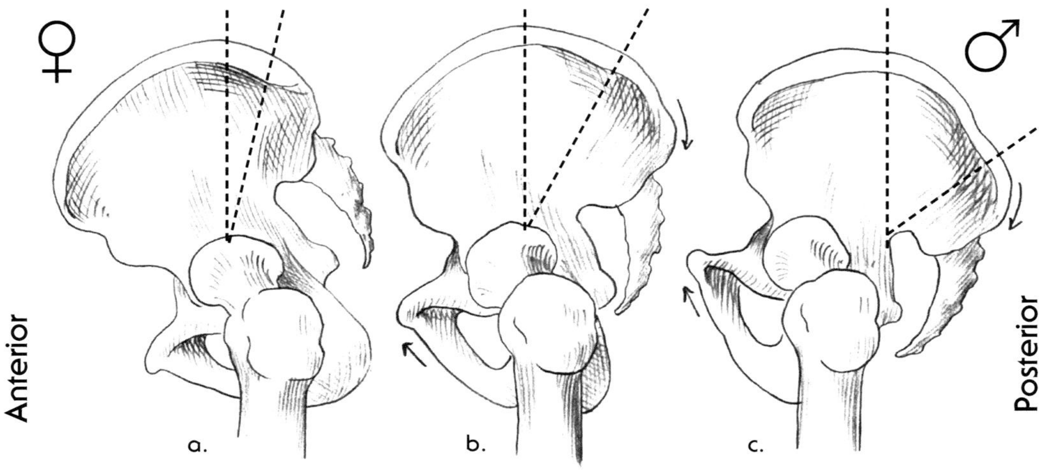

Figure 6-15
Illustration of the range of normal angles of pelvic tilt.
Sacral base angles are depicted by the dotted lines.
(a) The anterior tilt is a typical female feature. The sacral base angle approaches zero or perpendicular to the floor.
(b) This is a neutral pelvic tilt. This is considered normal but a range of angles between (a) and (c) is commonly found.
(c) This is a posterior tilt of the pelvis. The sacral base angle can be as high as 45 degrees. This is a typical male tilt. A central X-ray with A to P direction will give different appearances through each of (a), (b) and (c). The appearance on X-ray will change again with comparisons of recumbent and standing or seated views of the same individual.

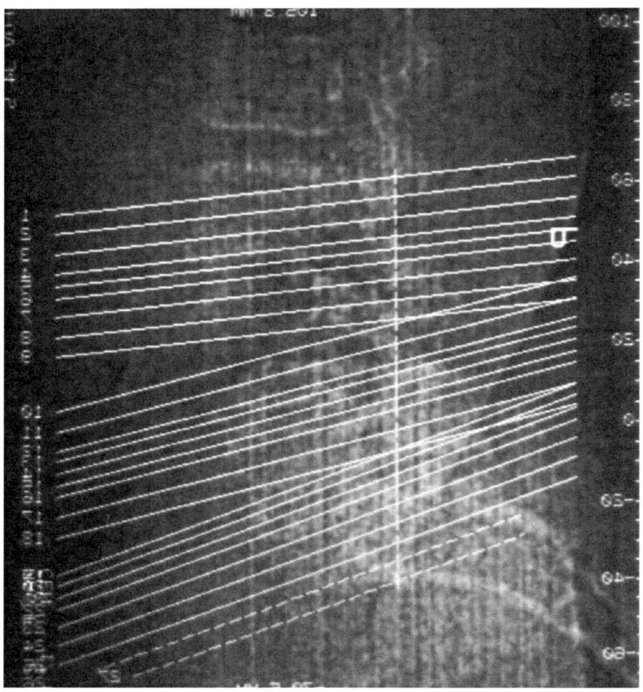

Figure 6-16
This lateral X-ray of the lumbar spine and pelvis have the planes of view of the CAT scan superimposed on it. Note the three different angles of views for the scans. Alignment and symmetry are important to evaluate, but the variety of angles of views can make this task more difficult.

Pelvic Tilt and Imaging

The normal pelvic tilt while standing can vary 45 degrees between the extremes of the anterior and posterior positions (**see Figure 6-15**).[14,15] The A-P X-ray can show a sacral base almost perpendicular to the central ray of the X-ray or one nearly parallel. The X-ray is really just a shadow picture. This complicates evaluation and diagnosis. This also gives a different appearance on imaging. **Figure 6-16** shows the slices of axial or cross-section pictures in advanced images (MRI or CT Scan). The tilt of the pelvis can change the picture of the pelvic joints. The irregular contours and angles of the sacroiliac joints make easy evaluation impossible. The standing or weight-bearing A-P X-ray can have a different tilt than a recumbent X-ray of the same person. The seated A-P X-rays of the pelvis change the angle yet again. In **Figures 6-17** and **6-18** the A-P X-rays of an anterior tilt and posterior tilt are shown. The diagnosis is the same for both individuals, but the appearance is different.

Figure 6-17
A-P X-ray of an anterior tilted pelvis.
This shows a superior subluxation of the left innominate.
Note the relative alignment of the pubic symphysis, this is because the pubic rami are parallel to the central ray.
(A) Right SI joint
(B) Right innominate
(C) Left innominate
(D) Left SI joint
(E) Pubic symphysis

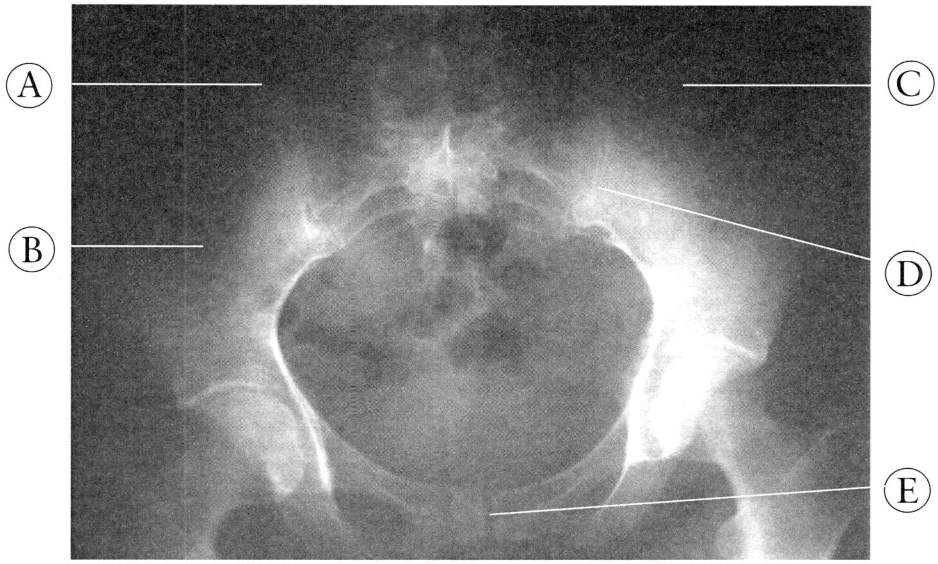

Figure 6-18
A-P X-ray of a posterior tilted pelvis.
This shows a superior left innominate, note the asymmetry of the SI joints and the misalignment of the pubic symphysis. This appearance is possible because the pubic rami are perpendicular to the central ray.
(A) Right innominate
(B) Right SI joint
(C) Left innominate
(D) Left SI joint
(E) Pubic symphysis

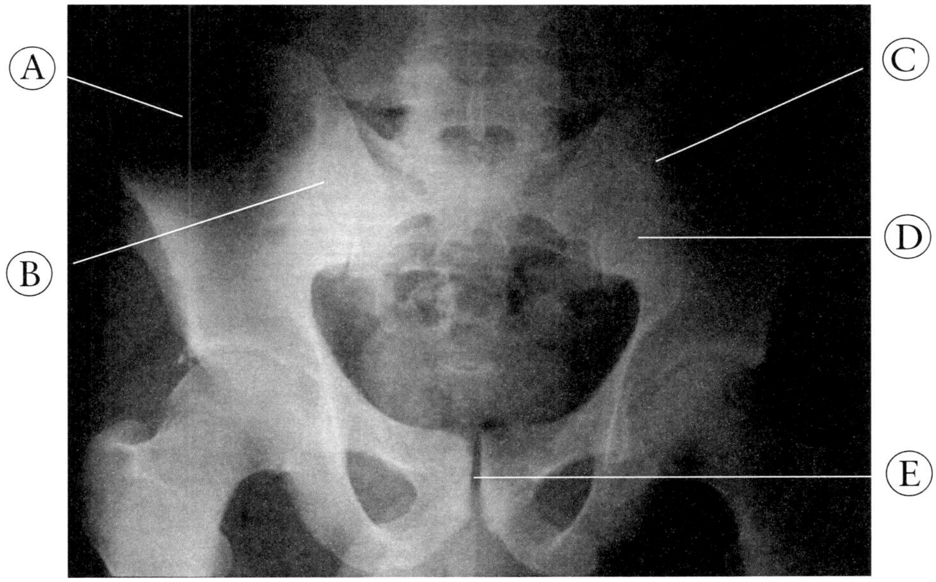

The Lumbosacral Relationship

The occurrence of even significant osteoarthritis in the lumbar spine can be a silent condition. An injury to the pelvis uncovers chronic degeneration and significant subluxations. Remarkable activity levels can be enjoyed with massive joint dysfunction of the lumbar spine. The recent onset of pain can be injury to the pelvic joints (see **Figures 6-19** and **6-20**).

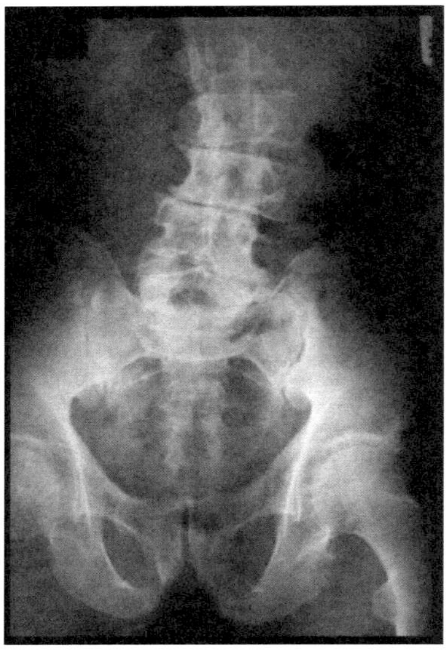

Right

a.

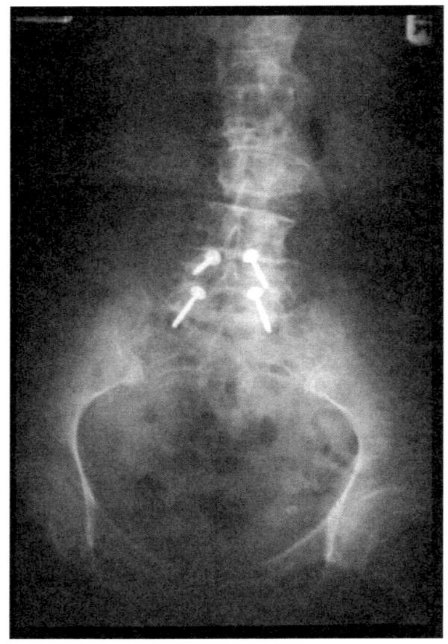

Right

b.

Figure 6-19 a & b

PELVIC TILT AND X-RAY APPEARANCE

A complete posterior rotation (right PI with ipsilateral superior pubis)

(a) Has a posterior tilt. The superior pubic rami are seen because they are generally perpendicular to central ray. Subject was an accomplished athlete for decades, and was still working out when film was taken.
(b) Has an anterior tilt and the pubic rami are generally parallel to the central ray. Note: in both cases spinal segments were not tender. The patients claimed very physically active lives and denied "years of pain." Both had the same complaint of right SI joint pain with right leg pain of recent onset. Note the spinal damage and the denial of pain and restriction of activity. Both patients complained of a recent on set of pain, "a" with lifting and "b" from a fall. Chiropractic adjustments to the pelvis restored both to their high level of activity.

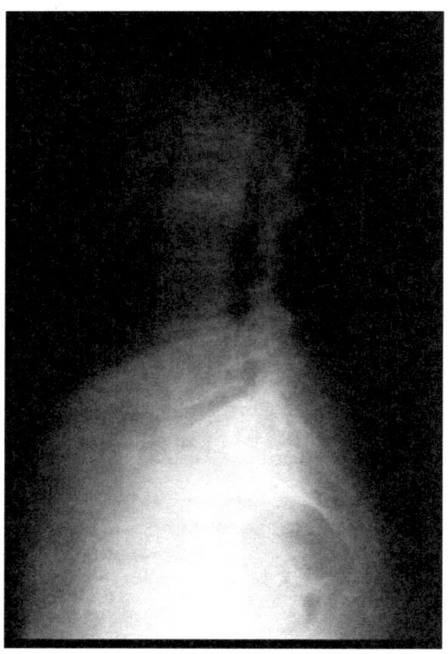

Right

a.

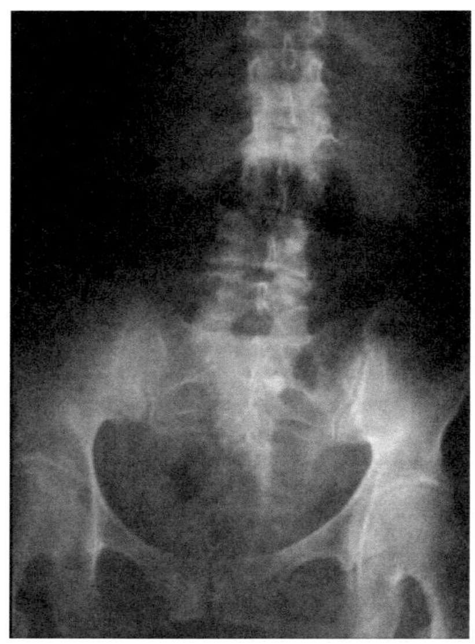

Right

b.

Figure 6-20 a & b

PELVIC SHEARING - non physiologic subluxations

Pelvic shearing in the presence of chronic degenerative osteoarthritis of the lumbar spine

These are A-P and lateral views of the lumbar spine and pelvis of a 72 year old woman who denies any history of back pain prior to a recent garden related event. Note fusion of L2-L3 and other changes of the lumbar spine. Subject is a skilled (and regular) ballroom dancer. Chiropractic adjustments to the pelvis restored her activity level.

PHYSIOLOGICAL SUBLUXATIONS OF THE PELVIS

The pelvic motion that normally takes place is maintained by the integrity of the pelvic ligaments. If the pelvic joints (or any joint for that matter) get stuck in a normal motion pattern, the integrity of the ligaments are not severely challenged. Usually a chiropractic manipulation with a short course of treatment will resolve the problem This injury pattern is within the physiological limits of the ligaments. It is characterized by limited motion caused by muscle guarding, pain and reduced symmetry of gait.

Figure 6-21 shows an axial plane MRI scan of an individual who complains of right hip and leg pain. The scan is taken with the **R** (in the middle on the left edge) indicating the patient's right and the **L** indicating the patient's left. The top is anterior while the bottom is posterior, with the ilium (or innominates) and sacrum appearing in cross-section (like a slice of bread). This is a perfect example of how subluxations of the pelvic girdle can manifest themselves on MRI. Notice the right ilium (on the left side of the scan) is more posterior to the sacrum than the left one; also the sacrum is narrower on the left than it is on the right. This would indicate sacral lateral flexion or tipping to the left, with the apex of the sacrum angled to the left. Note the asymmetry of the psoas muscles. This is an indication of muscular guarding patterns. This imaging should be preceded by a physical examination. This makes physical examination necessary and the imaging secondary. Very few studies on "low back pain" include the pelvic girdle in the investigation. Almost all "low back pain" is viewed as being disc related. This is not supported by MRI studies of the lumbar spine of 'normal" individuals. There is a large portion of the population that have damaged discs that are asymptomatic.[16,17]

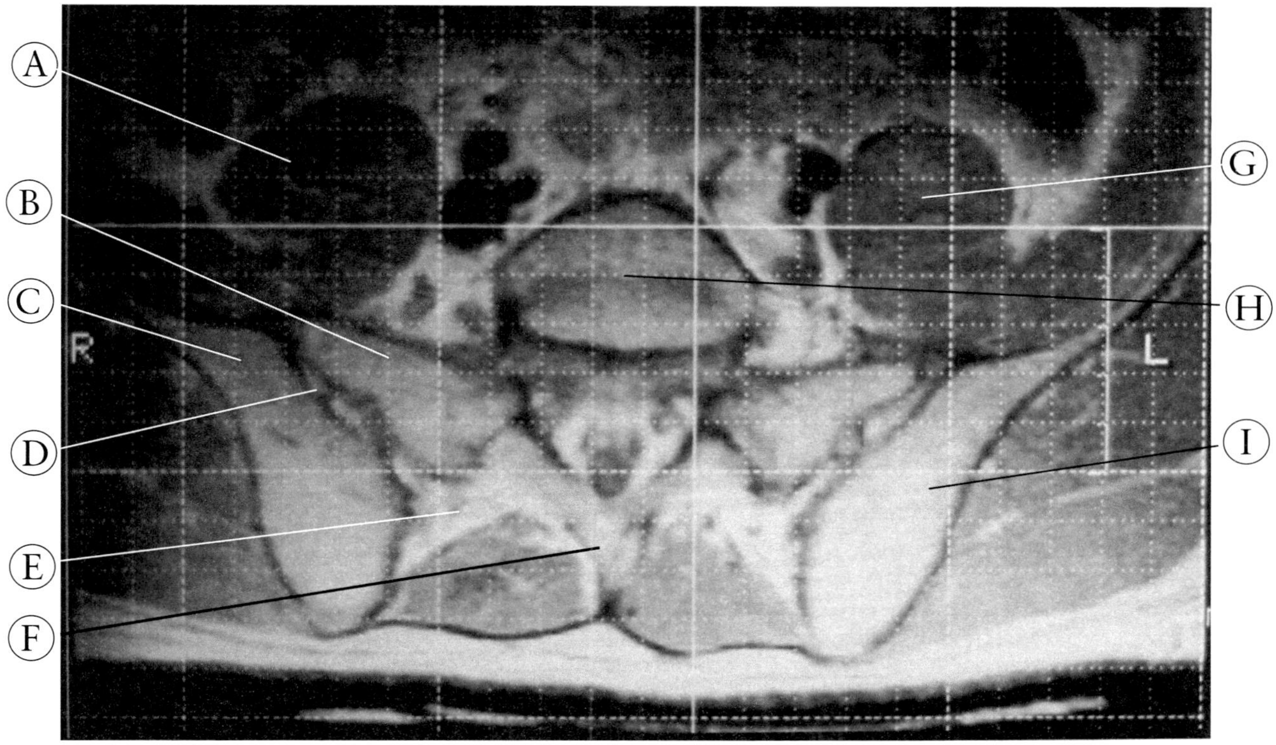

Figure 6-21
MRI axial view of the pelvis.

The subluxation of the sacrum is seen at the right sacroiliac joint with the right sacral ala anterior of the ilium. Using the grid to evaluate, the sacrum appears rotated or the ilium has moved posteriorly. Also note the difference in the diameter of the right and left psoas, indicating spasm of the right psoas.

(A) Right psoas
(B) Right sacral ala
(C) Right ilium
(D) Synovial portion of SI joint
(E) Fibrous portion of SI joint
(F) S1 spinous
(G) Left psoas
(H) Base of sacrum
(I) Left ilium

Note the common explanation by radiologists of this subluxation complex is: 'poor patient positioning'. The X-ray technicians say that the patient is flat on their back with arms at the side aligned with the grid as best as possible, 'the twists and misalignments are in the patient'.

These studies show that a damaged disc is not necessarily a cause of pain. This makes a thorough examination of all related regions extremely necessary. I find a large portion of patients with "hip" and "low back pain" are suffering from a lower leg injury. The proximal fibular-tibial joint controls the tension of the Tensor Fascia Lata (TFL), or the Illio-Tibial Band (ITB). Subluxation of the proximal "Fib-Tib" joint can cause unrelenting pain in the lateral tract of the leg and hip region. I have treated more than a dozen patients over the years that have had spinal surgery for relief of leg pain, some more than once, when they had an injured leg. No examination before or after the surgery was performed on the leg. I do not believe I can do anything to the lumbar spine (chiropractically or surgically) that would address the injured leg. Rational care is necessary to treat injured patients.

Figure 6-21 is an example of a subluxation complex of the pelvic girdle. It results in a recognizable pain pattern, and should be viewed as a clinical entity stressing the central nervous system, the peripheral nerves and the joints causing proprioceptive guarding of some or all

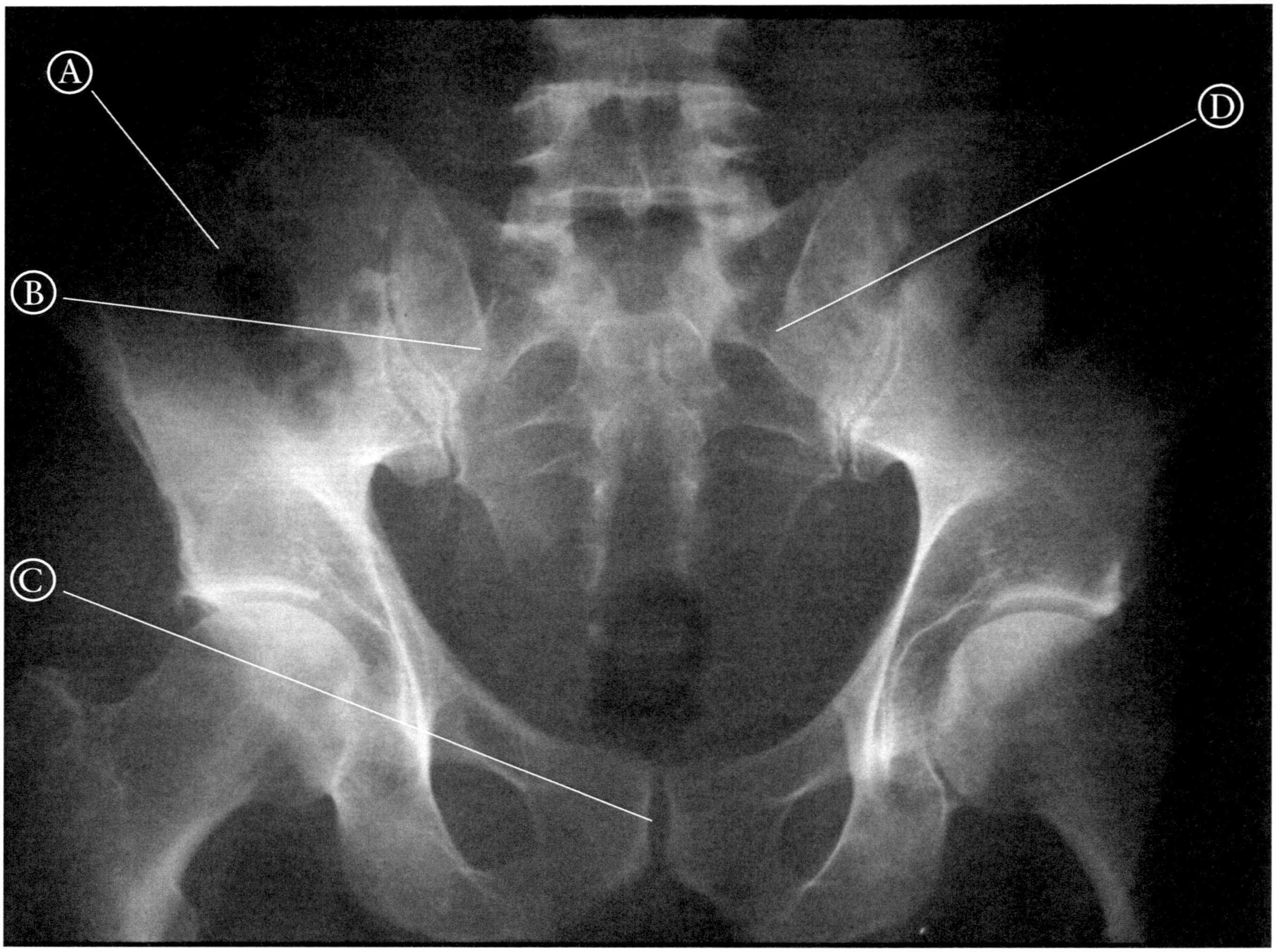

Figure 6-22

POSTERIOR OR FLEXION ROTATION OF ONE INNOMINATE

(a complete negative theta X of the right innominate or a right PI subluxation)

This is a recumbent view of a posterior pelvic tilt with a complete posterior rotation of the right innominate. The right posterior superior iliac spine (PSIS) is inferior to the left. Note elevation of right pubic rami. Correction of subluxation resulted in immediate relief and ability to walk.

(A) Right innominate
(B) Right posterior superior iliac spine
(C) Subluxated pubic symphysis
(D) Left posterior superior iliac spine

of the muscles attached to the pelvic girdle. It is important to know that pelvic subluxation can be viewed on advanced imaging.

Advanced imaging usually focuses on the lumbar spine, and it is only in the last few panels in the study that part of the pelvic girdle can be seen. It is crucial to pay close attention to those details of the advanced imaging when patients present with low back pain, hip, pelvic complaints, thigh or leg weakness, or pain and tenderness in any of the muscles that attach to the pelvic girdle. This includes everything from the insertion of longissimus capitis at the base of the occiput to the insertion of the sartorius at the medial, superior tibia. (My own left sacroiliac joint dysfunction is expressed by burning under my left scapula from the unhappy iliocostalis insertions).

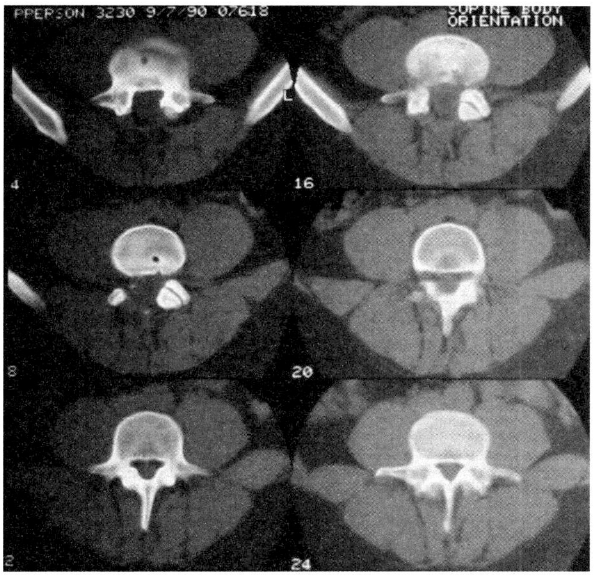

CAT Scan: Axial view

Figure 6-23 A & B
ROTATIONAL SUBLUXATIONS- physiologic subluxations
Positive and negative rotations on the X axis.
This 6 panel series shows right innominate posterior rotation relative to the left and or left anterior rotation. Note the sacral rotation, a subluxation, that accompanies this condition because of the oblique orientation of the sacroiliac joints. Also note the right side is on the reading left, and the top left panel is the most inferior view and bottom right the most superior.
(A) Posterior right ilium
(B) Left ilium

Left

Left

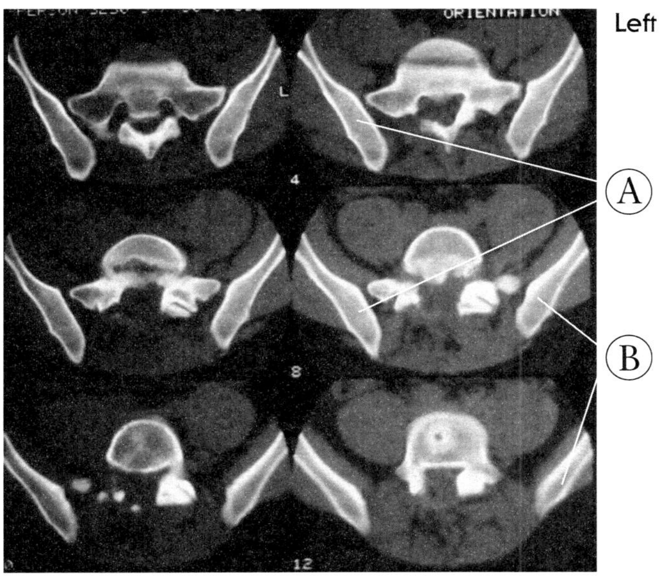

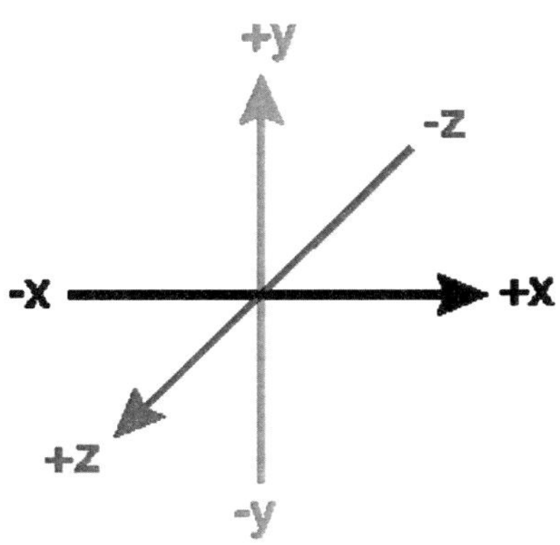

The Cartesian coordinate system
x-axis = Left/Right
y-axis = Down/Up
z-axis = Back/Front

Flexion/Extension Rotation

Flexion/extension (PI/AS) rotation of an innominate around the sacrum is a normal motion pattern of the sacroiliac joints. Hyper extension and hyper flexion injuries are common pelvic subluxation patterns. The posterior motion or position of the innominate is a normal flexion motion of the hip. The anterior motion and position of the ilium is an extension of the hip. These subluxation patterns are physiological subluxations, there is a normal motion pattern that the joint is stuck in. Muscular structures will be strained and ligaments will be sprained. If the degree of rotation is extreme, the pubic symphysis also subluxates as a result (see **Figure**

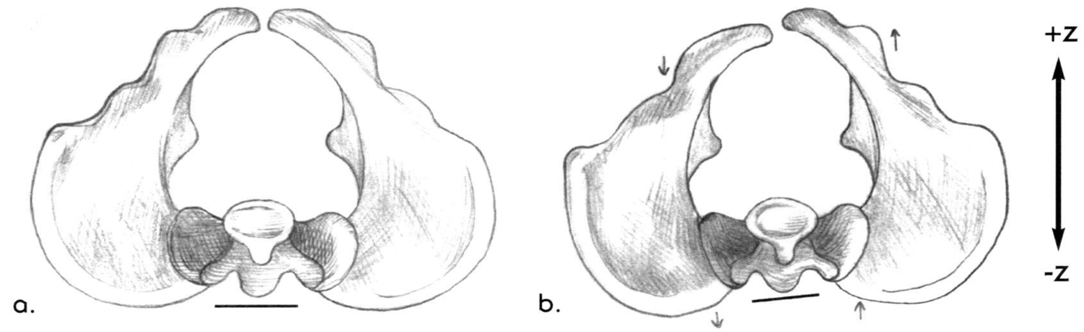

Figure 6-24
PELVIC SHEARING - non physiologic subluxations
This is an illustration of a theoretical view from above looking down on the whole pelvic girdle, not just a slice. In A the three joints of the pelvis are seen, the right and left sacroiliac joints and the pubic symphysis are aligned. In B the right pubic rami is anterior or ventral to the left and the sacrum is rotated. The shearing of the pelvis will have the appearance of positive and negative Z plane translations of one innominate relative to the other in the axial view. This type of injury involves sacral rotation as the right innominate shifts forward or anterior to the left. It is difficult to describe the axis of rotation in the varying pelvic tilts. Pubic symphysis shearing, tearing and SI joint ligament damage are very likely in this type of injury.

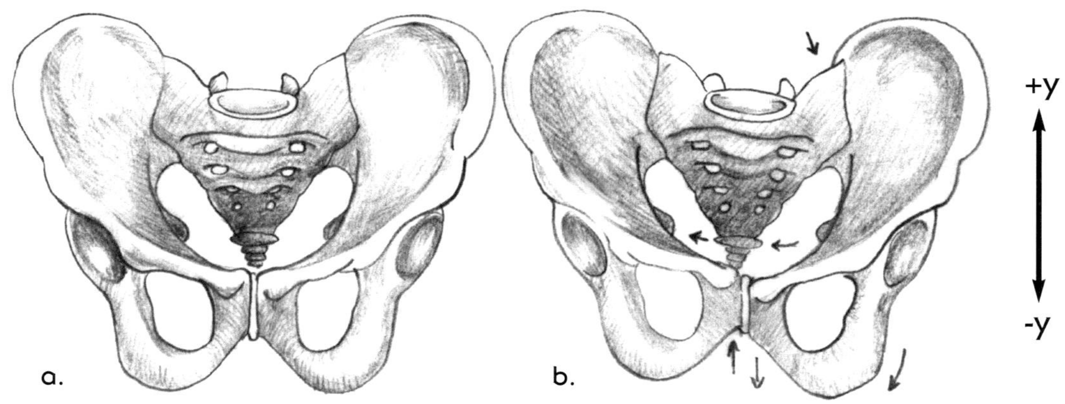

Figure 6-25
PELVIC SHEARING- non physiologic subluxations
(a) is an A to P view of a normal pelvis and (b) is the A-P appearance of a positive Y translation of the innominate on the left relative to the other. (Note the sacrum is tipped and the sacral apex is to the left of the pubic symphysis and the space between the ischial spine and the sacral border.) Also note the subluxation of the pubic symphysis, with the pubic rami on the left being elevated relative to other. I do not feel this an incidental finding. The psoas, iliacus and all the muscles attaching to the ischium and pubis will be adversely affected. This type of injury involves sacral shifting with the ala elevating with the superior innominate. This involves pubic symphysis and SI joint injury and intrinsic ligament damage because of the non physiologic displacement of the segments. Possible tearing of the pubic symphysis takes place. Axial imaging views will show the right iliac crest before the left in sequentially inferior views. Rotational displacement can be concomitant with Y or Z plane displacement. Combinations of these subluxation patterns in all planes can be present in one individual.

6-26). This is a more serious injury. Palpation and X-ray of the pubic symphysis reveals one ramus superior to the other. This might not be seen on the X-ray (**see Figure 6-22**), because of projection error on A-P Lumbopelvic views. Even on adanced imaging this can be difficult to determine (see **Figure 6-23**). This shows how important physical examination is for a proper diagnosis.

NON-PHYSIOLOGICAL SUBLUXATIONS

The phrase "non-physiological" is meant to describe subluxation patterns that are not part of the normal motion cycle of the joint. This indicates a ligament failure that is more severe, debilitating and persistent. Evidence from both dissection of cadavers and diagnosis and treatment of patients with pelvic trauma indicates

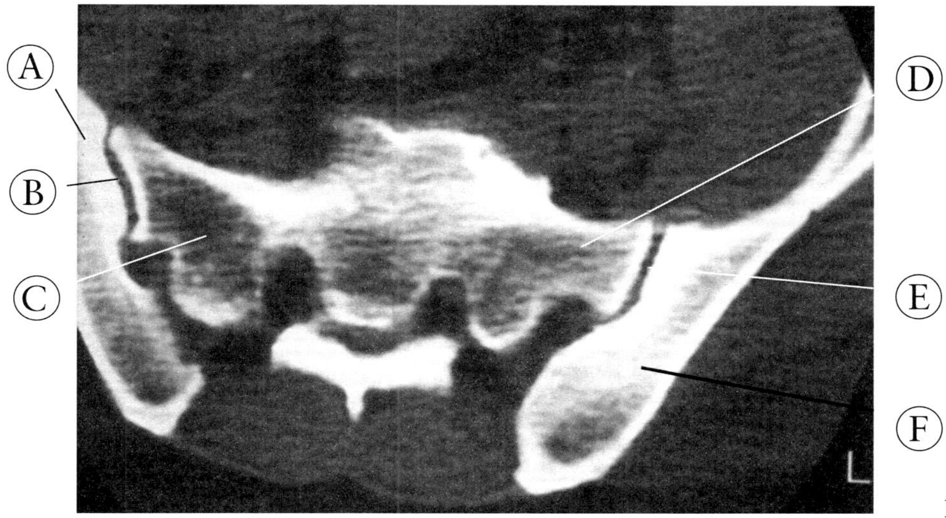

Figure 6-26
CAT scan of pelvis

This scan of the S2 level shows a subluxation complex of both SI joints. Note the difference in width between the right and left sides of the sacrum. This indicates that the sacrum is tipped. The left side is narrower and therefore a lower level of the sacrum, making the left sacral ala higher and the apex angled towards the left. The left ilium is posterior, larger and at a different angle than the right innominate. The left SI joint is subluxated with the sacrum anterior to the ilium.

(A) Right ilium
(B) Right SI joint
(C) Right side of the sacrum
(D) Left side of the sacrum
(E) Left SI joint
(F) Left ilium

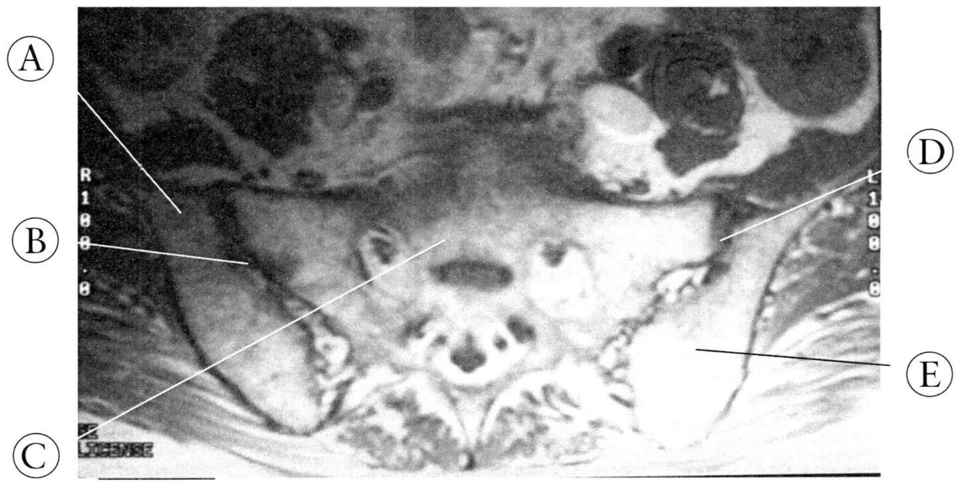

Figure 6-27
MRI of a subluxated pelvis.

The left innominate is posterior to the sacrum, the sacrum is rotated, the right side of the sacrum is anterior to the right ilium and the illi are asymmetrical. This is the appearance of significant pelvic distortion resulting in neurological deficit, altered gait and muscle atrophy.

(A) Right ilium
(B) Right SI joint
(C) Sacrum
(D) Left SI joint
(E) Left ilium

that the innominates can subluxate, independently of one another and the sacrum, in the planes Y, and Z. (in the Cartesian coordinate system). This condition results from a significant injury to the pelvis. The patient will have suffered a great amount of ligament failure.

Motor vehicle accidents and other high velocity events (skiing) are a major source of these types of injuries. I characterize these types of injuries as "Modern Injuries." These types of events were not happening 100 years ago. In the classes I teach at Life Chiropractic College West I find that nearly 100% of the students have been involved in one or more motor vehicle accidents. It is not so well known, however, that substantial subluxation of the innominate can involve the pubic symphysis as well as at the sacroiliac joints. Most physical examinations skip the anterior joints of the axial skeleton. The analysis of the relative positions of the pubic rami at the symphysis is the key to understanding many pelvic subluxation patterns. Variability in pelvic structure among individuals is surprisingly great, and can complicate diagnosis. In the Y axis, one innominate can translate unilaterally relative to the sacrum and opposing innominate primarily the +Y or superior direction. In the Z axis, either +Z, or -Z can occur. Both cause shearing at the sacroiliac joint and disruption of the pubic symphysis. These patterns of joint disruption exceed the physiological limits of the joints. They can be described as non-physiological subluxations. These injuries will not likely recover to a preinjury condition. The recovery to a functional, but limited, status will take many months to a few years.

Diagnosis of pelvic subluxation is further complicated by individual differences in the sacroiliac joint complexes. Wide variation occurs in the angles and curvatures of the joint complex itself. In some individuals the sacroiliac contact is flat, while in others it may exhibit ridged contours or deep sloping surfaces (**see Figure 6-7**). The result is that, particularly in X-rays, the same subluxation may look very different among individuals. Conversely, different subluxations may mimic one another, as noted in the example above (**see Figures 6-17** and **6-18**). These two individuals have the same diagnosis: a superior subluxation of the left innominate. The different pelvic tilts leave a completely different X-ray appearance. **Figure 6-17** is a female with an anterior pelvic tilt and **Figure 6-18** is a male with a posterior pelvic tilt (**see Figure 6-15**). Due to their variety, sacroiliac joints do not lend easily to any form of two-dimensional representation because, in the anatomical position, they are oriented obliquely in all three planes. To make matters even more confusing, the degree of obliqueness shows as much variation as the configuration of the joint surfaces. So, for the purpose of the following discussion, I will use supine and prone recumbent positions as my reference.

Pelvic Shearing: Non-physiological subluxations

Anterior To Posterior Pelvic Shearing

The +Z Or -Z Innominate

The sacroiliac joints narrow from superior to inferior, and from posterior to anterior, so that one innominate can translate in the Z axis relative to the other. **See Figure 6-24**, an illustration, showing the shearing in the anterior/posterior direction. This will typically leave the anterior pubic symphysis very painful on palpation. **Figures 6-26** and **6-27** are scans depicting a shearing of one innominate forward relative to the other which involves all three joints and rotation of the sacrum. These types of injuries do not respond well to side posture manipulation. On A-P Lumbopelvic X-ray of the anterior pelvis (**see Figure 6-15**) the subluxation appears

Figure 6-28
Subluxation of pubic symphysis
(A) Left pubic body
(B) Pubic symphysis

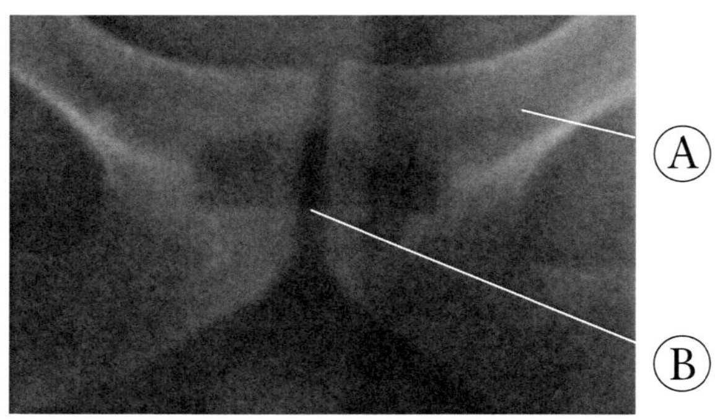

Figure 6-29
An Experiment with Imaging the Pubis Symphysis

This series of images demonstrates how subluxations of the pubic symphysis can be misrepresented or impossible to diagnose on standard x-ray views. The upper illustration shows schematically how the images were obtained, and how the visualization errors can be created.
Note the 2 middle pictures in the two right columns, these are very common subluxation patterns with motor vehicle accidents. The pubic joint will have extremely painful palpation for most patients. The X-ray findings do not correlate with the physical examination findings. This makes physical examination necessary and the imaging secondary. Very few studies on "low back pain" include the pelvic girdle in the investigation. Most "low back pain" is viewed as being disc related. This is not supported by MRI studies of the lumbar spine of "normal" individuals. These studies show a significant portion of the population has disc damage without symptoms. This makes a thorough examination of all related regions. I find a large portion of patients with "hip" and "low back pain" are suffering from a lower leg injury. The proximal Fibular-Tiblal joint controls the tension of the Tensor Fascia Lata (TFL), or the Illio-Tibial Band (ITB). Subluxation of the "Fib-Tib" joint can cause unrelenting pain in the lateral tract of the leg and hip region

Diagram of imaging apparatus. (Not to scale,)
View represents a mid-sagittal section as viewed from the "patient's" right side. This shows the relationship of the X-ray source, target structures, and X-ray film. Note that although the recording camera is positioned slightly below the "target," the shadow (and X-ray image) are two-dimensional, and are therefore accurately represented, even though the image of the target itself is subject to parallax (and depth-of-field focusing limitations). The camera is in fact at the same level as the shadow. That this is below the level of the target verifies the distortion of both the position and shape of the target structure introduced by the point-source X-ray and its position relative to any particular structure.

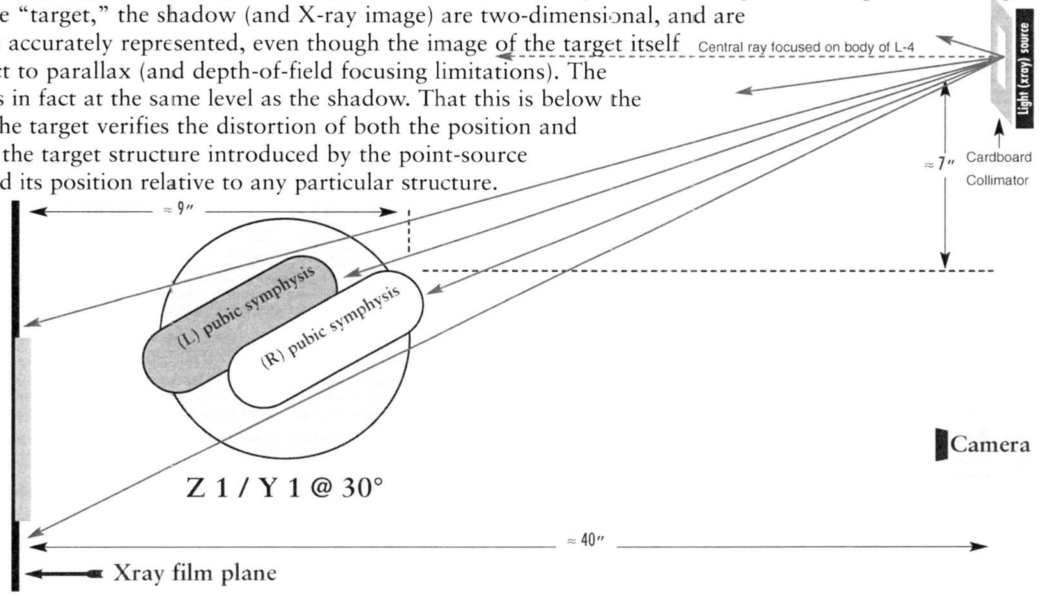

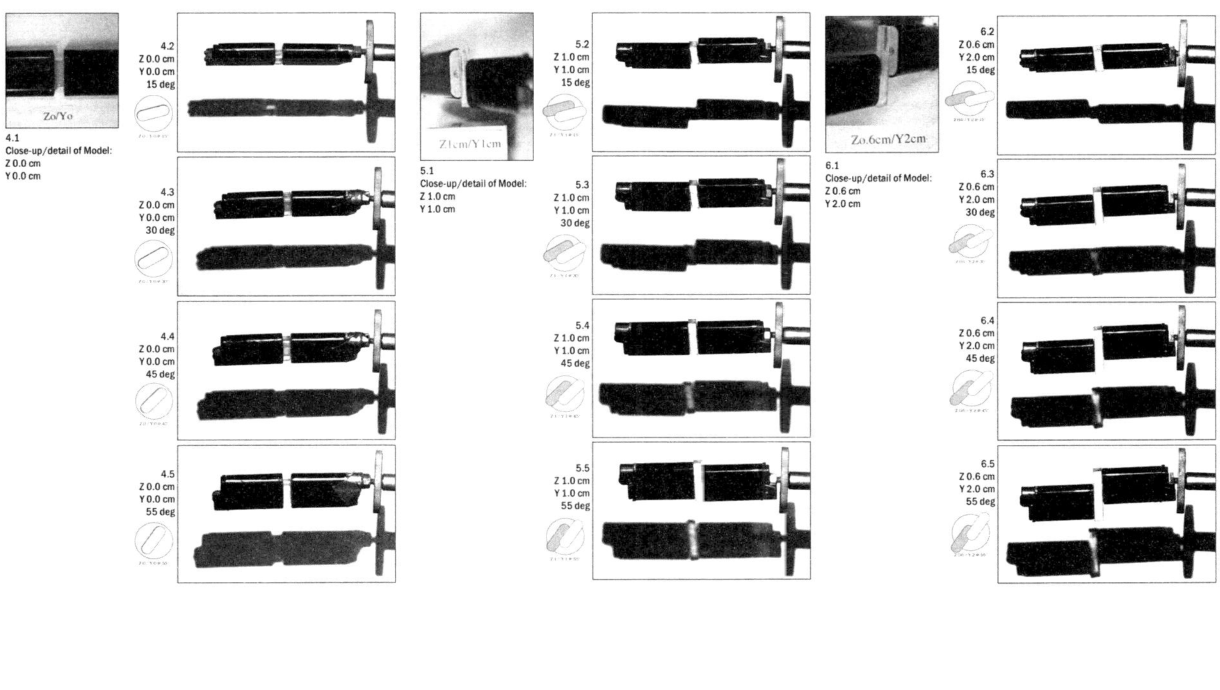

to be an inferior translation of the pubic rami. In a neutral or posterior pelvis (**see Figure 6-15**). the subluxation can be hard to see, although the pubic bone can appear larger on one side. (Translation away from the X-ray film should increase the shadow effect and project a larger image.)[18]

The +Y Or -Y Innominate

Displacement of the innominate superiorly to the sacrum (+Y Plane) is usually caused by a significant trauma such as a motor vehicle accident or falling on one ischium or one foot with the knee extended. This displacement of one innominate relative to the sacrum and other innominate is ligament failure.[19,20]

The illustration in **Figure 6-25b** shows translation of the whole innominate superiorly or in the positive Y axis. This results in one innominate being superior to the other. However, the same subluxation can appear to be different in standing AP X-rays, with different pelvic tilts. For instance, the +Y subluxation in an anterior pelvic tilt is not likely to be seen (**see Figure 6-19**). A physical exam of the pubic symphysis and the other joints and landmarks is the key to analyzing this condition. A superior pubic symphysis is surrounded by ridged, splinting musculature. The pubis can be very painful, tender or not, and palpation can refer pain to the SI joints. Comparison palpation and contact of the ischial tuberosities, iliac crests, ASIS and PSIS should indicate that one of the innominates is displaced in the positive Y, or superior direction. Often one innominate is closer to the rib cage in prone palpation.

Figure 6-26 shows an axial section of a CAT scan at the level of S2. This is an advanced diagnostic image of a chronic subluxation of the pelvis. The asymmetry of the illiums and psoas muscles, joint sclerosis and rotation are all signs of pelvic girdle distortion subsequent to trauma. In this case the patient had fallen off of a loading dock 15 years earlier, landing on an extended left leg. **Figure 6-27** is an MRI of the S2 level with the sacrum anterior to both illi. The left is worse than the right. This patient had been hit in a crosswalk by an automobile and suffered a gradual onset of left lower leg paralysis, including foot drop. The left innominate was superior to the right. Chiropractic adjustments to the pelvic girdle restored normal gait. In **Figure 6-29** there is a simplified view of an experiment showing how difficult it is too see

Pelvic Shearing: non-physiological subluxation of pelvis

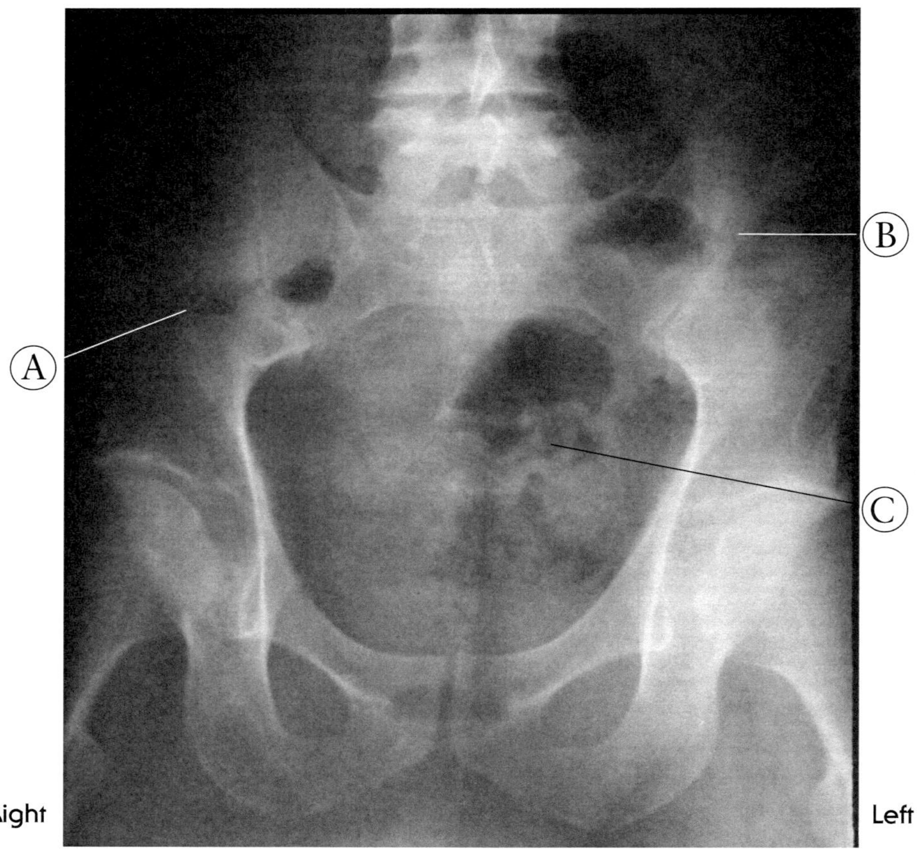

Figure 6-30
Standing A-P pelvic X-ray of a subluxated pelvis

This is an example of pelvic shearing, a non-physiological subluxation that must include ligament damage. The left innominate has superior (a +Y displacement) subluxation, but in the standing position appears lower. The acetabulum has moved up but the foot still has to be on the ground, angling and tipping the pelvis. Note the sacrum is in the left side of the pelvic rim.

(A) Right innominate (B) Left innominate (C Sacrum

pubic symphysis subluxation on A-P lumbopelvic views. I noticed years ago, in the anatomy lab, that the A-P pelvic X-rays of the specimens did not match with their visible appearance. This suggested there was a projection error with the A-P lumbopelvic view. A few years later I devised an experiment. I made plastic models of the aligned, moderately subluxated and significantly subluxated pubic symphysis. I put them in a mock 40° A-P lumbopelvic set-up with a collumated 90 Watt bulb. I put models in different positions spanning the range of the anterior and posterior pelvic tilts. The left column in **Figure 6-29** represents the normal alignment of the pubic bones. The middle column is with moderately misaligned pubic bones. The lower two frames give the false impression of alignment. The far right column represents significant subluxation of the pubic symphysis. The top two frames give the false impression of alignment. A physical examination is essential, imaging has limitations.

In **Figure 6-30** the X-ray shows minor pubic symphysis subluxation. On palpation it was a major subluxation with severe pain on palpation of the pubic symphysis and debilitating low back pain and altered gait. In **Figures 6-31, 6-32** and **6-33** the superior innominate is seen in multiple panels before the lower one is seen. Note the asymmetrical psoas muscles in each study. This is a sign of chronic neuromuscular guarding reflex. If the joints and ligaments of this major weight bearing structure are failing, I expect antalgia, altered and slow gait. **Figures 6-34** and **6-35** show X-rays of elderly, debilitated patients who used walkers. They were suffering from significant subluxations of the pubic symphysis. Chiropractic adjustments allowed them to stand and walk with more ease and less pain. The challenge is to get the temporary progress in care to persist when such ligament injury and instability is chronic. It is possible to have both innominates translate superiorly to the sacrum. This debilitating condition can cause coccygeal pain, testicular pain, pain with sitting, gynecological distress, pain with sex, and pain with urination. When the innominate subluxates superiorly to the sacrum the floor of the pelvis is stretched and inflamed. If both innominates are subluxated the symptoms can be severe. These are my clinical findings. Subluxation of the pelvis can be a significant health factor, adversely affecting many systems.

Superior subluxation of left innominate

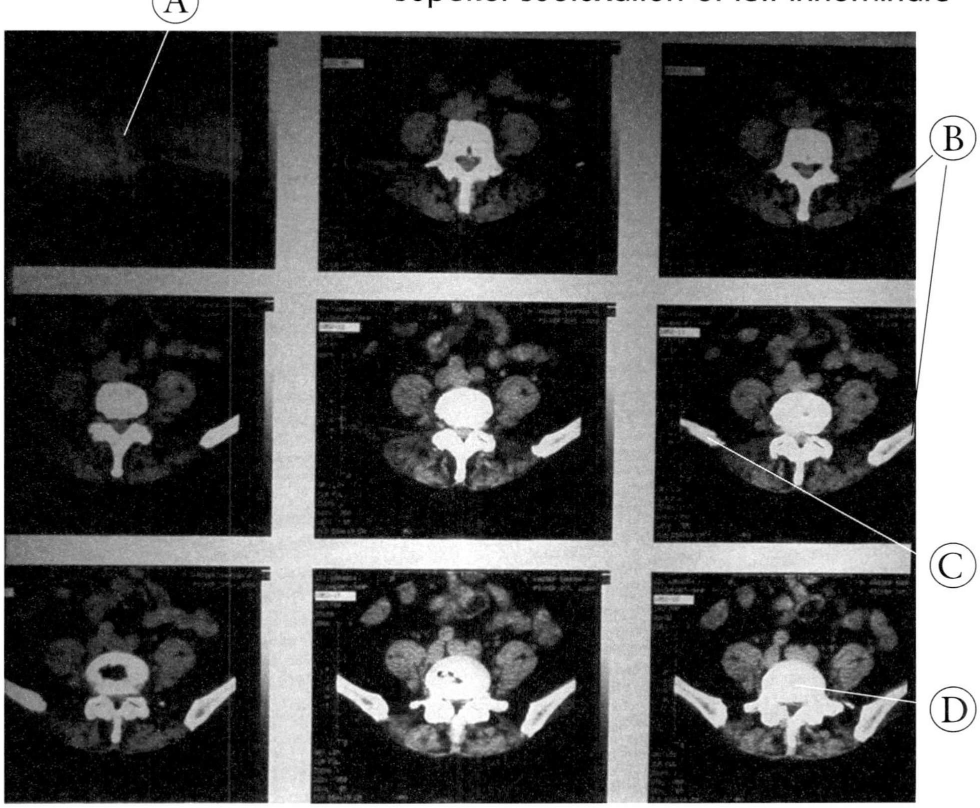

Figure 6-31
PELVIC SHEARING-non physiologic subluxations - V

This CAT scan shows the top of the left iliac crest in the upper right pane . The second far right panel shows the top of the right iliac crest. This indicates a 15mm difference in height. A superior or +Y subluxation of the left innominate is present. Symptoms included severe left buttock, hip and leg pain. The patient was referred to an orthopedic surgeon who recommended surgery of the lumbar spine.

(A) Planes of orientation of the scan shown with supine lateral lumbar X-ray
(B) Left iliac crest
(C) Right iliac crest
(D) L5

Superior subluxation of right innominate

a.

b.

c.

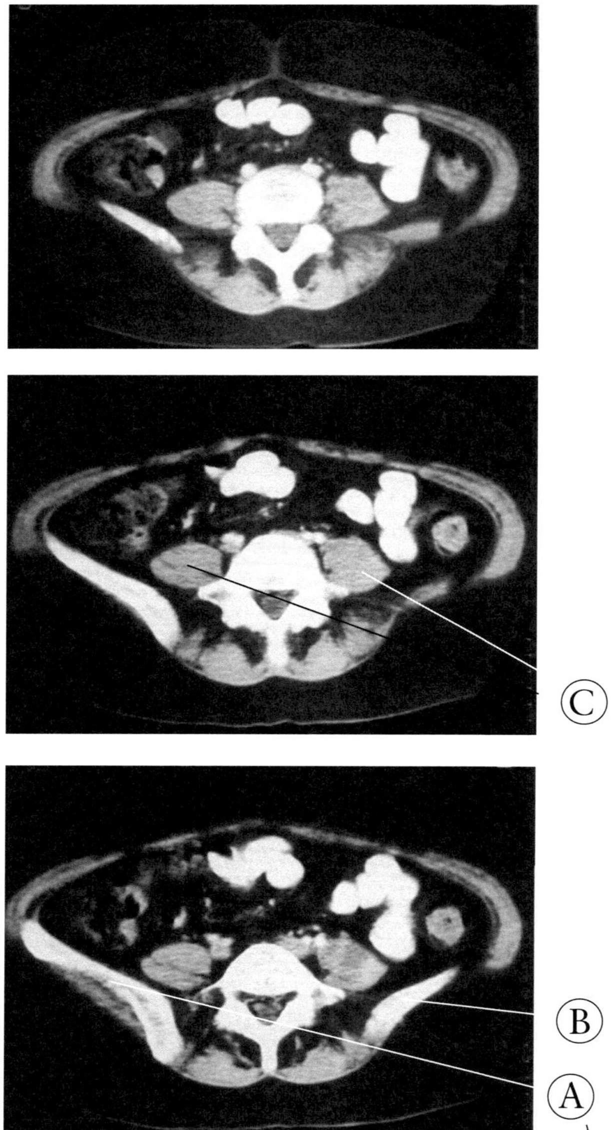

Figure 6-32 a, b, & c
PELVIC SHEARING - non physiologic subluxation
This is a CAT scan of top of pelvis with right innominate +Y or superior subluxation.The patient walks with a gait and has abnormalities that are improved with the correction of +Y right innominate translation.

(A) Right innominate
(B) Left innominate
(C) Psoas

a.

b.

c.

d.

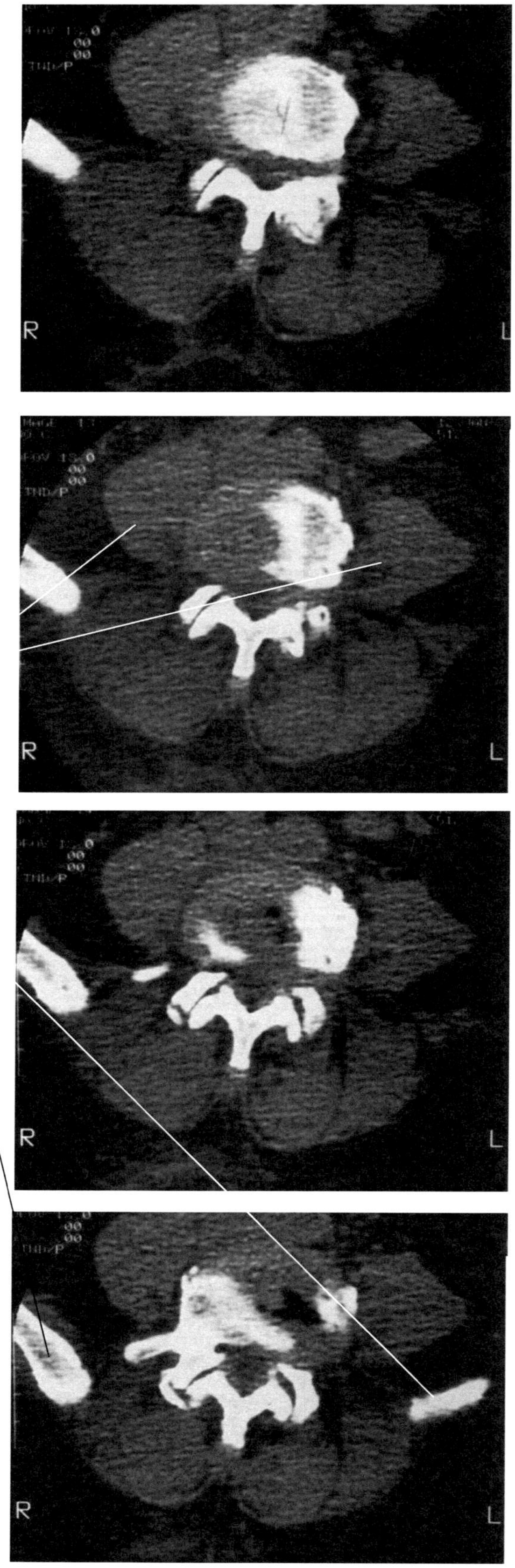

Figure 6-33 a, b, c, & d
PELVIC SHEARING - non physiologic subluxation
Right innominate has +Y translation. Note left rotation and lateral flexion of L4 & L5 due to superior elevation of right side of sacral ala. Note black spaces in discs in panels (b) and (d) of discs L4-L5 and L5-S1. Patient walked with cane and had obvious gait abnormality.

The Geriatric Pelvis

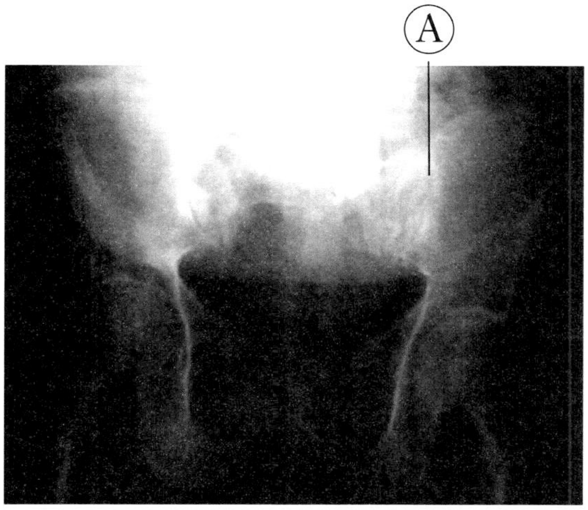

Figure 6-34
X-Ray of an 84 year old

Multiple injuries have rendered this 84 year old man unable to walk. Note the asymmetry of the sacroiliac joints and the misalignment of the pubic symphysis. This is an example of superior (+Y) and anterior (+Z) shearing of the left innominate. The muscles of the hip, thighs, abdomen and back were all rigid and painful. The patient was flexed at the hip as well as in knees and needed assistance to move. Correction of the pelvic subluxations allowed this individual to walk unaided.

(A) Left sacroiliac joint

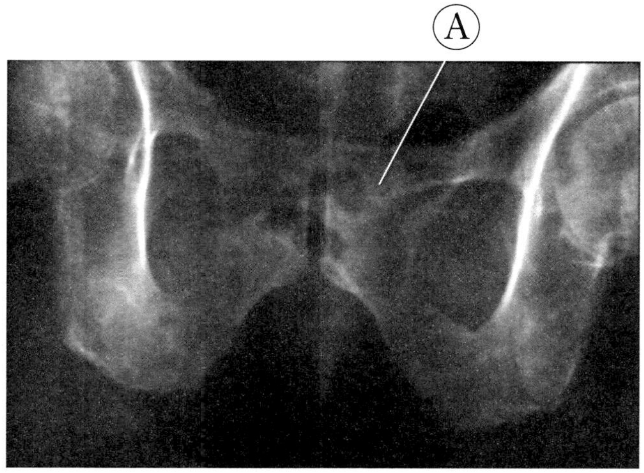

Figure 6-34 A
Detail from same study as Figure 6-34

Note shift of the left pubic bone upward relative to the right. This can result in spasms of the psoas, rectus abdominus and thigh muscles.

(A) Left pubic bone

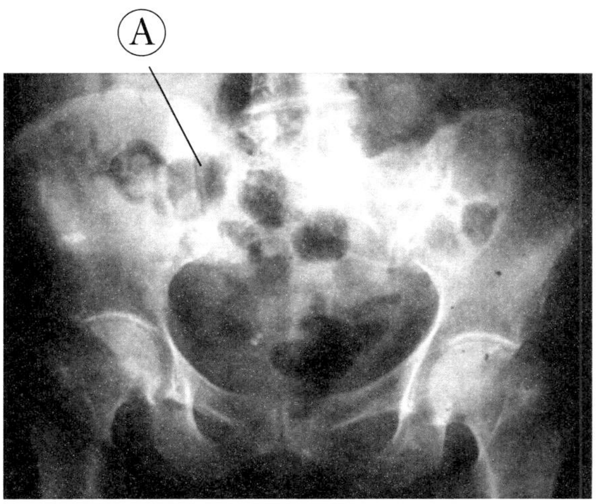

Figure 6-35
X-ray of an 82 year old

This 82 year old has a history of many falls, requires a walker and moves slowly in a flexed forward position. Note the asymmetry of the sacroiliac joints and pubic symphysis. This is an example of a superior (+Y) and anterior (+Z) right innominate with a significant left innominate posterior rotation.

(A) Right sacroiliac joint

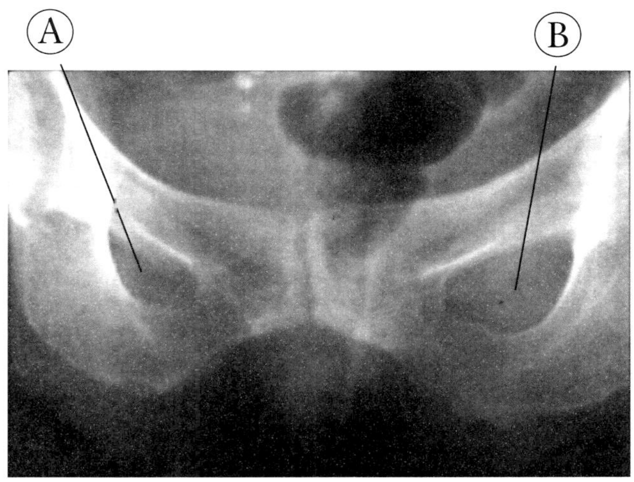

Figure 6-35 A
Detail from same study as Figure 6-35

Note the significant difference in the shape of the obturator foramen and the height of the pubic bones. This indicates rotation has taken place between the two innominates.

(A) Right obturator foramen
(B) Left obturator foramen

Intrasacral Subluxations

In Figure 6-3 (page 195, repeated on page 218) the normal sacral discs, appear to have pulpy nucleus pulposus in an aged person. In this study below the specimens shown here, Figures 6-36 to 6-41, have suffered injuries that have damaged their sacrums. The pulpy nature is gone and the discs have fused. In most of these individuals it is apparent they also damaged their lower spines. Note the loss of the

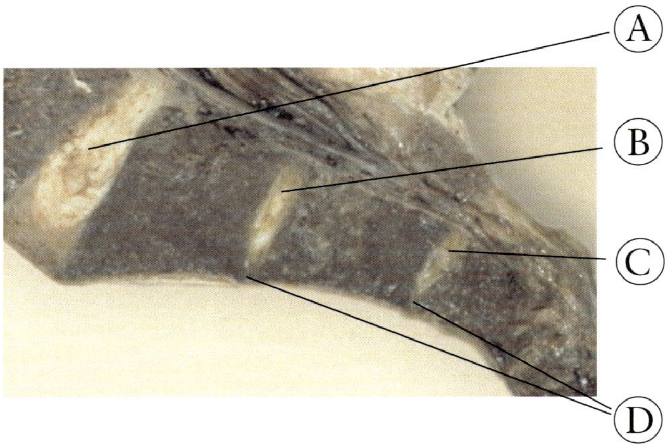

Figure 6-36
Damaged sacrum
Most individuals have sacral discs. This would indicate sacral motion is normal.
Note the L5-S1, S1-S2 and S2-S3 discs are all present with the beginning signs of degeneration. The annular walls are darker and the cortical borders of the sacral discs are thickened.
(A) L5-S1 disc
(B) S1-S2 disc
(C) S2-S3 disc
(D) Cortex of sacrum

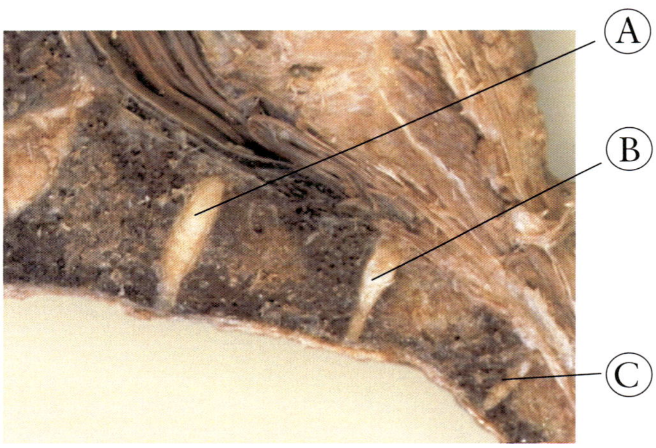

Figure 6-37
Damaged sacrum
Shown are sacral discs in an elderly specimen. Note the discs between the segments of S1 and S2, S2 and S3 and S3 and S4. The avascular structures confer motion and need motion to persist late into life.
Note the loss of anterior disc height at the S2-S3 disc and the angling of S3.
(A) S1-S2 disc
(B) S2-S3 disc
(C) S3-S4 disc.

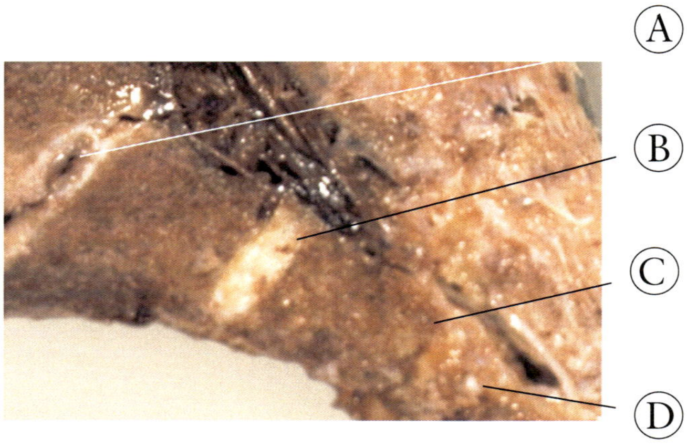

Figure 6-38
Damaged sacrum
A sacral disc with degenerative joints above and below. The L5-S1 is sheared and degenerating because of the subluxation of L5 posteriorly.
Note the appearance of S3 being slightly anterior to S2 suggesting an intrasacral subluxation.
(A) L5-S1 disc
(B) S1-S2 disc
(C) Site of S2-S3 fusion
(D) S3

Intrasacral Subluxations

normal kyphotic curve of the sacrums. This type of injury would interfere with sacral function (probably subluxating the sacroiliac joints) including it's motion of the lower end the spinal canal and walking. Altered joint mechanics in the sacroiliac joints has been associated with chronic low back pain.[22]

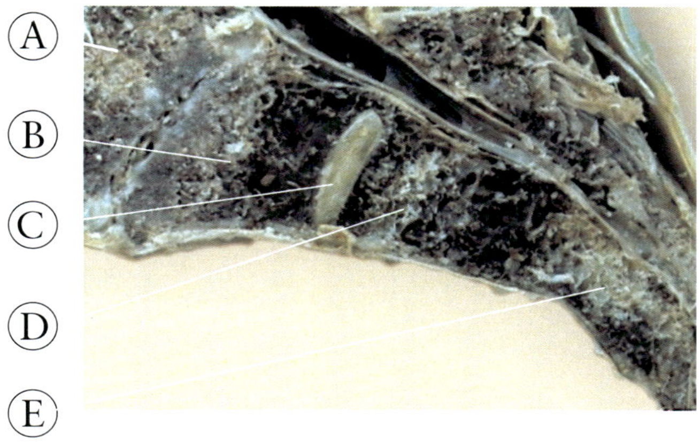

Figure 6-39
Damaged sacrum

This shows a sacral disc with end stage degeneration above and below. The L5-S1 joint has sheared and fused. L5 is posterior to the sacrum. The S1-S2 disc is dehydrated and the cortical bone has thickened. S3 is angled in ventral direction and the S2-S3 disc is gone.

(A) L5
(B) S1
(C) S1-S2 disc
(D) S2
(E) S3.

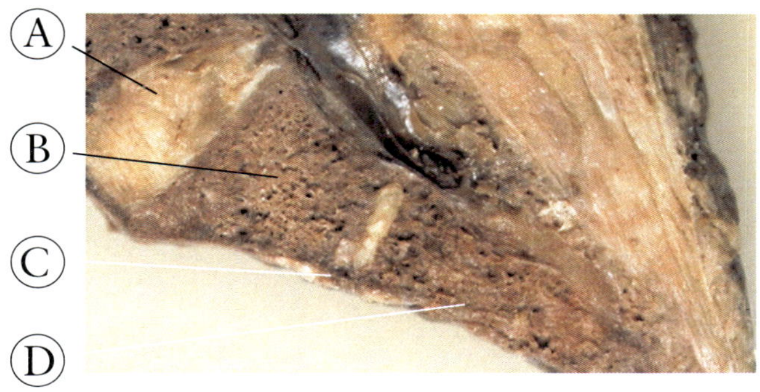

Figure 6-40
Damaged sacrum

This a picture of a sacral disc with a healthy L5-S1 joint and a fused S2-S3 joint. The L5-S1 disc is slightly wedged anteriorly. The S1-S2 disc is dehydrated and reduced in substance with a thickening of the cortical bone. S2 is angled in a dorsal direction.

(A) L5-S1 disc
(B) S1
(C) Thickened cortex
(D) S2

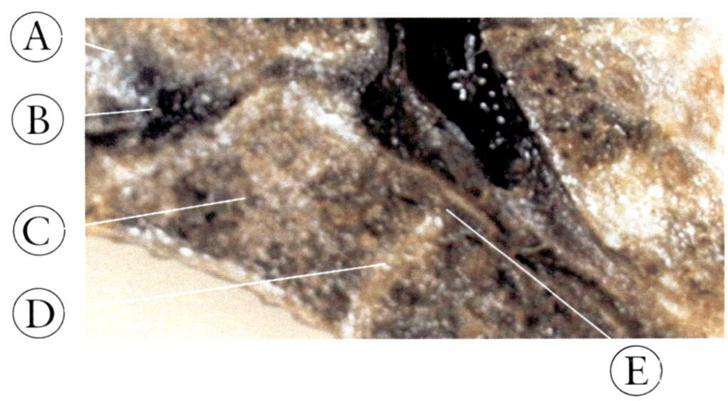

Figure 6-41
Damaged sacrum

This specimen has a significant subluxation of S1 anterior to L5 with fusion. The S1-S2 disc has barely persisted and the cortical bone has thickened.

(A) L5
(B) L5- S1 disc
(C) S1
(D) S1-2 disc
(E) Thickened cortex

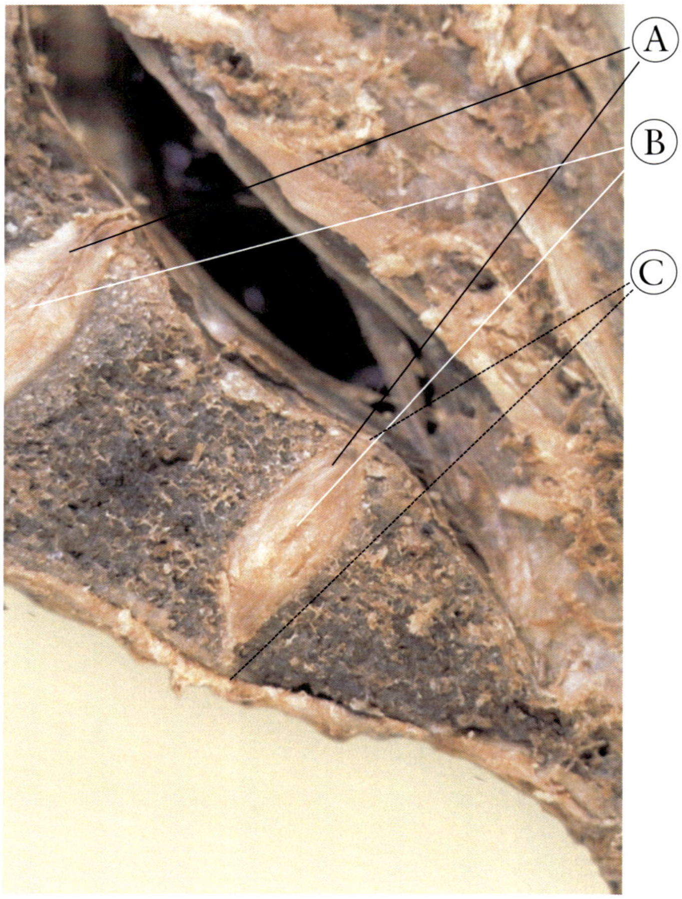

Figure 6-3 (repeated from page 195)

This is a view of the sacral discs of an 86 year old male.
The majority of elderly specimens had persistent sacral discs. The most persistent was the S1-S2 disc. The S2-S3 disc was less often observed. The S3-S4 disc was occasionally seen, about 25%. This view was slightly off the mid-sagittal plane. Note the presence of annular rings and a nucleus pulposus. The sacral discs are oval in shape in the A to P and coronal planes (Z and X planes). Note the continuous cortical bone that must be radio dense. This is significant evidence of sacral motion front to back and side to side.Discs require motion to persist (**see Figure 1-12b**). This is the anatomical explanation of the sacrum pumping the Cerebrospinal Fluid in the spinal canal. Sacral motion is likely to be connected to central nervous system physiology and function.

(A) Annulus fibrosus
(B) Nucleus pulposus
(C) Cortex of sacrum

ENDNOTES/REFERENCES

Chapter 1

1. Breig, A., *Adverse Mechanical Tension in the Central Nervous System*, Alquist and Wiksell, 1978,, pg 11
2. Louis, R. Spinal Stability as Defined by the Three-Column Spine Concept, *Anatomica Clinica*, 1985, 7:33-42.s, pg 34
3. Kaplan, F. S., Osteoporosis, *Clinical Symposium*, Vol. 35, Number5, pg 9
4. Sibonga JD. *Curr Osteoporos Rep. 2013* Jun;11(2):92-8. doi: 10.1007/s11914-013-0136-5. Spaceflight-induced bone loss: is there an osteoporosis risk? NASA Johnson Space Center, 2101 NASA Parkway, Houston, TX 77058, USA. Jean.sibonga-1@NASA.gov
5. Blau, J. N., Rushworth, G., Observations on the Blood Vessels of the Spinal Cord and Their Responses to Motor Activity, *Brain*, 1958, Vol. 81:354-363, pg 341
6. Marcus, M. L., Heistad, D. D., Ehrhardt, J. C., Abboud F. M., Regulation of Total and Regional Spinal Cord Blood Flow, *Circulation Research*, 1977, 1:128-134, pg 133
7. Hamamoto Y, Ogata T, Morino T, Hino M, Yamamoto H, Real-time direct measurement of spinal cord blood flow at the site of compression: relationship between blood flow recovery and motor deficiency in spinal cord injury. *Spine* 2007 Aug 15;32(18):1955-62.
8. Breig, *Advers. Mech Tension*, pg 38
9. Brieg, *Advers. Mech. Tension*, pg 11
10. Sayit E, Daubs MD, Aghdasi B, Montgomery SR, Inoue H, Wang CJ, Wang BJ, Phan KH, Scott TP., Dynamic changes of the ligamentum flavum in the cervical spine assessed with kinetic magnetic resonance imaging. *Global Spine J*. 2013 Jun;3(2):69-74. doi: 10.1055/s-0033-1337121. Epub 2013 Mar 19.
11. Brieg. *Advers. Mech. Tension*, Pg 17
12. Breig *Advers. Mech. Tension*, pg 39
13. Breig *Advers. Mech. Tension*, pg 11
14. Condon, B. R., Hadley, D. "Quantification of Cord Deformation and Dynamics During Flexion and Extension of the Cervical Spine using MR Imaging, *J. Computer Assisted Tomography*, 1988.12:947-955
15. Turnbull, I. M., Microvasculature of the Human Spinal Cord, *Journal of Neurosugery*, 1971, 35:141-147, pg 142
16. Turnbull, Microvasculature ..., pg 142
17. Sayit E, et al
18. Blau, pg 341
19. Marcus, pg 133
20. Sayit E, et al
21. Okada, Y., Ikata, T., Katoh, S., Yamada, H., Morphologic Analysis of the Cervical Spinal Cord, Dural Tube, and Spinal Canal by Magnetic Resonance Imaging in Normal Adults and Patients with Cervical Spondylotic Myelopathy, *Spine*, 1994, 19/20:2331-2335.
22. Morishita Y, Naito M, Hymanson H, Miyazaki M, Wu G, Wang JC., The relationship between the cervical spinal canal diameter and the pathological changes in the cervical spine., *Eur Spine J*. 2009 Jun;18(6):877-83. doi: 10.1007/s00586-009-0968-y. Epub 2009 Apr 9.
23. Nathan, H., Compression of the Sympathetic Trunk by Osteophytes of the Vertebral Column in the Abdomen: An Anatomical Study with Pathology and Clinical Considerations. *Surgery*, 1968, 4:609-625.
24. Nathan
25. Okada
26. Owen, J. H., Naito, M., Bridwell, K., Relationship Among Levels of Distraction, Evoked Potentials, Spinal Cord Ischemia and Integrity, and Clinical Status in Animals. *Spine*, 1990,15:846-81.
27. Owen, J. H., Naito, M., Bridwell, K., Oakley, D., Relationship Between Duration of Spinal Cord Ischemia and Postoperative Neurologic Defects in Animals. *Spine*, 1990, 15:846-851.
28. Ghosh, P., *The Biology of the Intervertebral Disc*, CRC Press, 1988, vol 1, pg 2
29. Kretch KS, Franchak JM, Adolph KE. Crawling and Walking Infants See the World Differently. Child Dev. 2013 Dec 16. doi: 10.1111/cdev.12206. [Epub ahead of print]
30. Blau, pg 341
31. Marcus, pg 133
32. Ghosh, vol 2, pg 66
33. Ghosh, vol 2, pg 66
34. Ando A, Suda H, Hagiwara Y, Onoda Y, Chimoto E, Saijo Y, Itoi E., Reversibility of immobilization-induced articular cartilage degeneration after remobilization in rat knee joints, Tohoku J Exp Med. 2011;224(2):77-85., *Child Dev*. 2013 Dec 16. doi: 10.1111/cdev.12206. [Epub ahead of print]

35. Hagiwara Y, Ando A, Chimoto E, Saijo Y, Ohmori-Matsuda K, Itoi E., Changes of articular cartilage after immobilization in a rat knee contracture model. *J Orthop Res.* 2009 Feb;27(2):236-42. doi: 10.1002/jor.20724.

36. Ghosh, vol 1, pg 32

Chapter 2

1. Hadley, L., M.D. *Anatomico-Roentgenographic Studies of the Spin*e, Charles C. Thomas, 1981., pg 264-5,
2. Henderson CN. The basis for spinal manipulation: chiropractic perspective of indications and theory. *J Electromyogr Kinesiol.* 2012 Oct;22(5):632-42. doi: 10.1016/j.jelekin.2012.03.008. Epub 2012 Apr 17.
3. Smith DL, Dainoff MJ, Smith JP. The effect of chiropractic adjustments on movement time: a pilot study using Fitts Law. *J Manipulative Physiol Ther.* 2006 May;29(4):257-66.
4. Passmore SR, Burke JR, Good C, Lyons JL, Dunn AS. Spinal manipulation impacts cervical spine movement and fitts' task performance: a single-blind randomized before-after trial. *J Manipulative Physiol Ther.* 2010 Mar-Apr;33(3):189-92. doi: 10.1016/j.jmpt.2010.01.007.
5. Jackson, R. *The Cervical Syndrome*, Charles C Thomas, 4th Edition, 1977, pg.82-83
6. Moodley M, Brantingham JW., The relative effectiveness of spinal manipulation and ultrasound in mechanical pain: Pilot study. *J Chiropr Med.* 2002 Autumn;1(4):184-8. doi: 10.1016/S0899-3467(07)60034-2.
7. Schmorl, G., Junghanns, H., *The Human Spine in Health and Disease*, Grune and Stratton, New York and London, 1971, pg 140
8. Schmorl, pg 140
9. Hadley, pg 264-5
10. Bar-Dayan Y, Weisbort M, Bar-Dayan Y, Velan GJ, Ravid M, Hendel D, Shemer J., Degenerative disease in lumbar spine of military parachuting instructors. *J R Army Med Corps.* 2003 Dec;149(4):260-4.
11. O'Neill TW, McCloskey EV, Kanis JA, Bhalla AK, Reeve J, Reid DM, Todd C, Woolf AD, Silman AJ., The distribution, determinants, and clinical correlates of vertebral osteophytosis: a population based survey., *J Rheumatol.* 1999 Apr;26(4):842-8.
12. Kasai Y, Kawakita E, Sakakibara T, Akeda K, Uchida A., Direction of the formation of anterior lumbar vertebral osteophytes., *BMC Musculoskelet Disord.* 2009 Jan 13;10:4. doi: 10.1186/1471-2474-10-4.
13. Hadley, pg 264-5
14. Bar-Dayan Y, et al.
15. O'Neill TW, et al.
16. Kasai Y, et al.
17. Hadley, pg 264-5
18. Hadley, pg 135-147
19. Jeon CH, Park JU, Chung NS, Son KH, Lee YS, Kim JJ., Degenerative retrolisthesis: is it a compensatory mechanism for sagittal imbalance?, *Bone Joint J.* 2013 Sep;95-B(9):1244-9. doi: 10.1302/0301-620X.95B9.31237.
20. Barrey C, Jund J, Noseda O, Roussouly P., Sagittal balance of the pelvis-spine complex and lumbar degenerative diseases. A comparative study about 85 cases., *Eur Spine J.* 2007 Sep;16(9):1459-67. Epub 2007 Jan 9.
21. Hadley, pg 135-147
22. Hadley, 135-147
23. Jackson pg. 59-60
24. Koreckij J, Alvi H, Gibly R, Pang E, Hsu WK., Incidence and risk factors of the retropharyngeal carotid artery on cervical magnetic resonance imaging., *Spine* (Phila Pa 1976). 2013 Jan 15;38(2):E109-12. doi: 10.1097/BRS.0b013e31827b0d4b.
25. Jackson, pg 82-83
26. Jackson, pg. 82-83
27. Jackson, pg 81-82
28. Jackson, pg 166
29. Hadley, pg 135-147
30. Christianson MS, Shen W., Osteoporosis prevention and management: nonpharmacologic and lifestyle options., *Clin Obstet Gynecol.* 2013 Dec;56(4):703-10. doi: 10.1097/GRF.0b013e3182a9d15a.
31. Traini T, Mangano C, Perrotti V, Caputi S, Coelho P, Piattelli A, Iezzi G., Human bone reactions around implants with adverse interfacial bone strain over 20 years., *J Biomed Mater Res B Appl Biomater.* 2014 Jan 17. doi: 10.1002/jbm.b.33109. [Epub ahead of print]
32. Shippen JM., The generation of loads in excess of the osteogenic threshold by physical movement., *Proc Inst Mech Eng H.* 2013 Jun;227(6):704-11. doi: 10.1177/0954411913481186. Epub 2013 Mar 19.

33. Condon, B.R., Hadley, D.M., Quantification of Cord Deformation and Dynamics During Flexion and Extension of the Cervical Spine Using MR Imaging, *Journal of Computer Assisted Tomography*. 12(6):947-955, November/December 1988 Raven Press, Ltd., New York

34. Owen (*"Levels"*)

35. Owen (*"Duration"*)

36. Jarzem, P. F., Quance. D. R., Doyle, D. J., Begin, L. R., Kostuik, J. P., Spinal Cord Tissue Pressure During Spinal Cord Distraction in Dogs, Spine, 1992, 85:S227-S234.

37. Zhang S1, Nicholson KJ1, Smith JR1, Gilliland TM1, Syré PP2, Winkelstein BA3., The roles of mechanical compression and chemical irritation in regulating spinal neuronal signaling in painful cervical nerve root injury., *Stapp Car Crash J*. 2013 Nov;57:219-42.

38. Vavasour IM1, Meyers SM2, Macmillan EL3, M√§dler B4, Li DK5, Rauscher A6, Vertinsky T7, Venu V7, Mackay AL8, Curt A9. Increased spinal cord movements in cervical spondylotic myelopathy. Spine J. 2014 Jan 23. pii: S1529-9430(14)00113-2. doi: 10.1016/j.spinee.2014.01.036.)

39. Jackson, pg 47

40. Zhang S1, et al

Chapter 3

1. Breig, A., *Adverse Mechanical Tension*, pg. 11-12

2. Louis, pg 39-40

3. Adams MA, Dolan P, McNally DS., The internal mechanical functioning of intervertebral discs and articular cartilage, and its relevance to matrix biology. *Matrix Biol*. 2009 Sep;28(7):384-9. doi: 10.1016/j.matbio.2009.06.004. Epub 2009 Jul 5.

4. Kroeber MW, Unglaub F, Wang H, Schmid C, Thomsen M, Nerlich A, Richter W. New in vivo animal model to create intervertebral disc degeneration and to investigate the effects of therapeutic strategies to stimulate disc regeneration. Spine (Phila Pa 1976). 2002 Dec 1;27(23):2684-90.

5. Adams MA, Freeman BJ, Morrison HP, Nelson IW, Dolan P. Mechanical initiation of intervertebral disc degeneration. *Spine* (Phila Pa 1976). 2000 Jul 1;25(13):1625-36.

6. Jackson, pg 82-83

7. Xiuqing.C., Bo, S., Shizhen, Z., Nerves Accompanying the Vertebral Artery and their Clinical Relevance, *Spine*, 1988, 12:1360-1364., pg 363-364,

8. Turnbull, I. M., Blood Supply of the Spinal Cord: Normal and Pathological Considerations, *Clinical Neurosurgery*, 1973, Vol. 20: 56-84 Pg. 71

9 Bodes-Pardo G, Pecos-Martín D, Gallego-Izquierdo T, Salom-Moreno J, Fernández-de-Las-Peñas C, Ortega-Santiago R, Manual treatment for cervicogenic headache and active trigger point in the sternocleidomastoid muscle: a pilot randomized clinical trial. *J Manipulative Physiol Ther*. 2013 Sep;36(7):403-11. doi: 10.1016/j.jmpt.2013.05.022. Epub 2013 Jul 8.

10. Wang L, Zhang L, Tang Y, Qiu L., The value of high-frequency and color Doppler ultrasonography in diagnosing congenital muscular torticollis., *BMC Musculoskelet Disord*. 2012 Oct 26;13:209. doi: 10.1186/1471-2474-13-209.

11. Simons, David G., Travell, Janet G., Simons, Lois S., *Myofascial Pain and Dysfunction*, Lippincott Williams and Wilkins, Second Edition, 1999, pg 308-314

12. Simons, David G., et al

13. Miyazaki M, Hymanson HJ, Morishita Y, He W, Zhang H, Wu G, Kong MH, Tsumura H, Wang JC.Kinematic analysis of the relationship between sagittal alignment and disc degeneration in the cervical spine., *Spine* (Phila Pa 1976). 2008 Nov 1;33(23):E870-6. doi: 10.1097/BRS.0b013e3181839733.

14. Wang M, Gourab K, McGrady LM, Rao RD., Alteration of load sharing of anterior cervical implants with change in cervical sagittal alignment., *Med Eng Phys*. 2008 Jul;30(6):768-73. Epub 2007 Nov 26.

15. Louis, pg. 39-40

16. Jentzsch T, Geiger J, König MA, Werner CM, Hyperlordosis Is Associated With Facet Joint Pathology At The Lower Lumbar Spine., *J Spinal Disord Tech*. 2013 Sep 27. [Epub ahead of print]

17. Jackson, pgs 60 and 82

18.Safain MG, Talan J, Malek AM, Hwang SW., Spontaneous atraumatic vertebral artery occlusion due to physiological cervical extension., *J Neurosurg Spine*. 2014 Jan 17. [Epub ahead of print]

19. Yoshimura K, Iwatsuki K, Ishihara M, Onishi Y, Umegaki M, Yoshimine T., Bow hunter's stroke due to instability at the uncovertebral C3/4 joint., *Eur Spine J.* 2011 Jul;20 Suppl 2:S266-70. doi: 10.1007/s00586-010-1669-2. Epub 2011 Jan 30.

20. Horowitz M, Jovin T, Balzar J, Welch W, Kassam A., Bow hunter's syndrome in the setting of contralateral vertebral artery stenosis: evaluation and treatment options., *Spine* (Phila Pa 1976). 2002 Dec 1;27(23):E495-8.

21.Jackson, pg 11-12

22. Zhang L, Zeitoun D, Rangel A, Lazennec JY, Catonné Y, Pascal-Moussellard H., Preoperative evaluation of the cervical spondylotic myelopathy with flexion-extension magnetic resonance imaging: about a prospective study of fifty patients., *Spine* (Phila Pa 1976). 2011 Aug 1;36(17):E1134-9. doi: 10.1097/BRS.0b013e3181f822c7.

23. Breig pg. 17

24. Zhang L, Zeitoun D, Rangel A, et al.

25. Breig, pg 22

26. Zhang L, Zeitoun D, Rangel A, et al

27. Grönqvist J, Häggman-Henrikson B, Eriksson PO., Impaired jaw function and eating difficulties in whiplash-associated disorders., *Swed Dent J.* 2008;32(4):171-7.

28. Kubein-Meesenburg D, Thieme KM, Weber S, Fanghanel J, Dumont C, Spassov A, Hahn W, Ihlow D, Nagerl H., Mandible, maxilla and cervical spine--a functional unit?, *J Physiol Pharmacol.* 2008 Nov;59 Suppl 5:75-80.

29. Kubein-Meesenburg D, Thieme KM, Dumont C, Ihlow D, Nägerl H., The movement structure of the mandible and alignment of the neck., *Ann Anat.* 2007;189(4):387-9.

Chapter 4

1. Nathan

2. Ruch, W., Autonomic Neuroanatomy of the Vertebral Subluxation Complex, *Somatovisceral Aspects of Chiropractic,* Masarsky and Masarsky ED., Churchill Livingston , 2001, Chapter 4

3. Owen (*"Levels"*)

4. Owen (*"Duration"*)

5. Fujita, Y., M.D., Yamamoto, H., M.D. "An Experimental Study on Spinal Cord Traction Effect," *Spine*, 1989, Vol. 14, 7:698-705.

6. Elliott MB, Barr AE, Clark BD, Amin M, Amin S, Barbe MF., High force reaching task induces widespread inflammation, increased spinal cord neurochemicals and neuropathic pain., *Neuroscience.* 2009 Jan 23;158(2):922-31. doi: 10.1016/j.neuroscience.2008.10.050. Epub 2008 Nov 7.

7. Marchand A1, Belleville G, Fleet R, Dupuis G, Bacon SL, Poitras J, Chauny JM, Vadeboncoeur A, Lavoie KL.Treatment of panic in chest pain patients from emergency departments: efficacy of different interventions focusing on panic management. *Gen Hosp Psychiatry.* 2012 Nov-Dec;34(6):671-80. doi: 10.1016/j.genhosppsych.2012.06.011. Epub 2012 Jul 25.

8. Poirier-Bisson J1, Marchand A, Pelland ME, Lessard MJ, Dupuis G, Fleet R, Roberge P.,Incremental cost-effectiveness of pharmacotherapy and two brief cognitive-behavioral therapies compared with usual care for panic disorder and noncardiac chest pain., *J Nerv Ment Dis.* 2013 Sep;201(9):753-9. doi: 10.1097/NMD.0b013e3182a2127d.9. Nathan. page 93

Chapter 5

1. Louis,

2. Pal, G.P., Sherk, H.H., The Vertical Stability of the Cervical Spine, *Spine*, 1988, 5:447-449.

3. Schmidt H, Heuer F, Claes L, Wilke HJ., The relation between the instantaneous center of rotation and facet joint forces - A finite element analysis., *Clin Biomech (Bristol, Avon).* 2008 Mar;23(3):270-8. Epub 2007 Nov 7.

4. Smit TH, Odgaard A, Schneider E., Structure and function of vertebral trabecular bone., *Spine* (Phila Pa 1976). 1997 Dec 15;22(24):2823-33.

5. Cheung JT, Zhang M, Chow DH., Biomechanical responses of the intervertebral joints to static and vibrational loading: a finite element study., *Clin Biomech (Bristol, Avon).* 2003 Nov;18(9):790-9.

6. Ghosh, Vol. 2 pg 2

7. Wu Y, Cisewski S, Sachs BL, Yao H., Effect of cartilage endplate on cell based disc regeneration: a finite element analysis., Mol Cell Biomech. 2013 Jun;10(2):159-82

8. Zhu Q, Jackson AR, Gu WY., Cell viability in intervertebral disc under various nutritional and dynamic loading conditions: 3d finite element analysis., : J Biomech. 2012 Nov 15;45(16):2769-77. doi: 10.1016/j.jbiomech.2012.08.044. Epub 2012 Oct 4.

9. Jackson AR, Yuan TY, Huang CY, Brown MD, Gu WY., Nutrient transport in human annulus fibrosus is affected by compressive strain and anisotropy., Ann Biomed Eng. 2012 Dec;40(12):2551-8. doi: 10.1007/s10439-012-0606-4. Epub 2012 Jun 6.

10. Ghosh, vol. 2, pg. 3

11. Ghosh, Vol. 2, pg. 2

12. Wu Y, Cisewski S, Sachs BL, Yao H., Effect of cartilage endplate on cell based disc regeneration: a finite element analysis., *Mol Cell Biomech.* 2013 Jun;10(2):159-82

13. McMillan DW, Garbutt G, Adams MA., Effect of sustained loading on the water content of intervertebral discs: implications for disc metabolism., *Ann Rheum Dis.* 1996 Dec;55(12):880-7.

14. Ghosh, vol. 2, pg 34-35

15. Accadbled F, Laffosse JM, Ambard D, Gomez-Brouchet A, de Gauzy JS, Swider P., Influence of location, fluid flow direction, and tissue maturity on the macroscopic permeability of vertebral end plates., *Spine* (Phila Pa 1976). 2008 Mar 15;33(6):612-9. doi: 10.1097/BRS.0b013e318166e0d7.

16. Jackson AR, Huang CY, Gu WY., Effect of endplate calcification and mechanical deformation on the distribution of glucose in intervertebral disc: a 3D finite element study., *Comput Methods Biomech Biomed Engin.* 2011 Feb;14(2):195-204. doi: 10.1080/10255842 2010.535815.

17. Ghosh, vol. 1 pg. 2

18. Ghosh, vol. 1, pg 32

19. Ghosh, vol. 1, pg. 32

20. Zander T, Krishnakanth P, Bergmann G, Rohlmann A., Diurnal variations in intervertebral disc height affect spine flexibility, intradiscal pressure and contact compressive forces in the facet joints., *Comput Methods Biomech Biomed Engin.* 2010 Oct;13(5):551-7. doi: 10.1080/10255840903337855.

21. Adams

22. Adams

23. Schmidt H, Galbusera F, Rohlmann A, Shirazi-Adl A., What have we learned from finite element model studies of lumbar intervertebral discs in the past four decades?, *J Biomech.* 2013 Sep 27;46(14):2342-55. doi: 10.1016/j.jbiomech.2013.07.014. Epub 2013 Aug 3.,

24. Hadley, pg. 127- 157

Chapter 6

1. Browning, James, E., *Pelvic Pain and Pelvic Organic Dysfunction, Somatovisceral Aspects of Chiropractic*, (chapter 8), Masarsky and Masarsky (ED). Churchill Livingston, 1999

2. Browning, James, E.

3. Pool-Goudzwaard, A., Gnat, R., Spoor, K., Deformation of the innominate bone and mobility of the pubic symphysis during asymmetric moment application to the pelvis, *Manual Therapy*, Feb. 2012 (1), 66-70

4. Blau, pg 341

5. Marcus, pg 133

6. Hamamoto Y, Ogata T, Morino T, Hino M, Yamamoto HReal-time direct measurement of spinal cord blood flow at the site of compression: relationship between blood flow recovery and motor deficiency in spinal cord injury. *Spine* 2007 Aug 15;32(18):1955-62.

7. Gosh, vol. 2 pg 2

8. Wu Y, Cisewski S, Sachs BL, Yao H., Effect of cartilage endplate on cell based disc regeneration: a finite element analysis., *Mol Cell Biomech.* 2013 Jun;10(2):159-82

9. Zhu Q, Jackson AR, Gu WY., Cell viability in intervertebral disc under various nutritional and dynamic loading conditions: 3d finite element analysis., : *J Biomech.* 2012 Nov 15;45(16):2769-77. doi: 10.1016/j.jbiomech.2012.08.044. Epub 2012 Oct 4.

10. Jackson AR, Yuan TY, Huang CY, Brown MD, Gu WY., Nutrient transport in human annulus fibrosus is affected by compressive strain and anisotropy., *Ann Biomed Eng.* 2012 Dec;40(12):2551-8. doi: 10.1007/s10439-012-0606-4. Epub 2012 Jun 6.

11. Leadbetter RE1, Mawer D, Lindow SW. *J Obstet Gynaecol.* 2006 Jan;26(1):20-3.The development of a scoring system for symphysis pubis dysfunction.

12. Leadbetter RE1, Mawer D, Lindow SW. *J Matern Fetal Neonatal Med.* 2004 Dec;16(6):349-54.Symphysis pubis dysfunction: a review of the literature.

13. Sizer, Phillip, S.; Phelps, Valerie; Thompson, Kirk; Disorders of the Sacroiliac Joint, *Pain Practice*, Volume 2, Number 1, 2002 17-34, Pages 21-25

14. Giles, L,G,F.; Anatomical basis of low back pain. Pg. 126-167, William and Wilkins; Baltimore MD. 1989

15. Lewis, K.; *Manipulative Therapy in Rehabilitation of the Locomotor System*, pg 44-45, Butterworth-Heinemann Ltd, Oxford

16. Boden, S. D., Davis, D. O., Dina, T. S., Patronas, N. J., Wiesel, S. W., Abnormal Magnetic-Resonance Scans of the Lumbar Spine in Asymptomatic Subjects, *The Journal of Bone and Joint Surgery*, 1990, 3:403-408.

17. Jensen, M. et al, Magnetic Resonance Imaging of the Lumbar Spine, *N Engl J Med* 1994; 331:1525-1526

18. Ruch WJ, An analysis of pubis symphysis misalignment using plain film radiography. *J Manipulative Physiol Ther.* 2005 Jun;28(5):330-5.)

19. La ban, M.M., Meerschaert, J.R., Taylor, R.S., Tabor, H.D., Symphyseal and sacroiliac joint pain associated with pubic symphysis instability, *Arch Phys Med Rehabil*, 1978, Oct:59(10) :470-2

20. Walheim, G.G., Olerud, s., Ribbe, T., Motion of the pubic symphysis in pelvic instability, *Scand. J. Rehabil. Med.*, 1984: 16(4):163-9

21. Vleeming, A.,Stoeckart, R., Snijders, Ch. J., van Wingerden, J.-P., and Dijkstra, P.F., The sacro-iliac joint- anatomical, biomechanical and radiological aspects, Journal of Manual Medicine, 1990, 5:100-102.

GLOSSARY

A

abdominal oblique muscles: internal and external
The external obliques originate at the lower eight ribs and insert at the iliac crest and linea alba (midline aponeurosis). Contraction of both compresses the abdomen. Contraction of one side alone bends the vertebral column laterally. Also rotates vertebral column. Innervated at the branches of thoracic nerves T7-T12 and iliohypogastric nerve.
The internal obliques originate at the iliac crest, inguinal ligament, and the thoracolumbar fascia and insert at the cartilage of the last three or four ribs and linea alba. Contraction acts as external oblique. Innervated at the branches of thoracic nerves T8-T12, iliohypogastric nerve, and ilioinguinal nerves. A disruption in the pelvic girdle will cause these muscles to partially or fully contract causing a disruption in the spinal curve and muscle guarding.

absolute motion
A localized movement that affects the entire vertebral column. A movement in the cervical region globally affects the rest of the spine.

acetabulum
A deep, cup-shaped depression on the anterolateral surface of the pelvis, formed internally by the os pubis, superiorly by the ilium, posteroinferiorly by the ishium, and anteroinferiorly by the pubis. The head of the femur articulates here.

adaptive response
An adaptive response to subluxation is muscle guarding and a concomitant shortening of muscles and ligaments. An adaptive response, either anticipated or observed, is reason for care.

A to P
Anterior to posterior direction in taking and viewing X-rays.

adhesions
A joining of parts normally free to move independently to each other. This occurs as a response to injury, edema, or irritation due to subluxation.

A.L.L.
Anterior longitudinal ligament

altered weight bearing
In the vertebral curve, normal weight bearing at each joint is balanced between three points, two facets and one body. Altering the weight bearing capacity of one or more points will alter the shape of the joint, alter the motion of the joint, and alter the surrounding tissue.

annulus fibrosus
The outer concentric layers of fibrocartilage which contains the nucleus pulposus in the intervertebral disc. Tearing or herniation of the annulus fibrosus changes the hydraulic capacity of the segments and can be concomitant with subluxation.

anterior
At or near the front of the body; ventral

anterior longitudinal ligament
A broad ligament that extends from the occipital bone to the sacrum. It supports the vertebral column and unites the vertebrae anteriorly.

anterior spinal artery
Supplies blood to the major substance of the spinal cord. Subluxation can block the anterior spinal artery and will cause the spinal cord to become hypoxic.

anterolisthesis
Anterior displacement of a vertebra with loss of joint integrity.

antero/posterior
Directed from the front toward the back.

apex
1. The outermost point of a convexity.
2. The apex of the sacrum is at the bottom where it joins with the coccyx.

arachnoid
The inside covering of the thecal wall. The presence of a subdural space indicates a pathology.

arthritis
Inflammation of a joint. The most common arthritic inflammatory condition of the spine is characterized by subluxation.

articulation
A joint. Indicates motion between two or more bones. Tissues associated with articulation depend on motion for their health.

atlantoaxial
Pertaining to the joint or space between the atlas and axis, the first two cervical vertebrae.

atlas
The first cervical vertebra, C1, having a two-point weight bearing system, lacking a body, and articulating superiorly with the occipital condyles of the occipital bone, which permits nodding of the head. The atlas articulates differently with C2, the axis, at the inferior articular facets.

autonomic nervous system
A division of the nervous system comprised of a series of reflex areas that control involuntary motor functions and innervate the heart, glands, viscera, and smooth muscle.

avascular
Lacking a direct supply of blood; oxygen, carbon dioxide, nutrients, and waste, all diffuse through connective tissue via motion.

axial
1. Pertaining to the axis, C2. 2. Pertaining to the axial plane of the Cartesian coordinate system, the Y plane. 3. Pertaining to the axial skeleton, consisting of the bones of the skull, hyoid, ribs, sternum, and vertebral column.

axial loading
A mechanism of injury to the cervical spine in which an axially directed load exerts a longitudinally compressive force that results in a fracture of a mid-cervical vertebral body. This compression can be from the top-down or from the bottom-up.

axis
The second cervical vertebra, C2, is the first three-point weight bearing system in the vertebral column. The dens of the axis projects through the atlas, C1, and makes a pivot on which the head and atlas rotate, permitting side-to-side rotation of the head. The axis articulates superiorly with the atlas at the two superior articular facets and inferiorly with C3 at the two inferior articular facets and the body of the vertebra via the intervertebral disc.

B

brain stem
The portion of the brain immediately superior to the spinal cord, made up of the medulla oblongata, pons, and midbrain. The brain stem is contiguous with the spinal cord and subject to forces initiated in the vertebral column. The blood supply to the brain stem is dependent on the integrity of the vertebral artery.

buckling
Deformation of an architectural structure due to rapid acceleration or deceleration of only part of the structure. This would be a good replacement term for "whiplash".

C

calcified
Crystallized and hardened tissues caused by the infiltration of tricalcium phosphate, calcium carbonate, and magnesium salts. They are deposited in the framework formed by the collagenous fibers of the matrix of a tissue. This can be a normal response to stress or a response to abnormal stress.

calcification
The process of deposition of mineral salts within a tissue or structure.

canal stenosis
The narrowing of the spinal canal. 1. A congenital condition, a narrower canal than normal, can be a silent condition until injury occurs. 2. A developed or acquired spinal canal stenosis is a result of subluxation of vertebrae and the subsequent widening endplates.

capillaries
A tiny, thin-walled blood vessel that connects arterioles and venules through which materials are exchanged between blood and tissue cells.

capillary bed
A network or plexus of capillaries in a region of localized high metabolic activity. Blood flow is linked to the motion of the tissue, which act as a pump.

capsule
Joint capsule. The membrane that encloses a joint to form a closed cavity. It is primarily collagen fibers with a synovial membrane covering the inside and it is embedded with nerve endings of various types. Distress of this structure can result in reflex guarding of the muscle and tendon complexes that are involved.

cartilage
A specialized connective tissue composed of a homogenous, highly polymerized hyaline matrix containing nucleated cells and chondrocytes that lie in cavities or lacunae in the matrix. The matrix is white or gray, semiopaque, consisting chiefly of proteoglycans and collagen fibers, and is produced by cells called chondroblasts which give way to the chondrocytes.

The matrix is avascular and relies on movement to maintain its health and integrity. Hyaline cartilage is smooth in appearance and is found at the articulating facets of the vertebrae. Fibrocartilage is fibrous in appearance due to interlacing fibrous tissue strands in the matrix. It is found as transitional material from bone to the intervertebral disc material as well as the pubis symphysis.

Cartesian coordinate system
A three-dimensional coordinate system in which the coordinates of a point are its distances from three intersecting perpendicular straight lines or planes. These are described as the X, Y and Z axes or planes. It is used to describe position in human anatomy.

caudae equinae
Nerve rootlets of the spinal nerves that arise off the terminal portion of the spinal cord in the lower thoracic region. It is named by the Latin for horse's tail, which it resembles. These hair-like fibers form the lumbar, sacral and coccygeal nerve roots.

cavitation
The formation of a cavity in the intervertebral disc by pathological processes. The degeneration of tissues of the disc can be initiated by shearing, loss of movement, and hyperloading which interrupts the nutrient pump.

central nervous system
The part of the nervous system that is condensed and centrally located; the brain and spinal cord.

cerebellum
The portion of the brain lying posterior to the medulla and pons, concerned with coordination of movement. Damage can cause ataxia (lack of muscle coordination), disturbance of gait, and severe dizziness. The position of the cerebellum in the occiput can be changed with vertebral column changes. The blood supply is vertebral artery dependent.

cerebrospinal fluid
This plasma like fluid continuously circulates through the ventricles of the brain and spinal canal surrounding the spinal cord in the subarachnoid space. The motion of the vertebral column and sacrum is the supposed mechanism of circulation.

cervical
Of or pertaining to the neck.

cervical curve
An essential architectural feature of the human spine. Changes in the shape of the cervical spine result in central nervous system deformation and joint pathology. The cervical curve is lordotic or the convex side of the curve is ventral.

cervicogenic
Symptoms produced from problems in the neck, i.e. cervicogenic headaches, unilateral cervicogenic deafness.

chronic
Long-term or frequently recurring.

chronic inflammation
A long-term, localized protective response to tissue injury designed to destroy, dilute, or wall off an infecting agent or injured tissue. Characterized by redness, pain, heat, swelling, and sometimes loss of function. Loss of joint integrity generates an inflammatory response.

clavicle
The collarbone. The medial end of the clavicle, the sternal extremity, is rounded and articulates with the sternum. The broad, flat, lateral end, the acromial extremity, articulates with the acromion of the scapula. These articulations are primarily ligaments and capsules and form the only bony articulation of the pectoral girdle to the chest.

clivus
The anterior portion of the occipital bone. It forms the front part of the foramen magnum. The dens of the axis attaches to the clivus.

coccyx
The lowermost element in the backbone. It is the fusion of the three or four coccygeal vertebrae and is triangular in shape. Articulates superiorly with the sacrum. The sacrococcygeal ligament is contiguous with the sacrotuberous ligaments.

compression fracture
A fracture due to impact loading in which the bone has been crushed. Seen in the vertebral bodies of osteopenic patients.

conductivity
The capacity of a tissue to conduct current.

congenital stenosis
A narrowing of an opening or passage due to inherited variations.

contracture
1. A permanent shortening of a soft tissue, such as a muscle or tendon, so that it cannot passively attain its normal length.
2. A state of diminished or loss of compliance of a normally pliant tissue. A shortening with a decrease range of motion, a common feature of chronic subluxation.

conus medularis
The distal termination of the spinal cord. It is tapered and ends at the level of the intervertebral disc between the first and second lumbar vertebrae in the adult.

coronal
1.The frontal plane. It divides the body into anterior (front) and posterior (back) portions. 2.The X plane in the Cartesian coordinate system.

cortex
1. The dense bone that forms the external surface of a bone called cortical bone. 2 The outer part of an organ.

cortical bone
The dense outer wall of a bone.

costotransverse
Pertaining to the ribs and transverse processes of the vertebrae. The transverse process is posterior to the rib and articulates with the neck of the rib.

costo-vertebral
Of or pertaining to a rib and a vertebrae. The typical costo-vertebral joint (T2-T10) is a three joint complex made up of the head of the rib, superior and inferior demifacets and the intervertebral disc.

CNS
Central nervous system.

cross section
1. A section formed by a plane cutting through an object, usually at right angles to an axis. 2. The Z plane of the Cartesian coordinate system.

cranium/cranial
The cranium can be defined as the bones of the skull that protects the brain and the organs of sight, hearing, and balance, including the frontal, parietal, temporal, occipital, sphenoid, and ethmoid bones. Cranial can be defined as a subdivision of the superior body cavity formed by the cranial bones and containing the brain.

D

degeneration
The deterioration of the cells of a tissue by alteration of the tissue. A pathological process of a progressive nature.

degenerative joint disease
A chronic joint disease characterized by a degeneration of articular cartilage, hypertrophy of bone, and formation of new bone in the subchondral areas and margins of the joint, particularly the weight-bearing joints. The most common pathological feature of this condition is subluxation and resulting loss of joint space.

dehydration
The removal or reduction of water from the body or from a substance.

demifacet
A thoracic vertebral body structure that articulates with the heads of the ribs.

dens
A toothlike process projecting upward from the body of the second cervical vertebra that articulates with the anterior arch of the atlas. It acts as a pivot around which the atlas rotates.

dentate ligament
A narrow fibrous band situated on each side of the spinal cord throughout its entire length and separating the anterior from the posterior roots of the spinal nerves. The inner border is continuous with the pia mater. The outer serrated border is fixed at intervals to the dura mater.
The dentate ligament is used to support the spinal cord in the cerebrospinal fluid. Synonym: denticulate.

desiccated
Dried, friable, easily crumbled.

deviation
1. A variation from normal. 2. Displacement of one of the body's masses relative to the others. When at rest, it is no longer aligned with one or more coordinate system planes.

disc
The intervertebral disc.

DJD, D.J.D.
Degenerative joint disease.

DISH
Diffuse Idiopathic Skeletal Hyperotosis

dorsal
Relative to or situated on the posterior or back surface; opposite of ventral. Synonym: thoracic.

dura
The dura mater. The outer wall of the thecal sac.

E

eburnation
A radiodensity feature on X-ray that is a product of degeneration of the cartilage at the articulating surface of a bone. This exposes the underlying subchondral bone which then converts into a dense, smooth, ivory-like substance. This is a common feature of degenerative changes in an articulation.

endplate
The bony cortex on the superior and inferior surfaces of each vertebral body as well as the cartilage that defines the disc from above and below, separating it from the adjacent vertebral body.

epidural adhesion
An adhesion between the vertebral canal wall and the dura mater in the epidural space. This can be due to subluxation and the resulting chronic inflammation, a feature of degenerative joint disease and mechanical distress. It can also be seen as a result infectious insult or post operative finding.

epidural space
The outermost space covering the brain and spinal cord located on or over the dura mater and inside a mostly bony encasement.

erector spinae
This is the largest muscular mass of the back and consists of three groupings: iliocostalis, longissimus, and spinalis. These groups, in turn, consist of a series of interlapping muscles. The iliocostalis group is laterally placed, the longissimus group is intermediate in placement, and the spinalis group is medially placed. The proprioceptive links are to the sacroiliac joints and the position of the ilium relative to the ribs and vertebrae.

esophagus
A muscular collapsible tube that lies behind the trachea. The posterior wall of the esophagus is adhered to the anterior surface of the vertebral column. It is 23 to 25 cm long and begins at the end of the laryngopharynx, passes through the mediastinum anterior to the vertebral column, pierces the diaphragm through the esophageal hiatus, and terminates in the superior portion of the stomach. It is innervated by recurrent laryngeal nerves and the cervical sympathetic chain.

extension
The straightening of a joint so that the two adjacent segments are moved apart, thereby decreasing the joint angle. Relating to the vertebral canal, when the head and or spine is tipped backward the canal length is shortened.

extremity
1. A distal or terminal portion. 2. An arm or leg.

F

facet
The posterior zygopophyseal joints of the spine, true diarthrodial articulations. They are endowed with articular cartilage and synovial capsules, with a shape and planar geometry specific to the area of the spine in which they occur. These capsules are imbedded with proprioceptors.

facetal capsule
Ligamentus type enclosures of the gliding articulations of the vertebral column. They have a synovial lining on the inside. The capsules are innervated with proprioceptors that will respond to altered positions (subluxations). Threshold irritation can cause reflex splinting and constant noxious neurological stimuli.

fascia
A sheet or band of connective tissue that envelops muscles and muscle groups, usually of similar function. Fascia is pervasive and interconnects with the body tissues.

femur
The longest and heaviest bone in the body. Its proximal end articulates with the acetabulum of the hipbone.

fibrocartilage
Cartilage that contains dense, parallel bundles of collagenous fibers in the matrix. The bundles are separated by narrow clefts containing chondrocytes. This type of cartilage is found in the intervertebral discs, the pubis symphysis, and at the attachments of tendons and ligaments to bone.

fibrous
Containing or composed of fibers.

filum terminale
The thread-like attachments of the conus medularis to the bottom of the thecal sac. They are contiguous with the pia mater.

Fish body
A deformed vertebra whose shape resembles the profile of a fish. It can be congenital or acquired, i.e. a result of a compression fracture.

flexion
The act of bending or condition of being bent. In the spine, it can refer to forward bending, head moving towards knees, elongating the spinal canal and spinal cord.

foramen magnum
A large opening in the base of the anterior inferior part of the occipital bone that lies between the cranial cavity and the spinal canal. The spinal cord/brain stem passes through this opening.

foramen
An opening, orifice, perforation, or passage through which nerves or blood vessels pass. Usually found in bones.

fusion
1. The normal process for bone formation. 2. The end stage of the degenerative process of joint pathology, i.e. the end stage of degenerative joint disease.

G

glycoprotein
A conjugated protein whose non-amino acid component is a sugar(s). Glycoproteins are a major component of the nucleus pulposus of the intervertebral disc.

gravitational load
The force applied by the mass of the body on the joints and tissues due to gravity. The load increases inferiorly.

guarding
A description of a functional aspect of muscle tissue, a muscle spasm i.e. to protect a distressed joint complex. this is a neurological reflex.

H

herniation
A rupture of an intervertebral disc so that the nucleus pulposus protrudes outside the annulus fibrosus. Trauma and other excessive forces on the disc can result in a loss of annulus fibrosus integrity.

hydration
Combining or causing to combine with water.

hydraulic
Operated by a fluid under pressure, i.e. an intervertebral disc. A hydraulic system transmits force.

hydrophilic
Having an affinity for water. The nucleus pulposus of the intervertebral disc is hydrophilic due to glycoproteins and other components.

hyoid bone
A single U-shaped bone that is a component of the axial skeleton but does not articulate with any other bone. It is located in the neck between the mandible and larynx. It supports the tongue and provides attachment for some of its muscles and for muscles of the neck and pharynx.

hyperkyphosis
A kyphosis of the thoracic spine greater than normal range.

hyperload
The loss of normal three point weight bearing can result in all the weight being supported by one point or joint leading to excessive loading. This will cause an alteration of the tissue, bone and ligament, to accommodate this change in weight bearing.

hypertonic
A condition of muscle and tendon tension that is significantly greater than normal resting tone. It can be directly related to noxious proprioceptive input from the joint distress,

subluxation. Hypertonic muscles at rest should be a neurological finding. It leads to loss of joint space and reduced articular excursion.

hypertrophy
An increase in size or volume of a part or organ produced by enlargement of existing cells, not by an increasing number of cells.

hypokyphosis
A kyphosis of the thoracic spine lesser than the normal range.

hypolordotic
A curvature of the cervical and lumbar spine less than the normal range.

I – J

iliacus
The iliacus originates at the iliac fossa and inserts at the tendon of the psoas major. Action is to flex and rotate the thigh laterally and also flexes the vertebral column. Innervation is at the femoral nerve. Proprioceptive links are to the sacroiliac joint and the pubis symphysis.

ilium
The ilium is the largest of the three original bones of the hip. Its superior border, the iliac crest, ends anteriorly in the anterior superior iliac spine. Posteriorly, the iliac crest ends in the posterior superior iliac spine. The posterior inferior iliac spine is just inferior to it. The spines serve as points of attachment for muscles of the abdominal wall and erector spinae. Inferior to the posterior inferior iliac spine is the greater sciatic notch. The internal surface of the ilium seen from the medial side is the iliac fossa, a concavity where the iliacus muscle attaches. Posterior to this fossa is the iliac tuberosity, a point of attachment for the sacroiliac ligament, and the auricular surface, which articulates with the sacrum to form the sacroiliac joint.

imbibition
The flow of fluid through tissue via motion.

inferior
Lower in place or position.

inferior articular facet
A vertebral structural feature characterized in the cervical region by an anteroposterior position, in the thoracic region by an anteromedial position, and in the lumbar region by a lateral position.

inflammation
The reaction of living tissues to all forms of injury and irritation. It is a vascular and neurological process characterized by heat, redness, swelling, pain, and loss of function.

innominate
The hip bone. In early life it is three bones, the ilium, ischium and pubis. The three bones fuse as the individual reaches adolescence.

intercostal
Between the ribs.

interspinous ligament
Thin, almost membranous ligaments that connect adjacent spinous processes with fibers running anterosuperiorly from the apex of the spinous process below toward the root of the spinous process above. It is embedded with proprioceptors and other nerve structures.

intervertebral disc
Composed of a nucleus pulposus (center) and an annulus fibrosus (outer wall). It is largly composed of water and therefore a hydraulic system and it transmits force to the vertebral body. It is, therefore, not a shock absorber but allows a flexible vertebral column (this is essential to spinal cord vascular function).

intervertebral foramen
Openings that are along the lateral border of the intervertebral canal. They are formed anteriorly by the intervertebral disc, the lower portion of the vertebral body above, and the upper portion of the vertebral body below; posteriorly by the posterior zygapophyseal joint and ligamentum flavum; and superiorly and inferiorly by the a vertebral pedicle. The spinal nerve roots and vascular components of the spinal column pass through these openings.

intrathecal
Running through the thecal sac into the subarachnoid space between the arachnoid mater and the pia mater.

intrathecal adhesions
An adhesion between the arachnoid mater and pia mater. This is a product of inflammation and will cause an interruption of normal thecal and spinal cord dynamics or motion. It can also impede the flow of cerebrospinal fluid and entrap neurological and vascular structures.

ischial tuberosity
The blunt, inferior aspect of the ischium on which the body rests in the sitting position. Origin of the superficial transverse perineus, ischiocavernosus, inferior gemellus, quadratus femoris, semimembranosus, and semitendinosus muscles.

ischium
The inferior and posterior of the three bones that make up the innominate. It contains a prominent ischial spine, a lesser sciatic notch below the spine, and an ischial tuberosity. The rest of the ischium, the ramus, joins with the pubis and together they surround the obturator foramen.

I.V.D.
Intervertebral disc.

I.V.F.
Intervertebral foramen.

K

kyphosis
Pertaining to a kyphotic curve.

kyphotic curve
A normal architectural feature of the human vertebral column in the thoracic and sacral regions. It is characterized by the concavity of the curve facing the ventral or anterior surface. Alteration of the kyphotic curve changes the shape of the central nervous system and other associated tissues.

L

lamina
The flat bone that forms the roof of the posterior vertebral arch. In a typical vertebra, it is a paired structure on either side of the midline that unites posteriorly to form the spinous process.

laminectomized
The surgical removal of the posterior bony arches of one or more vertebrae in order to expose the neural elements in the spinal cord. A laminectomy allows inspection of the spinal canal as well as identification and removal of pathologic tissues from the cord and roots.

larynx
The voice box. It is a short passageway that connects the pharynx with the trachea. It lies in the midline of the neck anterior to the fourth through sixth cervical vertebrae, C4-C6. Intrinsic and extrinsic muscles act on the pharynx, they are; for the intrinsic: cricothyroid, posterior crycoarytenoid, lateral crycoarytenoid, arytenoid, and thyroarytinoid and for the extrinsic: omohyoid, sternohyoid, sternothyroid, and thyrohyoid.

lateral
On the side. Opposite of medial.

lateral flexion
A flexion to either side.

lateralisthesis
A displacement lateral to normal position.

ligament
A cord, band, or sheet of fibrous connective tissue linking two or more bones, cartilages, or other structures together. A ligament imparts stability, usually to a joint, preventing excessive motion in certain directions. It is embedded with proprioceptors and other nerve structures.

ligamentum flavum
Any of a series of bands of yellow elastic tissue attached to and extending between the ventral portions of the laminae of two adjacent vertebrae, from the junction of the axis and the third cervical vertebra to the junction of the fifth lumbar vertebra and the sacrum. They assist in maintaining the erect position of the spine and serve to close the spaces between the vertebral arches.

lordosis
Pertaining to a lordotic curve.

lordotic curve
A normal architectural feature of the human vertebral column in the cervical and lumbar regions. It is the angle formed by perpendicular lines drawn from the superior endplate of L1 and the inferior endplate of L5. Alteration of these curves changes the shape of the central nervous system and other tissues.

lumbar
Pertaining to the lower region of the spine, specifically the lower five vertebrae, L1-L5.

lumbar curve
An essential architectural feature of the human spine. Changes in the shape of the lumbar region of the spine result in central nervous system deformation and joint pathology. The lumbar curve is lordotic or the convex side of the curve is facing the ventral or anterior surface.

lumbosacral aponeurosis
A band of thick fascia connecting the lower thoracic region and lumbar spine with the sacrum. Synonym: thoracolumbar fascia.

luxation
A complete dislocation of an articulation.

M

magnetic resonance imaging
An imaging technique that employs radio frequency waves and a strong magnetic field to produce clinically useful images. The resulting image gives excellent soft tissue contrast without bony artifact. There is also excellent imaging of medullary bone.

mandible
The lower jawbone. The bone comprises the tooth-bearing, horseshoe shaped body and two upright plates of bone, the rami, each of which is surmounted by two processes, an anterior process called coronoid and a posterior, or condyloid process and articulates with the temporal bone.

marginal osteophytes
A horizontal bone extension of the vertebral endplate. It is the response of the body to a shearing of the intervertebral disc usually as a result of trauma. This ossification process is a response to stress due to altered architecture.

mastication
Chewing.

mastoid process
A rounded projection of the temporal bone posterior to the external auditory meatus. Origin of the occipitalis and digastric muscles and insertion of sternocleidomastoid, splenius capitis, and longissimus capitis muscles.

medial
Near the midline of the body.

medullary bone
The marrow part of bone, the space within the diaphysis of a bone.

meningeal
Pertaining to the meninges.

meninges
The supportive and enclosing tissues of the central vervous system; the dura mater, the arachnoid, and the pia mater and other structures. They impart motion to the central nervous system.

midsagittal
A vertical plane at the midline that divides the body into left and right portions.

military neck
Loss of the cervical curve. It is a straightening rather than a reversal.

MRI
Magnetic resonance imaging.

myelopathy
Any disorder of the spinal cord or nervous tissues, usually producing signs and symptoms of cord dysfunction.

Ⓝ

necrosis/necrotic
The death of a cell or group of cells comprising a tissue or tissues as a result of injury or disease.

nerve root
One of the two bundles of nerve fibers that emerge from the spinal cord to join together as a spinal nerve. These bundles are the dorsal and ventral nerve roots.

nerve rootlets
Hair-like fibers extending from the spinal cord. They converge laterally and gather into a nerve root.

neuron
A nerve cell consisting of a cell body, dendrites, and an axon.

neutral position
Normal anatomical position; body is erect and facing observer, arms hanging at the sides with palms turned forward.

neurovascular bundle
A grouping of nerves and blood vessels that both innervate and supply blood to a given region.

nonmarginal osteophytes
An osteophyte forming on the vertebral body not at the endplate. This ossification process is a response to stress due to altered architecture.

nucleus pulposus
The central, semielastic, spongy zone of the intervertebral disc. It is a hydrodynamic structure that has a greater fluid content than the rest of the disc and is composed of glycoproteins and interlaced collagen fibers.

Ⓞ

osmotic
The pressure that develops when two solutions of different concentrations are separated by a permeable membrane.

ossification
Formation of or conversion into bone.

osteoarthritis
A progressive joint disorder characterized by a deterioration of the articular cartilage and reactive new bone formation in the subchondral regions. Although the name implies an inflammation, this process is not primarily inflammatory, therefore, it can more accurately be called degenerative joint disease. This condition can occur as a result of the pathogenesis of subluxation.

osteophyte
A projection or outgrowth of bone; a bone spur. The tissue attaching or inserting into bone can be under mechanical distress causing its calcification and forming the outgrowth.

osteoporosis
A common bone disorder characterized by decreased density of normally mineralized bone resulting in bone fragility. Causes of osteoporosis are post-menopausal, age-related, disuse, dietary deficiencies, chronic illness, neoplasm, endocrine abnormalities, genetic disorders, and idiopathic problems.

Ⓟ – Ⓠ

para-spinal phyte
Ossification of the soft tissue structures that surround the vertebral body. This ossification process is a response to stress due to altered architecture.

parasthesia
A condition of altered sensation.

pedicle
A bony process projecting backward from the body of a vertebra, which connects with the lamina on either side.

pelvis/pelvic girdle
The bony, basin-shaped ring that provides the weight-bearing for the trunk and lower extremities while protecting the lower abdominal viscera. It consists of the two innominate bones that articulate posteriorly with the sacrum. Distally, the pelvis articulates with the proximal end of the femurs at the acetabuli. The pelvic ring is joined posteriorly by the sacroiliac joint and anteriorly by the symphysis pubis. More than half of an individuals muscle mass arises from the pelvis.

pelvic shearing
A non-physiologic displacement of the innominates relative to each other in the Y and/or Z planes. Significant ligament injury occurs in both the sacroiliac joints and the pubis symphysis.

parasagittal
A vertical line that does not pass through the midline and that divides the body or organs into unequal left and right portions.

pharynx
The throat. It is a somewhat funnel-shaped tube about five inches long that starts at the internal nares and extends to the level of the cricoid cartilage. It lies just posterior to the nasal cavity, oral cavity, and larynx, and is just anterior and attached to the cervical vertebrae. The muscles that act on the pharynx are, in the circular layer, the inferior, middle, and superior constrictors, and in the longitudinal layer, the stylopharyngeus, the salpingopharyngeus, and the palatopharyngeus.

pia mater
The inner membrane of the thecal sac. It invests or covers the spinal cord and roots into cord matrix. The pia mater supports and shapes the spinal cord.

PIIS
posterior inferior iliac spine

P.L.L.
Posterior longitudinal ligament

pons
Lies directly above the medulla and anterior to the cerebellum. It connects the spinal cord with the brain and parts of the brain with each other. The longitudinal fibers of the pons belong to the motor and sensory tracts that connect the spinal cord or medulla with the upper part of the brain stem.

posterior
Rear, back, or dorsal surfaces of the body.

posterior impression
An anatomical feature of the intervertebral disc. The indented posterior surface helps to give shape to the spinal canal.

posterior longitudinal ligament
A ligament that runs on the posterior surfaces of the vertebral bodies, extending from the axis down through the entire length of the vertebral column, and fanning out at the vertebral margins to reinforce the intervertebral discs.

proprioception
The sensation of position and change of position of the body and its parts. Proprioception is transmitted through special organs, most of which are in muscles, tendons and joint tissues.

proprioceptive reflex
An automatic response of muscle and tendon initiated by stimuli that arise from joint distress. The reflex mechanism itself is mediated by sensory afferent stimulation of motor neurons of the involved musculature. Since there is a direct connection at the spinal cord level with no higher motor neuron involvment, its a reflex. This occurs in spinal cord lesion victims below the lesion as do the standard neurological reflexes.

protrusion
The state of being thrust beyond a boundary forward or laterally.

pseudo-joint
Common in degenerative changes. A false joint is formed where two bones rub together when they should be apart. The most common occurrence in the spine is the spinous processes in the lumbar region.

PSIS
The posterior superior iliac spine.

psoas major
The psoas major originates at the transverse processes and bodies of the lumbar vertebrae and inserts at the lesser trochanter of the femur. The action flexes and rotates the thigh laterally and also flexes the vertebral column. Innervated at the lumbar nerves L2-L3. It has a proprioceptive link to the sacroiliac joints and pubis symphsis. The lumbar nerve roots exit the spine into the psoas and the lumbar plexus is in the belly and tendons of the muscle. The psoas attaches to the diaphragm.

pubic body
The medial portion of the pubic bone. Each side joins with the fibrocartilaginous disc called the pubis symphysis.

pubis symphysis
The pubis symphysis has annular rings and a spongy center, is avascular, and motion is a major component of its physiology. This joint can tear and subluxate and suffer major stability problems. Misalignment of this joint automatically misalign one or both sacroiliac joints. Proprioceptive links are to the psoas, iliacus, all the hip muscles, medial and anterior muscles of the thigh and the abdominal and erector groups.

R

rectus abdominus
The rectus abdominus originates at the pubic crest and pubis symphysis and inserts at the cartilage of the fifth to seventh ribs and the xiphoid process. Action is to compress the abdomen to aid in defecation, urination, forced expiration, and childbirth. It also flexes the vertebral column. Innervation is from the branches of thoracic nerves T7-T12. Proprioceptive innervation is between pubic bone and lower rib cage. Unilateral rectus abdominus splinting can be a sign of pubis symphysis subluxation.

recumbent position

The body position of lying down on a horizontal surface.

retro

Abbreviation for retrolisthesis.

retrolisthesis

Any posterior displacement of a vertebra in relation to the one below it causing stress and probable tearing of the annulus fibrosus and nucleus pulposus. Also, the altered biomechanics and loss of normal motion resulting from a retrolisthesis is the etiology of almost all degenerative or arthritic changes to the disc, vertebral body, facet, and other associated tissues.

retropulsion

The process of being pushed posteriorly. This term is used in the description of vertebral body fractures to refer to fragments that have fallen back into the spinal canal.

rib

A curved, slightly twisted strip of bone that forms part of the skeleton of the thorax. There are twelve pairs of ribs. The head of each rib articulates with one of the twelve thoracic vertebrae. The other end is attached to a section of cartilage. The first seven pairs, the true ribs, are connected directly to the sternum by their costal cartilages. The next three pairs, the false ribs, are attached indirectly to the sternum. Each is connected by its cartilage to the rib above it. The last two pairs, the floating ribs, end freely in the muscles of the anterior body wall.

rootlets

Nerve rootlets.

rotation

The turning or moving of a part around its axis of rotation. The unit of measure is degrees or radians.

S

sacral ala

The wing-like projections evolving from the region of S1. They are analogous to the transverse processes. They form the fibrous area of the sacroiliac joint.

sacral apex

The inferior aspect of the sacrum, articulating with the superior portion of the coccyx.

sacral base

The superior aspect of the sacrum, articulating with the inferior portion of L5.

sacral disc

The disc between scaral segments. As the sacrum ages, it begins to fuse, becoming for all practical purposes, a single but flexible bone. When these bones, S1-S5, articulate, the intersacral discs remain in place and act just the same as the intervertebral discs of the other vertebrae. The cortex of the sacrum is contiguous but this must be a flexible structure. Physiological function of intrasacral discs necessitates motion as the only mechanism of nutrition and waste elimination. The sacral discs do what the intervertebral discs do: confer flexibility. There is only one mechanism for fluid and nutrient exchange for the intervertebral disc and that is imbibition through motion. This must also be true for sacral disc physiology and function.

sacroiliac joint

The paired articulations between the sacrum and the iliac bone in the pelvis. These two joint complexes are different in each individuals. Some of the factors are the size of the joint, size of each portion, shape of each portion, and orientation of each portion to each other. These factors could explain the different responses to the same treatment with the same diagnosis.

sacroiliac ligament (anterior and posterior)

Anterior: This ligament is contiguous with periosteum of ilium and sacrum. This is one of the structures involved with S.I. joint injuries, sustaining a sprain with either physiological or non-physiological subluxations.

Posterior: This ligament is contiguous with and attached to the lumbosacral fascia from above and the medial attachment of the gluteus maximus muscle from below. It connects the sacrum and the ilium behind and forms the chief connection between these bones.

sacrospinous ligament

The ligament from the lateral edge of the sacrum to the spine of the ischium. This ligament along with the sacrotuberous ligament is primarily responsible for conferring motion to the sacrum. As the leg swings forward for heel strike, the innominate nutates with the ilium moving posterior and the ischial tuberosity moving forward and via the sacrotuberous and sacrospinous ligaments, moves the ipsilateral side of the sacrum forward.

sacrotuberous ligament

The ligament from the lateral edge of the sacrum to the ischial tuberosity. Fibers of the sacrotuberous can be contiguous with the tendon of the biceps femoris. Unilateral shortening of the ligament can rotate and or angle the sacrum between the ilium creating a contralateral stretching and irritation to various structures, this could be a factor in a number of syndromes. The sacrotuberous ligament, along with the sacrospinous ligament, confer motion to the sacrum with motion of the leg.

sacrum

The sacrum is a triangular shaped bone formed by the partial fusion of sacral vertebrae. It articulates laterally with the ilium, superiorly with L5, and inferiorly with the coccyx. The sacrum is five separate segments in the child and S1-S5 are fused by age 25 to form, for all practical purposes, a single but flexible bone.

sagittal

A vertical plane that divides the body into left and right portions.

Schmorl's node

A punched-out area in the endplate of a vertebral body that is surrounded by repaired compact bone. It is due to a prolapse of the nucleus pulposus into the vertebral body through the endplate and into the medullary bone. On a lateral X-ray a Schmorl's node is seen as a radiolucency in the upper or lower margin of the body of the affected vertebra surrounded by compact bone.

sclerosis

A hardening and/or thickening of a tissue or organ, usually due to an increase in fibrous tissue.

segment

A portion of a larger body or structure.

shearing

A type of deforming force applied in the axial plane to the spine resulting in angular deformation. Involves numerous ligament, joint, muscle and nervous tissue structures besides the vertebrae.

SI joint

Sacroiliac joint

sinuvertebral artery

A small branch or arterial twig off the vertebral artery that enters the intervertebral foramen. It supplies blood to the thecal sac and spinal cord. Loss of lordotic curve and subluxation of numerous cervical vertebrae can cause translation of the cord, thecal sac, and nerve roots into the anterior wall of the spinal canal and the intervertebral foramen. Chronically compressed sinuvertebral artery could cause negative sympathetic syndrome.

soft tissue

The nonosseous tissue of the body, including intervertebral discs, tendons, muscle, connective tissues, nerves, vascular structures and ligaments.

spasm

Involuntary musculature contraction. It can be due to proprioceptive sensory bombardment, peripheral nerve entrapment or central nervous distress, all of which can be due to subluxation.

spinal canal

A continuous channel running longitudinally through the vertebral column. The anterior wall is formed by the posterior surfaces of the vertebral bodies and intervertebral discs and by the posterior longitudinal ligament. The posterior wall is formed by the vertebral laminae, the ligamentum flava and the intervertebral foramina. Canal length (flexion increases 5-7 cm the length over extension) and shape (side bending and rotation create a concave-convex formation of the lateral surfaces of the canal) are affected by the shape or posture of the spinal column. The anatomic relationship with the spinal cord and caudae equinae determine the shape of the lower central nervous system. A kyphosis of the cervical spine is a flexion deformity that affects the entire length of the canal, spinal cord, brain stem and nerve roots.

spondylolithesis

The anterior displacement of a vertebra in relation to the lower vertebra.

spondylosis

Degenerative disease of both the disc and the zygapophyseal joints of the spine. Symptoms include pain and restriction of movement. Spondylosis produces a characteristic appearance on radiographs that includes narrowing of both the disc space and the neural foramina, as well as the presence of osteophytes. The most common etiology is subluxation.

spinal column

The spinal column includes the vertebral column, spinal cord, meninges, nerves, ligaments, and cerebrospinal fluid.

spinal cord

The portion of the central nervous system enclosed in the vertebral column. It begins as a continuation of the medulla oblongata at the inferior part of the brain stem and extends from the foramen magnum of the occipital bone to a tapered end at the junction of L1-L2. It consists of nerve cells and bundles of nerves connecting all parts of the body to the brain. The spinal cord changes it shape with the changing shape of the spinal canal and meninges. The spinal cord can increase in length 3-5 cm going from full extension to flexion. With flexion and spinal cord lengthening, the dentate ligaments stretch and narrow, pulling the edges of the cord with them. Acting together, they pull the from the right and the left and increase the coronal diameter. The anterior to posterior diameter decreases, making the cord appear oval on axial view. Pia mater invests the spinal cord with roots into the cord matrix. The subarachnoid space is the CSF filled space between the pia mater covering of the spinal cord and the inside of the thecal sac covered with the arachnoid mater.

spinal laminar junction

A radiographic line. The vertebral lamina unite posteriorly to form the spinous process. At the point of junction there is a white line which is the posterior wall of the vertebral canal.

spinous process
That part of a vertebra that projects posteriorly from the arch, producing a lever arm for introduction of motion by attaching muscle groups.

spurring
An osteophyte, beak, or lip, on the articular margin of a bone. Endplate spurs are all disc related, posterior as well as anterior and lateral.

stairstepping
In a radiograph, stairstepping has the appearance of stairs due to repeated subluxations from disc to disc, resulting in a sequential loss of alignment in a series of vertebrae.

stenosis
A narrowing of an opening or passage, such as the spinal canal, can be congenital or acquired. It is a common finding with chronic subluxation with involved segments.

sternum
The breastbone. It measures about 15 cm in length and is located in the median line of the anterior thoracic wall. The sternum consists of three basic portions: the superior manubrium, the medial body, and the inferior xiphoid process. The manubrium articulates with the medial ends of the clavicles as well as the first and second ribs. The body articulates directly or indirectly with the second through tenth ribs. The xiphoid process provides the insertion point for the rectus abdominus and transversus abdominus muscles.

subarachnoid adhesions
An adhesion occurring between the arachnoid and pia mater. See intrathecal adhesions.

subarachnoid space
The space between the arachnoid and pia mater. It contains circulating cerebrospinal fluid and large blood vessels. Obliteration of the anterior subarachnoid space seen in advanced imaging by the spinal cord taken in the supine position can be a sign of central nervous system tethering and distress. Loss of space due to fibrous adhesions or stenosis is considered pathological and relate to severe neurological conditions.

subdural space
Theoretical or potential space between the dura mater and arachnoid mater. It looks and acts like a single tissue, hence the term, theca. These two layers of tissue are normally adhered together.

subluxation
Loss of joint alignment and integrity. This describes an injury to the joint structures such as the ligaments, discs, joint capsules, supporting tendons, and fascia. Subluxation is the most common etiology of osteoarthritis and is characterized by immobilization, inflammation, pain and muscle spasms.

superior
Situated above or towards the upper part of the body; opposite of inferior.

superior articular facet
A vertebral structural feature characterized in the cervical region by a posterosuperior position, in the thoracic region by a posterolateral position, and in the lumbar region by a medial position.

supine
Lying on the dorsal surface with the face upward.

sympathetic chain
Long nerve complexes on each side of the vertebral column from the base of the skull to the coccyx. It is the extravertebral portion of the central nervous system containing part of the autonomic nervous system.

sympathetic nervous system
One of the two subdivisions of the autonomic nervous system, having cell bodies of preganglionic neurons in the lateral gray columns of the thoracic segment and first two or three lumbar segments of the spinal cord. It is primarily concerned with processes involving the expenditure of energy. Paravertebral ganglia as well as spinal nerve roots have been observed to be adversely affected by chronic degenerative processes of the vertebral column.

synovial joint
A joint in which there is a space between the articulating bones. A synovial joint is freely movable and is classified as a diarthroses. They are surrounded by a capsule and held together by ligaments. Disruption of normal relationships (subluxation) causes inflammation, muscle guarding and limited range of motion leading to arthritic changes if allowed to become chronic.

(T)

tendon/tendinous
A band of dense fibrous tissue that forms the termination of a muscle and attaches it to a bone. When the muscle contracts, it pulls on the tendon, which moves the bone. The tendons are embedded with proprioceptors and other neurological structures.

tethered cord syndrome
A collection of signs, symptoms and complaints that are the result of central nervous system distress from chronic elongation of the neural canal in the vertebral column. Characterized by translation of the spinal cord into the anterior canal wall obliterating the patency of the anterior spinal artery. Also known as filum terminale syndrome or cord traction syndrome.

theca/thecal
The theca or thecal sac refers to part of the meninges, the dura mater and the arachnoid mater.

thoracic
Pertaining to the thoracic region of the spine, T1-T12.

thoracic curve
An essential architectural feature of the human spine. Changes in the shape of the thoracic region of the spine result in central nervous system deformation and joint pathology. The thoracic curve is kyphotic or the concave side of the curve is ventral.

thoracolumbar fascia
A thick, broad tissue anchoring the erector spinae, abdominal muscles, and latissimus dorsi. It connects the lower thoracic area, lumbar spine, sacrum, and iliac crests.

thorax
The chest.

three-point weight bearing
The three-point weight bearing system in the vertebral column is based on weight distributed between three points, the body of the vertebra and the two articular facets. This system works for each joint in the vertebral column from C2 to S1. Disruption of the three-point weight bearing system alters the dynamics of the joint and associated tissues and leads to osteoarthritis. See also altered weight bearing.

trabecula
The trabecula of the arachnoid are delicate fibrous threads connecting the inner surface of the arachnoid to the pia mater.

trachea
The windpipe. It is a tubular passageway for air about 12 cm in length and 2.5 cm in diameter. It is located anterior to the esophagus and extends from the larynx to the fifth thoracic vertebra where it divides into right and left primary bronchi. The cartilaginous layer consists of sixteen to twenty incomplete rings of hyaline cartilage that look like a series of letter C's stacked one on top of the other. The open parts of the C's face the esophagus and permit it to expand slightly into the trachea during swallowing. The solid parts of the C's provide a rigid support so the tracheal wall does not collapse inward and obstruct the air passageway.

tractioned
Stretching or elongating a tissue, i.e. spinal cord from deformation of spinal column.

transverse abdominus
The transverse abdominus originates at the iliac crest, inguinal ligament, lumbar fascia, and cartilages of the last six ribs and inserts at the xyphoid process, linea alba, and pubis. Action is to compress the abdomen. Innervation is from the branches of the thoracic nerves T8-T12, the iliohypogastric and ilioinguinal nerves.

transverse processes
A bony process projecting from the base of the neural arch of the vertebra at the junction of the pedicle and the lamina. They serve as points of insertion and origin for the splenius cervicis, iliocostalis cervicis, longissimus thoracis, longissimus cervicis, longissimus capitis, and intertranversarii muscles.

trochanter
Either of the two bony protuberances that project from below the neck of the femur. These are known as the greater and lesser trochanters. The psoas major muscle inserts at the lesser trochanter. The gluteus medius, gluteus minimus, piriformis, obturator internus, superior gemellus, and inferior gemellus insert at the greater trochanter.

U

urogenital
The region of the pelvic floor below the pubis symphysis, bounded by the pubis symphysis and the ischial tuberosities and containing the external genitalia.

V

vascular
Pertaining to or containing many blood vessels.

vasoconstriction
A decrease in the size of the lumen of a blood vessel caused by the contraction of the smooth muscle in the wall of the vessel.

ventral
Pertaining to the anterior or front side of the body; opposite of dorsal.

vertebral artery
This vessel is the first and largest branch of the subclavian artery. It enters the foramen in the sixth cervical vertebra and ascends through the foramina in the transverse processes of all the vertebrae above this. It passes through the atlas, beneath the posterior occipitoatlantal ligament, pierces the dura mater and arachnoid, and enters the skull through the foramen magnum.

vertebral canal
A canal formed by the foramina of the vertebrae that contains the spinal cord and meninges. The canal is formed by the posterior aspect of the vertebral body, the medial portion of the pedicles, and the anterior surface of the lamina.

vertebral column
The flexible supporting column of the axial skeleton composed of vertebrae separated by intervertebral discs and bound together by ligaments. The meninges act as a supporting soft tissue structure for the inside of the vertebral column. Synonym: spinal column.

visceral
Pertaining to the viscera; a collective term for the internal organs.

Ⓦ – Ⓩ

whiplash
A term for an injury in which the cervical spine is unexpectedly and violently forced or "whipped" in one direction then suddenly in the opposite direction.

zygapophyseal joint
Of or pertaining to the lateral articulating joints of the spine. See facet.

INDEX

A

Abdominal
complaints, 205
oblique muscle
internal, 193
external, 193
tissues, lining, cavity, 194
Absolute motion, 2, 3, 6; see also Global motion
Acetabulum, 194, 196, 212
Adaptive response, 100, 102
Adhesions
epidural, 22
fibrous, 89
intradural, 16
subarachnoid, 23, 24, 89
A.L.L. (Anterior longitudinal ligament), 14, 17, 32, 41, 105, 109, 111, 119, 121, 163, 187
Altered weight bearing, 2, 17, 19, 26, 47, 53 54, 59 68, 70, 77, 95, 129, 134, 136, 180
Annular rings (Annulus Fibrosus), 14, 131, 134, 195, 199
Annulus fibrosus, see Annular rings
Anterior longitudinal ligament, see A.L.L.
Anterior spinal artery, 20, 22, 89
Anterolisthesis, 13, 14, 48, 76, 100, 106, 108, 112, 117, 162
Anteroposterior, 52, 122; see also A.L.L.
A-P (Anterior to posterior), 7, 110; see also Anteroposterior
alignment, 133
diameter of C5's body, 19
direction, central X-ray, 202
displacement of vertebrae, 190
sacral discs, coronal planes, 205
subluxations of the lumbar spine, 143
subluxation, lack of and DJD, 165
subluxation, sacrum, 161
view of normal pelvis, 207
X-ray in supine position, 208
Arachnoid, (see also Dentate ligament, arachnoid mater)
dura, 4
mater, 2, 4, 5, 23
trabeculae, 5, 23
Arthritis, 136
Articulation, 13
posterior, 2
rib-disc, 85
Atlanto-axial , 2
Autonomic nervous system, 86
Avascular
fibrocartilaginous disc, 195
intrasacral discs, 191
structures, 14, 131, 216
Axial
cut, 15
views, 9 25, 27, 90, 202, 205, 207, 209, 210
skeleton, 85
Axial loading, 109

B

Brain stem, 2, 7, 21, 44, 45
Buckling, 29

C

Calcified
A.L.L., 11; see also A.L.L.
discs, 17, 121
P.L.L., 14, 119; see also P.L.L.
Calcification
A.L.L., 14, 118
C4-5, C5-6, C6-7, 41
L2, 168, 169
L5 loss of disc height and, 165
T5 fracture and, 120
T6-7 to T11-12, 115
T9-10 & T10-11, 119
T11-12, 119
Canal stenosis, 9, 16, 17, 30, 45, 49, 51, 58, 61, 69, 71, 75, 78, 134, 171
spinal, 24, 25, 136
vertebral, 40
Capillaries, spinal cord, 11
Capillary bed, 196
hyaline, 199
SI joint, 197, 198
Cartilage, 197
deterioration, 14
lack of, C3-6 facets, 67
vertebral column, 2
Cartesian coordinate system, 206
Caudae equinae, 2, 7, 21, 179, 189, 195
Cavitation, 19, 49, 65 111, 117, 129, 145, 155, 158, 161, 163, 169, 173, 175-177, 179, 181, 187
Central nervous system, see C.N.S.
Cerebellum, 3, 4, 30, 44, 45, 81
Cerebrospinal fluid, 197
Cervical curve, 16, 17, 19, 20, 24, 27, 56, 87, 123
lordotic cervical, 38, 40, 42, 44, 46, 48, 50 52
loss of, 56
Cervicogenic, 29
Chronic
inflammation, 22-24, 89
lumbar subluxation, 129
neurological distress, 91
pelvis, subluxation, 208
posterior stairstepping, 176
spasm, the cause of some headaches, 29
Chronically degenerative, 14 58, 87, 134, 181, 203, 204
Clavicles, 32
Coccyx, 2, 5, 6
Compression fracture, 89, 100, 107, 112, 117, 120, 126, 132, 144, 145, 152, 160, 170, 174, 175, 184-186
Conductivity, 22, 89
Congenital stenosis, 9, 38, 72
Conus medularis, 2, 7, 189
and thoracic disc herniation, 88
Contracture
thoracolumbar fascia, 150, 161
Coronal, 131, 195
Cortex
of sacrum, 195, 216, 219
Cortical bone, 195, 196, 216, 217
Costo-transverse, 85, 87
Costo-vertebral, 85-87

CNS (Central nervous system)
anatomy and physiology, 1-10
and nutrient delivery, 7, 11, 14, 196, 199
effects of motion, 16, 194
proprioceptive input and, 193
subluxation and, 13, 20, 24, 27, 63, 205
Cranial
flexion, 7
Cross section
in advanced imaging, 204
of lumbar disc, 131
of sacrum, 205
Curve, see
cervical
lordotic
lumbar
thoracic

D

Degeneration, 1, 14, 16,17, 30, 32, 38, 39, 41, 44, 48, 50, 57, 64, 66, 67, 79, 101, 107, 108, 109, 110, 112-114, 118
of discs, 129, 130, 144, 147, 148, 156, 160, 165, 172, 181
end stages, 24, 60, 178, 180, 217
patterns, causes of, 25, 95, 134
initiated by immobility, 11
of sacrum, 153
of facets, 59
phase, 1, 77
advanced, 19
chronic, 203,204
beginning sings, 216
subluxation and, 58, 136, 164, 168, 181, 190
Degenerative joint disease, see DJD
Dehydration, 113, 129, 134
Demifacet, 85
Dens, 8, 57, 64
Dentate ligament, 4, 5, 7, 32
arachnoid mater, 7
Dessicated, 14
Disc, 129-131
Are Not Shock Absorbers, 131
DJD (Degenerative joint disease), 24, 26, 67, 111, 116, 151
Dorsal
abdominal lining, 194
cord nerve and vascular entrapment, 109
cortical bone covering, 196
spinal cord, surface, 64
Dura mater, 2, 4, 5, 23

E

Eburnation, 42
End plate, 12, 37, 45, 55, 57, 75, 98,108, 130, 131,132, 134, 135, 176, 183, 188, 189
Epidural adhesions, 22, 24
Epidural space, 7
Erector spinae, 136, 191, 193, 194
Esophagus, 32
Extension
flexion-extension, 3, 5, 6, 31
hip, 192
innominate femoral head, 206
lordotic curve, 6, 18
lumbar spine, 20,
spinal canal, 5
thecal sac, 5, 6
Extremity, upper, 19, 20

F

Facet, 2, 3, 13-15, 39, 42, 45, 49, 53, 59, 63, 67, 68
altered weight bearing, 90
articular, 129, 195
degeneration, 14, 30, 44, 66,77
gapping, 63, 200-01
height loss, 35, 55, 88, 151, 163
hypertrophy, 30, 42, 70, 105, 109, 111, 115, 119, 121, 129
inferior articulating, 15
jamming, 59, 67
separation, 6
sclerosis, 14, 67, 165
superior articulating, 15
uncoupling of, 134
weight bearing, 39, 49
zygopophyseal joints, 13
Facetal capsule, 134
Fascia, 134,
Fibro-cartilaginous disc, 195
Fibrous, 197
adhesions, 89
and cartilaginous, 195
mass, 88, 89
network, 88
portion of the SI joint, 197
SI joint, fibrous component, 197
Filum terminale, 7
Flexion, 3, 7, 17-21, 31, 51, 57, 104, 127
/extension, 5, 31, 206
cervical, 20-21, 189
cranial, 7
deformity, 17, 21
forward, 7, 17, 201
head, 1, 5, 10
lateral, 7, 205, 214
traumatic, 40
Foramen magnum, 6, 45, 64
Foramen
jugular, 4, 10
intervertebral (IVF), 6, 7, 30, 89, 136
Fusion, 17, 42
C5 and C6, 21, 26, 31, 38,
C6-7 fused with C7, 43, 63, 68-69
C6-7, 63, 68-69, 83
cervical spine, 11
complete, C5-C6, 68
L2-3, 204
L5-SI joint, 135, 162, 168, 169, 170, 216
L5 vertebra, 123, 145, 147, 149, 173, 175
S2-S3, 202, 203
S3, 4 & 5, 195
T6 to T9, 122
Vertebral bodies, 43

G

Glycoprotein, 130
Gravitational load, 129
Guarding (spasmed), 13, 39, 102, 206, 218, 225

H

Herniation, 87, 88, 96, 110-111, 114
multiple disc, 96, 98
posterior disc, 87, 88
thoracic disc, 87. 88
Hydration 16, 26, 98, 101, 113, 119, 129, 134, 196
Hydraulic function, 129
interruption, 129
system, closed, 129
Hyoid bone, 32
Hyperkyphosis, 29, 100, 109, 130, 132, 134, 138, 139
due to compression fracture, 126-127
from altered weight bearing, 29
osteoporosis and, 126, 127, 130
progressive spurring, 118, 122-123, 130, 132, 134
result of osteoporosis, 88, 129
thoracic spine, 21, 23-25, 29-30, 85
Hyperload, 14
Hypertrophy, 30, 42, 70, 105, 109, 111, 115, 119, 121, 129, 163, 163, 175
A.L.L., 105, 109, 121
of facets, 42, 43, 70
vertebrae, 129
uncinato process, 30

I – J

Iliacus muscle, 193, 219
Ilium, 193, 205, 208, 210
Imbibition, 86, 181
Innominate, 193, 181, 182, 189, 191-201
Intercostal
artery, 86
nerve, 86, 87
neurovascular bundles, 87
vein, 87
Interspinous C3-7, distance, 21
Intervertebral disc, 84,195, 199,
Intervertebral foramen, see I.V.F.
Intradural adhesions, 24
Intrasacral, 197, 198, 216, 217
Intrathecal, 24, 25, 108, 109
Intrinsic muscles, 134
Ischial tuberosities, 211
Ischium, 193
I.V.F. (Intervertebral foramen), 6, 7, 30, 89, 136

K

Kyphosis, 20, 21, 72, 81, 83
Kyphotic, 15
cervical, 13, 52, 54, 56, 58, 60, 62, 64, 66, 68, 70, 72, 74, 79
sacral, 1
thoracic, 80, 81, 86, 88, 91, 96, 98, 106, 108, 177

L

Lamina, 2, 6, 19, 22, 23, 30, 32, 51, 85
Laminectomized, 3
Larynx, 32
Lateralisthesis, 87
Ligament, see
A.L.L. (Anterior longitudinal ligament)
Dentate ligament
P.L.L. (Posterior longitudinal ligament)
SI (Sacroiliac) joint/ ligament
Sacrospinous ligament
Sacrotuberous ligament
Ligamentum flavum, 2, 22-24, 43, 82-83
Lordotic curve,1, 6, 18, 21, 29, 31, 36, 40, 44, 46, 50, 53, 160; see also cervical, lordotic
loss of, 21, 36, 54, 56, 58, 140, 141, 172, 178, 190
reversal, 21
Lumbar curve, 16, 17, 123, 135, 139, 144, 148, 152, 156
Lumbo-sacral aponeurosis, 136
Luxation, 13

M

Magnetic resonance imaging, see MRI
Mandible, 3, 32, 33
Marginal osteophytes, 95, 119
Mastication, 32
Mastoid process, 10, 29
Medullary bone, 131, 132
Meningeal, 2, 5, 7, 23
Meninges, 2, 5, 7, 23
Mid-sagittal, 13, 20, 26, 80, 195
Military neck, 20, 36, 54, 56, 58
MRI (magnetic resonance imaging)
cervical, 20, 21, 23, 26, 27, 30, 32, 37, 80, 82, 90, 93
lordotic, 191
pelvic, 205, 208
sacrum, 205, 208
thoracic, 25, 90, 125-127
Myelopathy, 19

N

Necrosis or necrotic, 66, 73
Nerve root, 7, 8. 10, 18, 23, 24, 31, 34, 86, 87, 89
Nerve rootlets, 4, 7, 23, 24, 89
Neutral position, 4, 18, 21, 22, 81, 82, 90, 104, 201
Neurons, 11, 88, 89
Neuro-vascular bundle, 195
Non-marginal osteophytes, 95; see also Osteophyte
Nucleus pulposus, 14, 130, 131, 132, 154, 171, 195, 199. 216

O

Osmotic, 133
Ossification, 109
Osteoarthritis, 14, 20, 29, 129, 136, 203-204
Osteophyte, 14, 20, 22, 30, 59, 82, 83, 89, 93, 95, 99, 114, 119; see also non-marginal osteophyte
Osteoporosis, 2, 17, 88, 118, 120

P – Q

Parasthesia, 20
Pedicles, 88, 129
Pelvis, 1, 85, 193, Chapter 6
Pelvic girdle, Chapter 6

Pharynx, 32
Pia mater, 5, 7, 24, 25
P.L.L. (Posterior longitudinal ligament), 8, 11, 20, 23, 26, 99, 85, 245, 247, 253, 254
Pons, 1, 2, 4, 7, 8, 30, 31, 57
Posterior longitudinal ligament, see P.L.L
Posterior superior iliac spine, see PSIS
Proprioceptive, 193, 199
  guarding, 134, 205
Protrusion
  disc, into cord, 87, 88
  into vertibral canal, 43
  L2-3 disc, into L2, 132, 133
Pseudo-joint, 166
  atlas & C2, 78
  spinous process contact forming, 166, 174
PSIS (posterior superior iliac spine), 209
Psoas, 149, 150, 205, 207, 214. 219, 224-227, 242, 245, 249, 254
  major hip flexors, 193
  pubic bone, 199-201, 215, 201
Pubis symphysis, 7, 205, 208, 211-213, 215, 219, 222, 235, 238, 241, 242, 245, 249, 254

R

Rectus abdominus, 215
Retropulsion, 126
Retrolisthesis, 14,
  lumbar, stair-stepped
  mid-sagittal, 14
  T11, 111
Rib,
  articulation, 85
  cage, 1
  severe radiating, 127
  spine relationship, 86
  thoracic spine, 85
Rootlets, see Nerve rootlets
Rotation, 206
  and joint sclerosis, 208
  C1 to C2, 15
  complete posterior, 204
  lateral flexation and, 7
  shearing and, 207
Rotational, 196
  misalignments, 29

S

Sacral ala, 205, 208, 214
Sacral apex or base, 150, 196, 207
Sacral base posterior, 179
Sacral disc, 21, 151, 163, 175
Sacroiliac joint, see SI joint
Sacrospinous ligament, 196
Sacrotuberous ligament, 196
Sacrum, 2, 134-36
Schmoral's node, 107, 117, 152, 171
Sclerosis, 86
  compression fracture with, 146
  facet, 14
  lower, 41
Segmental motion, 2
Sheared, 77
Shearing, 14
SI (Sacroiliac) joint/ ligament, 193
Soft tissue, 95
Spinal canal, 1-3
Spinal column, 1, 2, 4
Spinal cord, 1, 2,
Spinous process
  cervical, 6, 24, 30, 64, 79
  contact, and pelvic joints, 167
  lumbar, 143
  thoracic, 85
Spondylosis, 12, 136
Spondylolisthesis, 135
Spurring, 15, 17, 19, 104, 134, 165
Stairstepping, 12, 14
  cervical, 46
  lumbar, 168
Stenosis, 16, 17
  of spinal canal, 30
Sternum, 32
Subarachnoid adhesions, 24,25
Subarachnoid space, 5, 7, 24, 89
Subdural space, 4
Subluxation, definition of, 13,
Superior articulating facet, 15
Superior spinal laminar junction, 19
Supine, 20, 220
Sympathetic chain, 86, 87
  "Storm", 15
Sympathetic nervous system, see Sympathetic chain
Synovial, 85, 197, 205

T

Tendon or tendinous, 29, 136
Theca or thecal, 2-8, 23, 115
Thoracic, 85
  A-P, 3
  spine
    adhesions, 22, 23
    alignment with head, 23
    and weight bearing, 95
    and sympathetic chain, 87
    compression fracture, 89
    compression of vertebral bodies, 88 94
    cord tethering, 90
    cord tractioning, 23
    disc herniation, 88
Thoracic curve, 17, 96, 98, 102, 104, 106
Thorax
  and lumbar spine, 174
  and subluxation of pubic symphysis, 199
  muscles of, 193
Three point weight bearing, 2, 129
Trabecula
  arachnoid, 5
  of medullary bone, 132
Transverse abdominus muscle, 193
Transverse processes
  added stability and, 88
  as levers, 199
  of C1, 10
  rib articulations and, 90, 95
Trachea, 32
Tractioned
  cord, 24
  uterus, 194
Trochanter, 194

U

Urogenital, 194

(V)

Vascular
changes and alignment, 14, 15, 18, 25, 29, 30, 32
Vasoconstriction, 15
Vertebral canal, 8-9, 17, 24, 30
    changing length and tethering, 22, 57, 95, 124
    protrusions into, 43, 87
Vertebral artery, 15, 29
Vertebral column 1, 2, 16, 17
    absolute motion of, 6
    adhesions and, 24, 25
Visceral problems
    and pelvic subluxation, 194

(W) – (Z)

Whiplash, 30
    vulnerability to, 18, 52
Zygopophyseal joints, 13, 14

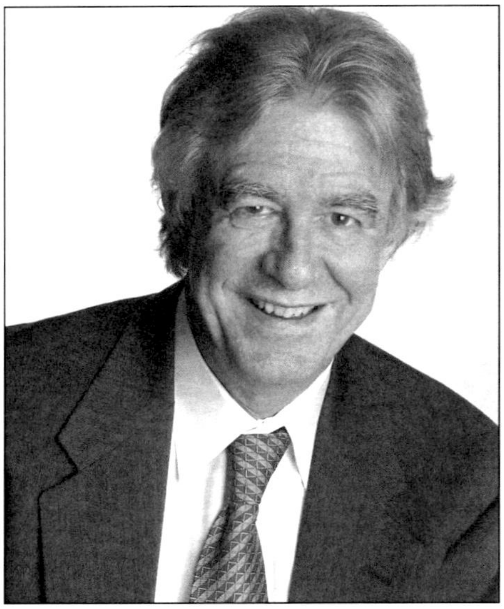

Biographical Information

William J. Ruch, D.C. graduated from the University of San Francisco with a B.S. in Biology and received his D.C. from Life Chiropractic College West in 1986.

Dr. Ruch spent seven years developing spinal and pelvic dissection procedures and has studied, photographed and X-rayed hundreds of human cadavers in the course of his research; his extensive photographic library of these studies form the core material for this book. He has taught dissection of the human spine at Life Chiropractic College West for over twenty years, during which time he amassed the extensive knowledge of spinal and pelvic pathophysiology upon which the text heavily relies.

He has maintained a private practice in Oakland, California for twenty-seven years. He has authored nine articles on clinical anatomy in the Journal of Clinical Chiropractic, *and has had cadaver specimen and X-ray photographs published in the book* Clinical Chiropractic *by G. Plaugher, Williams and Wilkins, 1993.*

Colophon:

Designed by William Ruch and Paul Marcus.
Typography and layout by Paul Marcus
Photo masking by Paul Marcus, Shereen Harris, and Olivia Destandau

Body copy set in Sabon and **Bold** 10pt on 12pt leading.

Captions set in Helvetica 9 pt on 11 pt.

Titles and headers set in ITC Serif Gothic Bold and **Black**.